COMPUTED TOMOGRAPHY OF THE

CORONARY ARTERIES

COMPUTED TOMOGRAPHY OF THE
CORONARY ARTERIES

Second Edition

EDITORS

Pim J de Feyter

Gabriel P Krestin

CO-EDITORS

Filippo Cademartiri

Carlos van Mieghem

Bob Meijboom

Nico Mollet

Koen Nieman

LAYOUT

Denise Vrouenraets

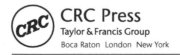

CRC Press
Taylor & Francis Group
Boca Raton London New York

CRC Press is an imprint of the
Taylor & Francis Group, an **informa** business

First edition published in the United Kingdom in 2005
Second edition published in the United Kingdom in 2008 by Informa Healthcare,

First published 2008 by Infroma UK Ltd

Published 2019 by CRC Press
Taylor & Francis Group
6000 Broken Sound Parkway NW, Suite 300
Boca Raton, FL 33487-2742

© 2008 by Taylor & Francis Group, LLC
CRC Press is an imprint of Taylor & Francis Group, an Informa business

First issued in paperback 2019

No claim to original U.S. Government works

ISBN 13: 978-0-367-45256-8 (pbk)
ISBN 13: 978-1-84184-657-6 (hbk)

Visit the Taylor & Francis Web site at
http://www.taylorandfrancis.com

and the CRC Press Web site at
http://www.crcpress.com

A CIP record for this book is available from the British Library.

Library of Congress Cataloging-in-Publication Data

Contents

Preface

Since the first edition of *Computed Tomography of the Coronary Arteries* was published in 2005, knowledge about CT technology has significantly increased, which prompted us to provide an updated version of the book.

Non-invasive coronary imaging using multi-slice CT has rapidly evolved as a diagnostic modality to detect or exclude the presence of significant coronary artery disease. In addition, multislice CT is able to provide important information about non-obstructive plaques and their tissue composition, including whether they are non-calcified, calcified, or mixed coronary plaques.

The technological improvements of CT scanners have been impressive and 64-slice CT has largely superseded four- and 16-slice CT scanners, while prototype 256- or 320-slice CT scanners have been introduced very recently.

Many reports have been published about the diagnostic performance of CT coronary angiography to detect significant coronary stenosis compared with invasive coronary angiography. These reports unanimously agree that CT coronary angiography can reliably exclude the presence of significant coronary artery disease but that the accurate detection of coronary obstructions, i.e. extent, location, and distribution, is still somewhat limited, and requires improvement in spatial and temporal resolution.

Cardiac CT has matured significantly and has attracted many radiologists and cardiologists to begin a cardiac CT program in their departments. We also believe that cardiac CT has a bright future and may become the most important non-invasive modality for the visualization of the coronary arteries.

The CT technique, although relatively straight forward, requires thorough understanding of the basic principles for accurate interpretation and clinical application of CT coronary images.

Many cardiologists and radiologists are not familiar with cardiac CT, and we believe that our book provides easy and understandable information about cardiac CT. The book is the result of close collaboration between both cardiologists and radiologists, and the contents are a reflection of the specific insights of each discipline. We clearly believe that for optimal interpretation and implementation of cardiac CT teamwork between radiologists and cardiologists is essential.

We hope that the second edition will again serve its goal as a concise, quick reference for understanding and interpreting CT coronary images.

Pim J de Feyter
Gabriel P Krestin

Acknowledgments

The editors wish to express their gratitude to the many individuals employed in both radiology and cardiology departments of Erasmus MC Rotterdam, who have supported us. Their help was indispensable to compile *Computed Tomography of the Coronary Arteries*.

This book would not have become a reality without the much appreciated skilful help of the members of the staff of Informa Healthcare Medical Books, with special thanks to Alan Burgess and Kathryn Dunn.

We would also like to thank Marcel Dijkshoorn and Berend Koudstaal for their assistance in patient preparation, data acquisition, and post-processing.

Finally, we would like to thank Denise Vrouenraets for her excellent secretarial assistance, enthusiasm, and encouragement.

CHAPTER 1

Basic principles

Cardiac imaging is currently one of the most rapidly advancing fields in clinical cardiology. Continuing technical innovations are expanding the applicability and usefulness of non-invasive imaging modalities such as ultrasound, nuclear imaging, positron emission tomography, magnetic resonance imaging and, most recently, computed tomography (CT). While CT became an essential imaging tool in general medicine early on, for a long time it was considered an unsuitable technique for imaging moving structures. However, current multislice spiral CT scanners, with rapid gantry rotation, are able to provide detailed and motion-free imaging of the heart and coronary arteries. It is undeniable that spiral CT has entered the arena of non-invasive cardiac imaging, and while its exact role in the clinical setting is still under investigation, expansive employment of cardiac spiral CT is anticipated by both cardiologists and radiologists.

DEVELOPMENT OF CARDIAC COMPUTED TOMOGRAPHY

Computed tomography is one of the many applications of X-ray radiation in clinical medicine. The technique was developed in the early 1970s by Godfrey N Hounsfield, and together with Dr Allan MacLeod Cormack, who contributed mathematical solutions, he received the Nobel Prize in Medicine for his work in 1979. These first computed axial tomography (CAT) scanners required long scan and reconstruction times to provide crude images (of the brain). Technical advancement led to faster imaging and reconstruction, whole-body scanners, improved image quality, and dynamic imaging protocols. In the interest of cardiovascular imaging, electron beam CT (EBCT) was introduced in the mid-1980s. EBCT is a non-mechanical CT technique that provides high temporal resolution owing to the absence of rotating scanner parts. In the early 1990s spiral CT allowed continuous data acquisition while the patient was moved through the gantry. In 1998 the first multislice spiral CT scanners with four detector rows were introduced. Because of their thin detectors, volumetric acquisition of data, and fast coverage, these scanners resulted in a breakthrough as regards angiographic applications and further propelled the development of advanced three-dimensional image processing applications. High temporal resolution, which is essential for imaging moving objects, was facilitated by accelerated rotation rates combined with dedicated reconstruction algorithms, and allowed almost motion-free imaging of the heart. Electrocardiogram (ECG)-gated contrast-enhanced CT angiography of the heart and coronary arteries improved with further development of faster rotation and shorter scan times by extending the number of detector rows, and further decreasing the thickness of the detectors.

COMPUTED TOMOGRAPHY BASICS

The process of (cardiac) CT can be divided into the following steps: data acquisition, image reconstruction, post-processing, evaluation and reporting, and data storage and exchange (Figure 1.1).

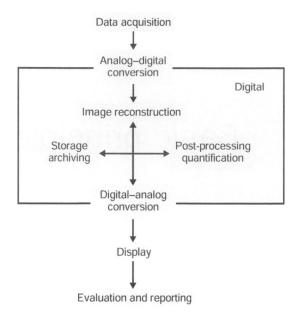

Figure 1.1 Schematic overview of the CT acquisition process.

Data acquisition

Data acquisition refers to the collection of X-ray transmission measurements through the patient. It requires an X-ray source that produces an X-ray beam, which is collimated into the shape of a fan or cone (Figure 1.2). When an X-ray beam passes through an object some of the photons are absorbed or scattered. The reduction of X-ray

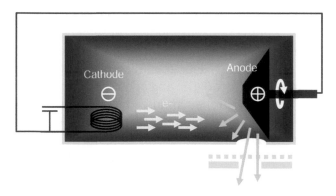

Figure 1.2 Roentgen tube. Within the electrical field electrons are released from the cathode and travel through the vacuum housing of the roentgen tube towards the anode. When the high-energy electrons collide with the anode, photons are emitted. The anode and the location of electron impact rotate to avoid over heating. Low-energy photons, which do not contribute to the image for mation, are filtered out. The remaining photons are then collimated to form a fan- or cone-shaped beam.

transmission, which is called attenuation, depends on the atomic composition and density of the traversed tissues, as well as on the energy of the photons. After passing through an object the partially attenuated X-rays are collected by X-ray detectors on the opposite side and converted from X-ray photons to electrical signals (Figure 1.3). These signals are then converted into digital data, after which the attenuation value is calculated. While the X-ray tube and detectors rotate around the patient, a large number of projections are collected from consecutive angular orientations.

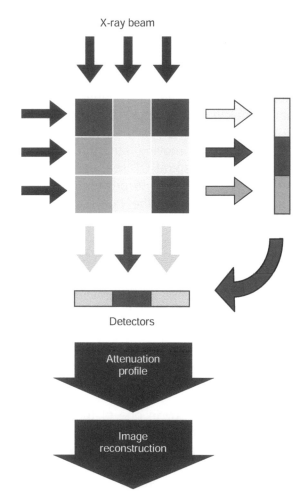

Figure 1.3 Depending on the traversed material, emitted photons are partially absorbed or scattered. The remaining photons are collected and measured by the detectors on the opposite side. T o calculate the attenuation throughout the plane, and reconstruct a CT image, a large number of attenuation profiles from consecutive rotational angles are required.

Image reconstruction

The reconstruction of images from the X-ray measurements involves the following steps (Figure 1.4). First, the measured X-rays are pre-processed, which is necessary to correct for beam hardening and scattered radiation. After pre-processing the raw data are filtered using convolution kernels. The filtering can result in very smooth to very sharp images based on the selected kernel. Depending on the reconstruction algorithm, projections from a 180° or 360° rotation are used for image reconstruction. Because spiral CT continuously acquires measurements at slightly varying longitudinal positions, an additional step is required before reconstruction. A complete set of projections at the selected plane position is created by interpolation of adjacent measurements in the longitudinal direction (Figure 1.5). The final step is to calculate the variation of regional attenuation within the image plane based on the collection of angular projections using back-projection reconstruction technique. The selected 'field of view' is divided into small image elements, called pixels. The density value of each pixel depends on the composition of the tissue it represents and is expressed in Hounsfield units (HU). The Hounsfield units are calculated from the attenuation measurements relative to the attenuation of water and range from −1024 to +3071 HU

$$\text{Hounsfield unit } (x,y) = 1000 \times \mu_{(x,y)} - \mu_{water} \, / \, \mu_{water} \, (\mu = \text{attenuation coefficient})$$

The result is a two-dimensional matrix of pre-selected size and detail, with each element representing the average attenuation of that location relative to water.

Image display

Contrary to continuous analog images (conventional X-ray), CT images are digital or numerical images (Figure 1.6). The attenuated X-ray that

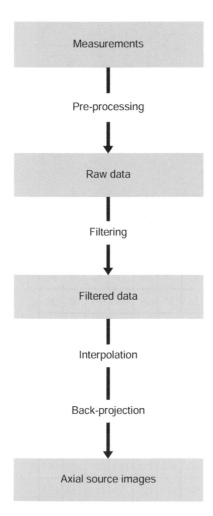

Measurements

↓

Pre-processing

↓

Raw data

↓

Filtering

↓

Filtered data

↓

Interpolation

↓

Back-projection

↓

Axial source images

Figure 1 . 4 CT image reconstruction.

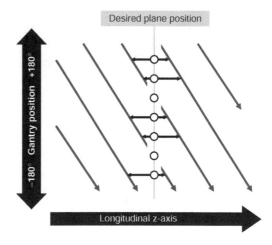

Figure 1 . 5 Interpolation of the spiral data. Because in spiral CT the table moves continuously, all projections are acquired at slightly different table positions. By weighted interpolation of the measurements a djacent to the plane position, weighted by the distance of the actual measurement to the reconstruction plane, a complete set of measurements is created and an image can be reconstructed using back-projection algorithms.

reaches the detector is transformed into an analog electrical signal and then converted into a discrete digital format that can be processed by computer. The CT images on screen are an analog visual representation of binary values that have been digitally processed. The image consists of a matrix of discrete attenuation values that are the result of sampling and computer processing. Theoretically this entire range of attenuation values (−1024 to +3071 HU) could be displayed in a gradually sliding scale from black to white. Unfortunately, the human eye is incapable of distinguishing these fine nuances. Therefore, it is important to adjust the display setting in such a way that the range of density values of the structure of interest are displayed with optimal contrast (Figures 1.7 and 1.8).

The window level indicates the density value at the center of the displayed gray scale, which determines the brightness of the image. The window width indicates which density values around the window level are within the gray scale display. Therefore, the width determines the image contrast. All matrix elements with attenuation values beyond the window limits appear as either saturated white or black on the screen. The density value of water is predefined at 0 HU. The density value of soft tissues, such as non-enhanced muscle and blood, varies between approximately −100 and +200 HU, while fat tissue is at the lower end of that scale and bone or other calcified tissues have higher attenuation values. Using routine intravenous contrast-enhancement protocols and contrast media, the attenuation

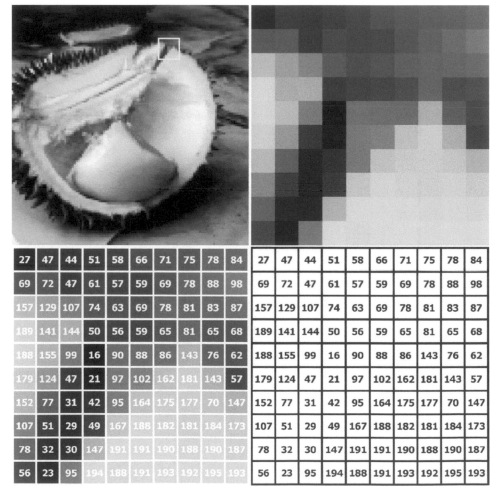

Figure 1 . 6 Digitization. Digitization of an (analog) image results in a numerical matrix.

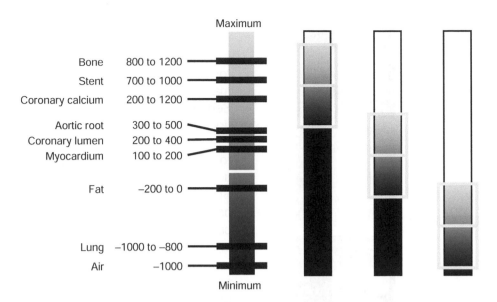

Figure 1 . 7 Tissue densities and window level and width settings. The tissue attenuation ranges of the various tissues in contrast-enhanced CT angiography are arranged on the first density scale. By setting the window level at a high-density level, structures such as bone tissue can be evaluated. An intermediate level around 200 HU allows differentiation of the vessels and their relation to the vessel wall and calcifications. A low window level setting allows appreciation of the lungs. Tissues with density values beyond the boundaries of the window width appear as either saturated white (higher density) or black (lower density).

value of the arterial blood is increased to a level between +200 and +400 HU. Metal has density values that overlap and exceed bone. Air and lung tissue have very low attenuation values. Taking the attenuation characteristics of the different tissue types into consideration, the window level of a contrast-enhanced CT image is set at around +250 HU and the window width at 400 HU. This allows appreciation of the contrast-enhanced blood and its relation to the surrounding tissues, with bone and other high-density structures displayed as saturated white, and fat and air displayed as saturated black. Depending on the users' interests and preferences, as well as the scanning conditions, these settings can be altered to allow optimal appreciation of the coronary luminal integrity.

Data storage

Data can be stored on film but, particularly if additional post-processing is anticipated in the future, digital storage is preferable. The size of a single CT image is approximately 500 kB. A complete cardiac study, including several reconstructions containing more than 250 slices each, will require at least 500 MB. Data can be archived on various magnetic and optical media. Alternatively, digital archiving using a picture archiving and communication system (PACS) may be preferred for convenient exchange and retrieval of data. To assure communication of imaging data between various imaging modalities, digital archives, evaluation workstations, printers, etc. from different manufacturers, a standard called DICOM (Digital Imaging and Communication in Medicine) has been developed.

COMPUTED TOMOGRAPHY SYSTEMS AND ACQUISITION MODES

Sequential and spiral CT

Originally, all CT scanners sequentially acquired axial slices according to the stop-and-shoot principle. In sequential scanning, during acquisition of a slice (or more slices with multidetector systems), the table remains stationary. After completion of the acquisition the table moves to a new (consecutive or overlapping) position to perform the next scan

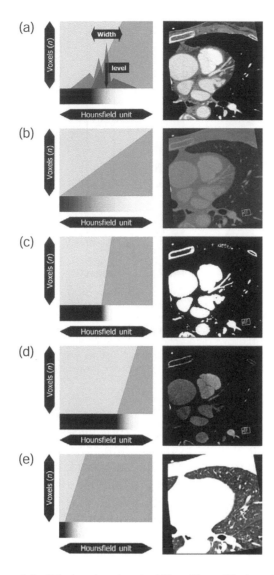

Figure 1.8 Window level and width settings. Display of a digital image can be manipulated by altering the window level and width. The histogram, which displays the pixel–density distribution, roughly consists of four tissue types: air and lung tissue, fat tissue, soft tissue, and dense tissue (a). The window settings deter mine how a measured and reconstructed density value is displayed on screen. T o evaluate the coronary arteries the level is set around the density value of the enhanced blood in the coronary arteries (a). Using a wide window results in low-contrast images, the entire range of density values are displayed with a slightly different shade (b). Because the human eye is incapable of distinguishing these fine nuances, the structures of interest are not clearly recognized. Selecting a very narrow width results in high-contrast images with completely saturated shading of the densities above and below the selected level (c). Increasing the level results in display of high-density structures, i.e. the contrast-enhanced structures and calcified tissue (d), and a low level results in brighter images and display of the low-density structures, i.e. the lungs (e), and completely saturated display of the other tissues.

(Figure 1.9). The disadvantage of this method is the relatively long scan time (Table 1.1). Spiral CT scanners allow for continuous tube-detector rotation and fast acquisition of data. This was made possible by the use of slip-ring technology. Sequential CT scanners rely on a physical connection in the form of cables between the rotating elements containing the roentgen tube and detectors and the stationary base, which necessitates unwinding of the wires after each acquisition. Spiral CT systems transmit energy and data between the rotating and stationary scanner parts via electrically conductive brushes and rotating rings. Instead of the stop-and-shoot (and rewind) principle of conventional, sequential scanners, spiral CT scanners are able to rotate continuously. During acquisition the table moves at a constant speed through the gantry (Figures 1.9 and 1.10). The path of the acquisition relative to the subject resembles that of a helix or

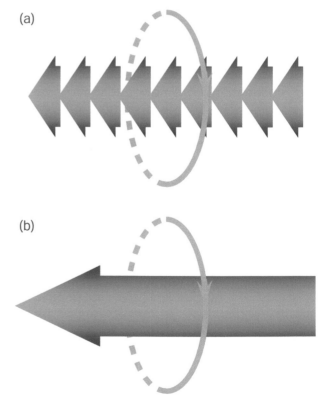

Figure 1 . 9 Sequential and spiral CT scanning. Sequential scanners acquire one (set of) slices, after which the table is advanced to the next plane position (a). Spiral scanners acquire data continuo usly while the table mo ves at a constant speed (b).

T ble 1 . 1 Triggered versus gated image acquisition and reconstruction

ECG synchronization	Prospective triggering	Retrospective gating
Reconstruction of multiple cardiac phases	Ð	Available
Multisegmental reconstruction algorithms	Ð	Available
Vulnerability to arrhythmia	Severe	Modest
Retrospective ECG editing	–	Available
Overlapped slice reconstruction	–	Available

ECG, electrocardiogram

spiral, hence the names: helical and spiral CT. Continuous acquisition ot data allows coverage of larger sections in the same amount of time. In particular angiographic applications, which demand temporary contrast enhancement, have benefited from this improvement in acquisition speed. Because the X-ray tube generates energy for an extended period more heat storage capacity is required. Also, the large amount of data that is being produced in a very short period requires expanded storage and processing capacity.

Electron beam CT

In mechanical CT, including multislice spiral CT, the roentgen tube and detector array physically rotate around the table. The extrafugal forces created during rotation restrict the rotation speed, and thereby the temporal resolution of mechanical CT. The electron beam CT (EBCT) was developed to image the heart. Instead of a physically rotating tube detector unit, EBCT generates and directs electrons along a stationary tungsten ring (Figure 1.11). Emitted X-rays from the target ring

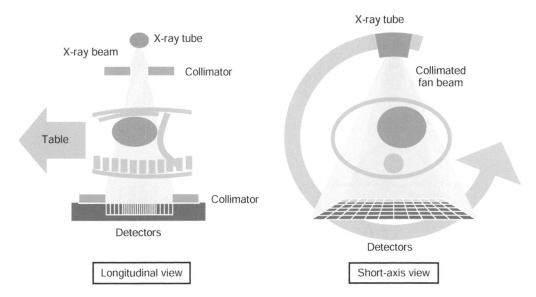

Figure 1 .01 Multislice spiral CT. The X-ray tube and the detectors rotate in an opposing position on the gantry around the patient. During continuous X-ray emission a collimated roentgen beam is passed through the patient and the attenuated radiation is collected while the patient on the couch is advanced continuously through the gantry. Instead of one detector row, several parallel detector rows acquire data, which allows accelerated scanning and a short scan time.

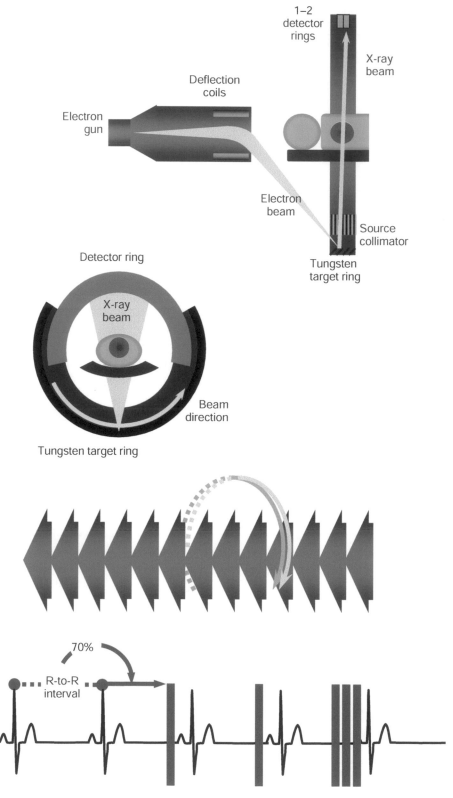

Figure 1 . 1 Electron beam CT (EBCT). An electron beam is generated and directed along a tungsten ring in the gantry below the patient couch. As the electrons hit the target ring, X-rays are created and a narrow fan beam is passed through the patient after collimation. One or more detector rings are positioned on the opposite side of the gantry to collect the attenuated radiation. After each image acquisition the patient couch is advanced 2– 3mm to the next position to per form the next scan. Newer types of EBCT can acquire between one and three or one set of images per heart cycle.

are collimated, and after passing through the patient collected by the stationary detectors on the opposite side. In the absence of rotating parts the temporal resolution of EBCT is 100 ms (potentially 50 ms), which was an enormous improvement of the resolution of mechanical CT at the time of development. Up to three acquisitions, each consisting of one or two axial slices, can be acquired per heart cycle, thus allowing retrospective selection of the most optimal data set. Although EBCT can be used for non-invasive coronary angiography, it is now most often used for quantification of coronary calcium.

Multislice CT

By increasing the number of detector rows, multiple channels of data can be acquired simultaneously (Figure 1.12). The advantage of multidetector or multislice CT acquisition is the increased longitudinal coverage that can be achieved per rotation (Figure 1.13). This is particularly useful for cardiac acquisitions, which deal with an inherently longer scan time compared with imaging of non-moving organs. Current state-of-the-art CT technology simultaneously

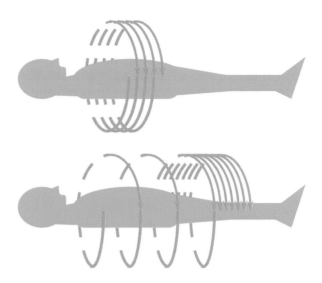

Figure 1 . 1 3ingle and multislice spiral CT scanning. Multiple detector rows allow for faster data acquisition and longer scan ranges within the same (breath hold) time.

acquires 64 slices. Most 64-slice scanners are physically equipped with 64 detector rows. Alternatively, one CT manufacturer offers a 32-detector system that allows 64-slice acquisition by double sampling in the longitudinal direction. By rapid, longitudinal alternation of the focal spot during acquisition, two partially overlapping sets of projections from slightly differing positions are acquired. Compared with systems with 64 detector rows, double z-sampling results in an improved longitudinal resolution at the penalty of a longer total scan time (Figure 1.14).

With the expansion of the number of detectors, the individual detector width decreased.

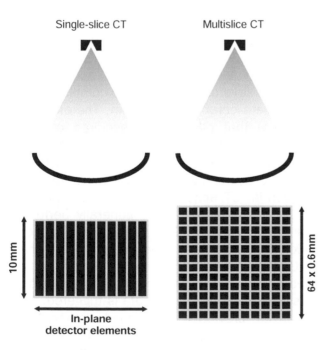

Figure 1 . 1 2ingle- versus multidetector row CT . A larger number of thinner rows of detectors improves spatial resolution and shortens the total scan time.

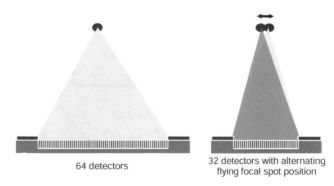

Figure 1 . 1 4ixty-four-slice CT using 64 detector rows or 32 detector rows combined with double sampling in the longitudinal direction.

From four- to 64-slice CT the detector width decreased from 1.0–1.25 to 0.5–0.6 mm. Combined with overlapping reconstruction of slices, this has improved the spatial resolution in the longitudinal direction. The through-plane resolution of current scanners approximates the in-plane resolution, resulting in isotropic voxel size, which is important for three-dimensional post-processing.

Dual-source CT

Dual-source CT scanners are equipped with two roentgen sources rotating at a 90° angle to each other (Figure 1.15). The advantage of dual-source CT is the improvement of the temporal resolution, which remains one of the most important limitations in cardiac CT. Additionally, assessment of ventricular function and valve function should be improved using dual-source CT. A potentially interesting application of dual-source CT is dual-energy CT. During scanning both tube detector systems operate using a different tube voltage (kV), which improves tissue differentiation.

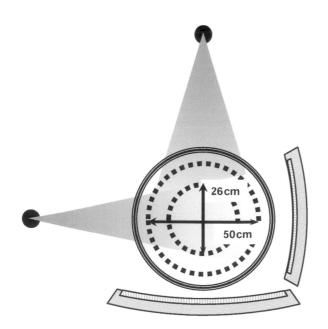

Figure 1 .51 Dual-source CT. Two tube detector systems are mounted at a 90° angle.

CARDIAC COMPUTED TOMOGRAPHY IMAGING

Requirements

A number of imaging aspects set cardiac CT apart from non-cardiac CT applications. The heart is an organ that is subject to displacement from voluntary movement, respiration, and cardiac contraction, all of which need to be neutralized during the data acquisition and image reconstruction. Additionally, because of the continuous motion of the heart, patient preparation and image reconstruction requires special attention. Injection of contrast medium is necessary to distinguish the coronary lumen from the vessel wall and other soft tissues, this is discussed in detail later. The coronary arteries are small, and the pathology under investigation even smaller. For these reasons cardiac CT and non-invasive coronary angiography challenges the performance capacities of current CT technology. Optimization of image quality and interpretability is only possible when the methodology of contrast-enhanced ECG-gated image acquisition and reconstruction, image post-processing, and display are well understood.

ECG-synchronized image reconstruction

Current CT technology requires acquisition of data over several heart cycles to combine to form a complete coronary angiogram. Therefore, it is essential that all data be acquired or reconstructed during the same phase-of cardiac contraction. Basically, there are two methods to obtain phase-consistent images (Figure 1.16). Sequential CT acquisitions, by conventional CT, EBCT, or multislice CT, are generally performed using prospective ECG triggering. The data acquisition is guided by on-line interpretation of the ECG. At the predicted moment of the desired cardiac phase, based on the duration of the previous cycles, acquisition of data is triggered. Apart from the previously mentioned drawbacks of sequential imaging, prospective ECG triggering is inherently more sensitive to heart rhythm irregularities. Spiral CT acquires data continuously,

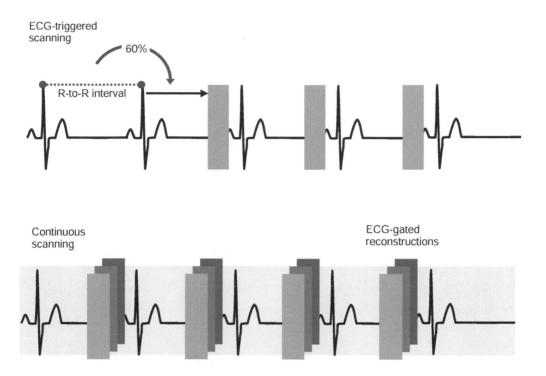

Figure 1 . 1 Electrocardiogram (ECG)-synchronized image reconstruction. Sequential scan protocols use prospective ECG triggering to synchronize the data acquisition to the motion of the heart. Based on the measured duration of previous heart cycles, the scan of one or more slices is initiated at a prespecified moment after the R-wave, for instance at 60% of the previous R-to-R intervals. Spiral CT scanners acquire data continuously and recor d the patient's ECG during the scan. Isocar diophasic images are reconstructed using retrospective ECG gating. The r econstruction window can be positioned anywhere within the R-to-R interval, and images can be created during any phase.

while recording the patient's ECG. From the raw scan data, the ECG serves to selectively gather the scan data that were acquired during a specified cardiac phase of each heart cycle. From this isocardiophasic raw data, all reconstructed images will show the heart in the same phase of contraction. This type of image reconstruction is called retrospective ECG gating. If data have been acquired continuously, the CT angiogram can be reconstructed during any cardiac phase (Figure 1.17). Three different ways to position the reconstruction window within the R-to-R interval on the ECG trace, and perform retrospective ECG-gated image reconstruction, are shown in Figure 1.18. However, the data used for reconstruction are acquired instantly but during a short period of time. The duration of this acquisition or reconstruction interval determines the temporal resolution of the scanner and varies between 83 and 150 ms, depending on the scanner's rotation speed and reconstruction algorithm. When the reconstruction window is placed during a phase of substantial cardiac motion, inconsistent attenuation profiles, due to displacement of structures during the acquisition, cause severe artifacts which may render the reconstructed images non-interpretable (Figure 1.19). Motion of the coronary arteries is continuous but relatively modest during the mid- to end-diastolic phase just before atrial contraction. Also, at the end of ventricular contraction the coronary arteries can be relatively stationary, which constitutes an alternative moment for motion-sparse coronary reconstruction (Figure 1.20). Severe coronary motion causes streak and blurring artifacts within the reconstructed slices. If images have been reconstructed during different cardiac phases, for instance when the gating has failed or due to varying R-to-R intervals as a result of arrhythmia, there will be an interrupted through-plane continuity of structures, while the in-plane image quality may be fine.

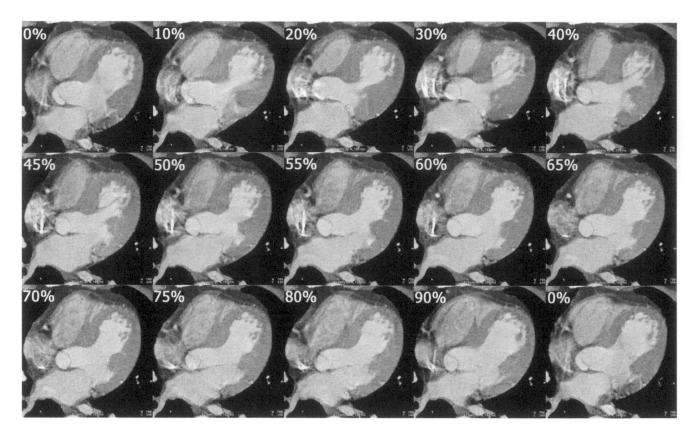

Figure 1 .71 Multiphasic reconstruction. Reconstruction of an axial slice through the left ventricle to detect the reconstruction window with the least motion artifact.

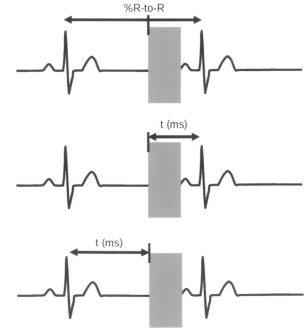

Figure 1 .81 Reconstruction window positioning. To ensure consistent isocardiophasic images and avoid interslice discontinuity, reconstruction must take place during the exact same phase within each heart cycle. The scanner's reconstruction software will allow different types of positioning with respect to the ECG. The position can be at a relative position as a percentage of the distance between the consecutive R-waves (R-to-R), or at an absolute time distance (t) with respect to the preceding or upcoming R-wave. There is little consensus about the most optimal method and, particularly in patients with an accelerating or varying heart rate, exploration of alternative methods can be worthwhile.

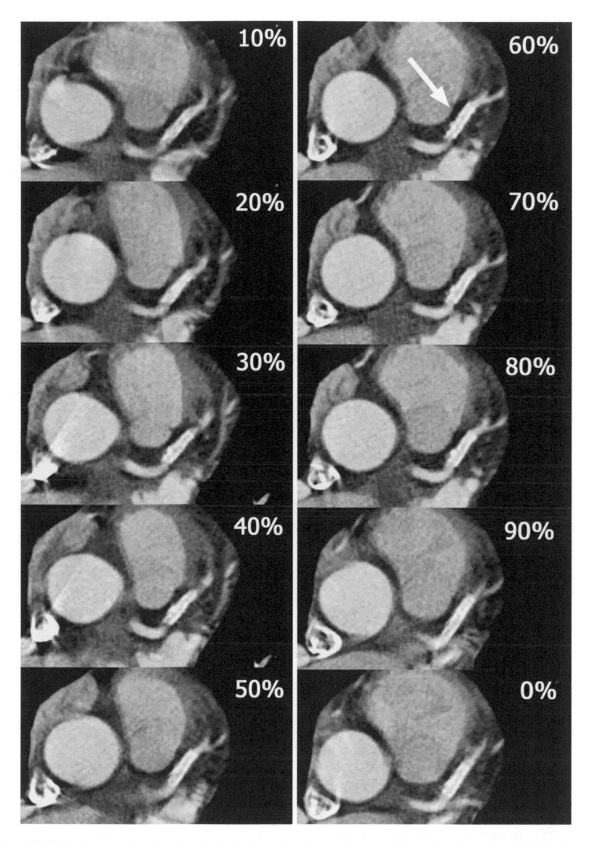

Figure 1 . 1 9 Multiphasic reconstruction of a stented left anterior descending artery. Reconstruction of an axial slice through the left anterior descending artery with a patent stent at ten different temporal positions within the heart cycle. Reconstruction window positioning is expressed as a percentage of the R-to-R interval.

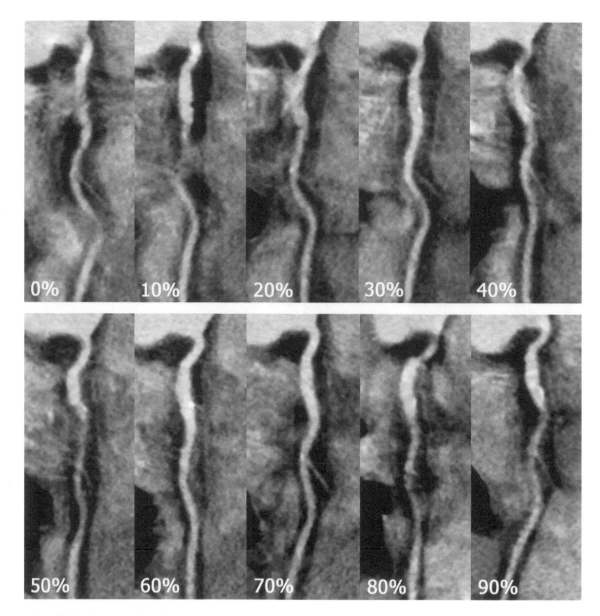

Figure 1 . 2 0 Multiphasic reconstruction of a right coronary artery. Ten reconstructions and curved multiplanar reformation of a diseased right coronary artery at different temporal positions within the heart cycle. Reconstruction window positioning is expressed as a per centage of the R-to-R interval. In addition to the mid to end-diastolic phase (60–70%), reasonable image quality could be obtained during end-systole (30%).

To reduce the radiation dose of cardiac CT, the roentgen tube output can be modulated during spiral CT acquisition. Because the coronary arteries are preferably reconstructed during the diastolic phase, tube output is decreased during the systolic using prospective ECG triggering (Figure 1.21). A good ECG signal is important to avoid misinterpretation and inappropriate triggering (Figure 1.22).

Displacement unrelated to cardiac contraction

To neutralize respiratory motion, the examination is performed during breath hold (5–15 s depending on the scanner). Additionally, the patient needs to be instructed not to make any other movements. There may be a subtle displacement of the heart due to a gradual shift of the diaphragm position while maintaining a breath hold.

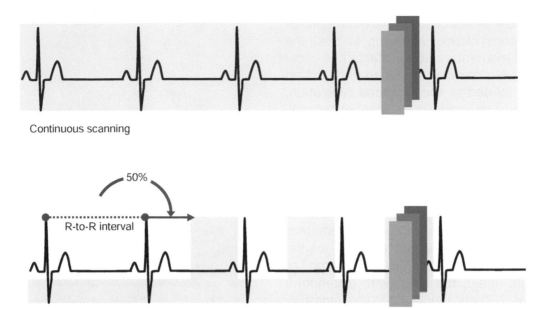

Figure 1.12 X-ray tube output modulation. While standard scan protocols require continuous output of the X-ray tube, more advanced protocols allow alternation of the output throughout the data acquisition procedure. Prospectively triggered by the ECG, the output of the roentgen tube is decreased during the systolic phase, when coronary evaluation is rarely per   formed, while nominal exposure is generated during the diastolic phase to ensure optimal image quality. The period of full exposure should be long enough for subtle variation of the reconstruction window position and the possibility to select the most optimal phase. Ideally, exposure during systole is sufficient for functional assessment of the ventricular per   formance. The exposure reduction is highest when the heart rate is low (at a constant scan pitch). Additionally, this application requires an ECG sign al that is free of noise or artifacts, as incorrect ECG signal reading can result in inadequate exposure during the diastolic phas   e, which in contrast to the positioning of the reconstruction window, cannot be edited after the acquisition of data.

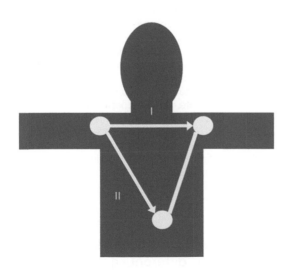

Figure 1.22 Positioning of the electrocardiogram (ECG) leads. The ECG electrodes are usually positioned around the left and right shoulder region at locations that are not affected by disturbing activity from the musculature underneath. The thir d lead is attached to the lower abdomen. In most patients either an Einthoven I or II configuration will result in a steep and high-amplitude R-wave, which is best interpreted by the scanner.

Gradual displacement of the heart causes discontinuity between the data that are acquired during consecutive heart cycles.

Heart rate, rotation speed, and temporal resolution

While the temporal resolution is of little concern when imaging non-moving organs, it is crucial in cardiac imaging. In cardiac CT the temporal resolution refers to the duration of the reconstruction window per heart cycle. It is comparable to the shutter time of a photo camera, and should ideally be infinitely short in order to avoid any motion artifacts on the image. Displacement of the object during the acquisition of projections (while the scanner performs a 180° rotation) results in inconsistencies, which the reconstruction algorithm is unable to handle well, resulting in smearing and blurring artifacts. The first step to avoid motion artifacts is selection of the most optimal phase for reconstruction. However, even at the most optimal moment motion artifacts can occur due to residual coronary displacement. Motion artifacts are related to the temporal resolution, which is in turn determined by scanner technology, reconstruction algorithms, and (preparation of) the patient.

Rotation speed

The rotation speed of the tube detector unit is one of the most important scanner parameters because it directly affects the temporal resolution. Four-slice CT with a rotation time of 500 ms could image the heart with a temporal resolution of 250 ms using a 180°-reconstruction algorithm. At a heart rate of 60 bpm, this would mean that the reconstruction window covers one-quarter of the entire cardiac cycle. The rotation time of 64-slice scanners varies between 330 and 420 ms, with a temporal resolution varying between 165 and 210 ms. Further acceleration of the rotation time is restricted by the excessive centrifugal forces involved with mechanical CT.

Multisegmental reconstruction algorithms

To improve the effective temporal resolution of CT, dedicated reconstruction algorithms have been developed. If a given z-position is scanned during at least two heart cycles, the data of both cycles can be combined. If the projections of 90° rotation of the first cycle are combined with the following 90° rotation of the next cycle during the same phase of cardiac contraction, then the effective temporal resolution is equal to one-quarter of the rotation time of the scanner (Figure 1.23). This could then be extended to three or four cycles to further reduce the effective temporal resolution (Figure 1.24). There are, however, a number of consequences and limitations to this approach. First of all, to sample each location two or more times the table speed needs to be sufficiently low. This means that either the heart rate needs to be fast, or the pitch needs to be lowered. Obviously this prolongs the scan time and increases the

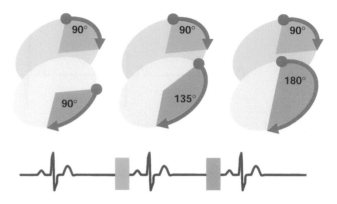

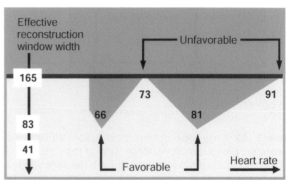

Figure 1.23 *Multisegmental image reconstruction. If the same section has been sampled twice, the data of the first and second acquisition can be combined to improve the effective temporal resolution. In the ideal situation the position of the second acquisition (during the same cardiac phase) is off-set by exactly 90° compared with the first. In this case the two 90° segments of projections can be combined to complete the necessary 180° of data (upper left example). The most unfavorable situation is when the tube is at the same position (or off-set by exactly 180°) during both acquisitions. In this case projections acquired during the same phase of both cycles overlap and no improvement of the temporal resolution is possible. The position at which the tube is during consecutive cycles depends on the rotation time and the heart rate of the patient. For a scanner with a rotation time of 330 ms, the effective temporal resolution using bisegmental reconstruction will depend on the heart rate with optimal heart rates of 66 and 81 bpm. At a heart rate of 73 or 91 bpm, the effective resolution will be equal to the nominal resolution of the 180° reconstruction algorithm (165 ms), as depicted in the graph.*

radiation dose. Second, the algorithm is only effective when different data are acquired during both cycles: ideally each of both 90° rotations provides a non-overlapping part of the total 180° projections needed for image reconstruction. Depending on the heart rate in relation to the rotation time of the scanner, multisegmental reconstruction algorithms

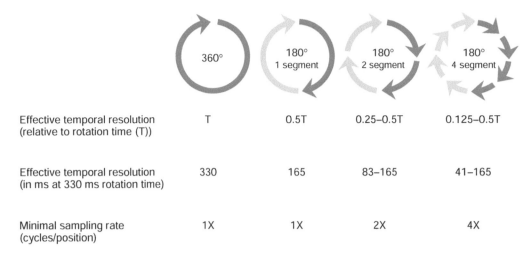

	360°	180° 1 segment	180° 2 segment	180° 4 segment
Effective temporal resolution (relative to rotation time (T))	T	0.5T	0.25–0.5T	0.125–0.5T
Effective temporal resolution (in ms at 330 ms rotation time)	330	165	83–165	41–165
Minimal sampling rate (cycles/position)	1X	1X	2X	4X

Figure 1 . 2 Reconstruction algorithms in cardiac multislice CT. In non-cardiac Imaging, data from an entire rotation are used for image reconstruction. For cardiac scanning a partial scan is used for image reconstruction. By combining data acquired at the same position during the same phase of two or four cardiac cycles, the effective temporal resolution can be reduced. Depending on the actual heart rate during acquisition and the rotation time of the scanner the effective temporal resolution varies between 50% and 25% (two segments) or 12.5% (four segments), of the rotation time of the scanner . Using these multisegmental reconstruction algorithms requires multiple sampling of the same position, with a shorter scan range and increased radiation exposure.

improve the effective temporal resolution by 0–50% (Figure 1.23). Finally, heart rate inconsistencies will result in coronary displacement between the two cycles and negatively affect the image quality.

Heart rate modulation

Even with newer CT equipment, high image quality with fewer motion artifacts is more often achieved in patients with a low heart rate (Figure 1.25). Therefore, to avoid motion artifacts heart rate modulating medication can be administered prior to the examination. Beta-blockers can be used orally, from 1 hour to several days before the examination, or intravenously at the time of the examination. When the use of beta-blockers is considered, the absence of contraindications and possible side-effects should be known with certainty. In case of an atrioventricular conduction delay, heart failure, or low blood pressure, beta-blockers are contraindicated. Prior to the examination, the patient's resting ECG should be examined and blood pressure measured. During examination the atrioventricular conduction may, in rare cases, be compromised or a symptomatic

drop in blood pressure may occur. However, using a low dose of metoprolol, i.e. 100 mg, this rarely occurs. In case of low blood pressure or mild conduction disorders an extended observation period is desirable. Alternatively, calcium channel blockers can be used when there are contraindications to beta-blockers.

The heart rate during the examination is also accelerated by anxiety. Explanation of the examination, expected sensations of the contrast medium, and reassurance are important to reduce this anxiety. Additionally, anxiolytic medication may be used, although this may have practical consequences if the patient is unaccompanied. Finally, abstinence from caffeine-containing beverages is recommended prior to the scan.

Dual-source CT

While the minimally required data for image reconstruction are collected by single-source CT in one-half of a rotation, simultaneous acquisition by a double roentgen-detector CT system requires only one-quarter of a rotation. By reducing the acquisition time per slice by half (Figure 1.26), the

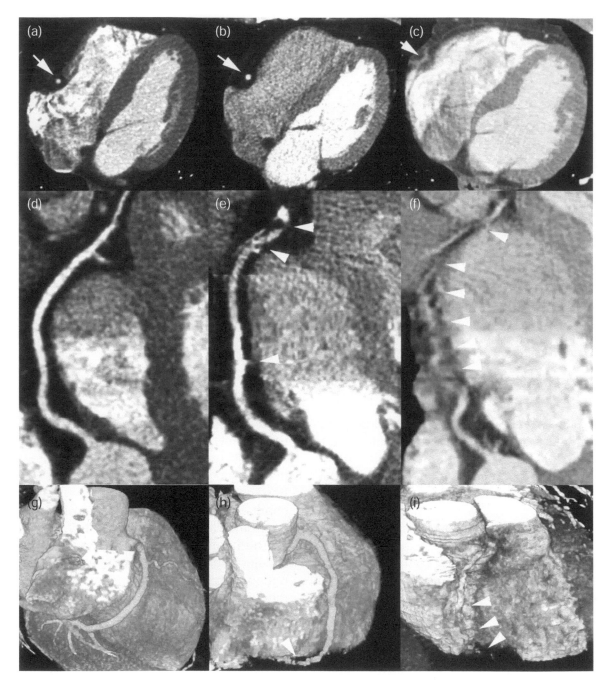

Figure 1 .52 Heart rate-related image quality. Representative cases of three patients with varying heart rates. The right coronary artery (arrows) is displayed at a heart rate of 49(A), 64(B) and 81(C) bpm [From reference 1, with permission.]

temporal resolution is improved by a factor of 2. At the time of writing dual-source CT is offered by only one manufacturer (Siemens). At a rotation time of 330 ms, the temporal resolution of the scanner is 83 ms. In patients with a faster heart rate the table speed can be increased (higher pitch), thereby reducing the total radiation dose. Depending on the pitch (0.2–0.43) and the volume scanned, the scan time varies between 7 and 13 s. Improvement of the temporal resolution should improve image quality, particularly in patients with a faster heart rate.

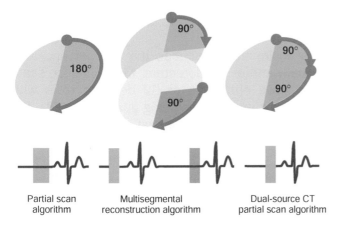

Figure 1 . 2 6 Monosegmental image reconstruction requires 180° of projections to reconstruct an image. Bisegmental reconstruction combines data from consecutive cycles and results in a reduction of the effective reconstruction window of between 0 and 50%, depending on the heart rate in relation to the scanner rotation speed. Dual-source CT acquires two 90° segments during the same heart cycle, reducing the reconstruction window by 50%, independent of the heart rate.

Spatial resolution

The spatial resolution refers to the degree of blurring in an image and the ability to discriminate objects and structures of small size. In CT we distinguish the in-plane (axial, xy, cross-sectional) resolution of an axial image, and the through-plane (longitudinal, z) resolution of the volume of axial slices (Figure 1.27). The spatial resolution of CT is affected by technical aspects of the scanner, the acquisition protocol, image reconstruction, and post-processing. With respect to the scanner, there are several important parameters that cannot be influenced by the operator. Spatial resolution is inversely related to the size of the focal spot of the roentgen tube, the distance between the tube and the detectors, and the size of the detector elements. Additionally, resolution improves with the number of acquired projections per rotation. The ability to distinguish details in the axial image is further influenced by the tube settings, motion, contrast enhancement, filtering, the image matrix size, size of the field-of-view, and display setting.

The slice sensitivity profile (SSP) describes the longitudinal resolution, and shows to what extent the reconstructed image is influenced by adjacent anatomy (Figure 1.28). For sequential

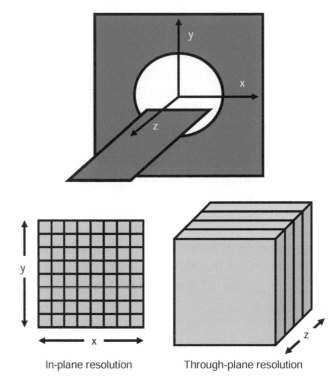

In-plane resolution   Through-plane resolution

Figure 1 . 2 7 The in-plane (xy) resolution represents the ability to distinguish details within the axial slice. The spatial resolution through the axial slices is called the through-plane (z or longitudinal) resolution.

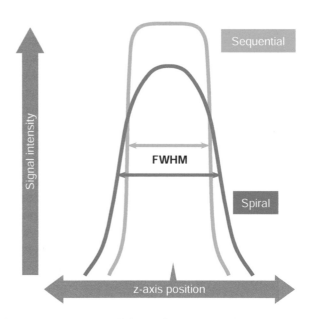

Figure 1 . 2 8 Slice sensitivity profile. Due to the interpolation of measurements the effective slice thickness (at full-width-half-maximum (FWHM)) of the reconstructed spiral CT images is slightly increased in comparison to the effective slice thickness of sequentially acquired CT images, at a constant individual detector width.

CT the width of the SSP and the longitudinal resolution are largely determined by the width of the detectors. In spiral CT the image is influenced by adjacent anatomy to a larger extent because of longitudinal interpolation of measurements. Increasing the pitch further widens the SSP and negatively affects the longitudinal spatial resolution. Therefore, the effective slice thickness, expressed as the width of the SSP curve at mid-level (full-width-half-maximum) is wider than the detector width.

When spatial resolution is insufficient compared with the size of the examined object, partial voluming will occur (Figure 1.29). This means that the attenuation by the different tissue components within an image element will be averaged.

Field of view and matrix size

The CT acquisition has a fundamental spatial resolution that depends on the scanner and the acquisition protocol. Although almost the entire area within the boundaries of the gantry is scanned, only that part where the patient is, or only a part of where the patient is, is selected for reconstruction. This reconstructed area is called the field of view. Reconstructed CT images contain a fixed number of image elements: 256×256, 512×512, or 1024×1024. Therefore, the resolution of the CT image is related to the field of view and the size of the matrix. For example, if the matrix size is 512×512 elements and the field of view is $25 \times 25 \, cm^2$, then the size of the pixels or image elements is $0.5 \times 0.5 \, mm^2$. If the fundamental sampling resolution of the scanner is sufficient, then the spatial resolution can theoretically be increased to $0.3 \times 0.3 \, mm^2$ by reducing the field of view to $15 \times 15 \, cm^2$. If coronary imaging is the purpose of the scan, the field of view is placed tightly around the heart to optimize the in-plane spatial resolution. If a specific structure within the heart needs to be examined in detail, an additional reconstruction with an even smaller field of view can be performed. This is limited by the fundamental spatial resolution of the scanner, beyond which further minimization of the field of view is without improvement of the spatial resolution (Figure 1.30).

Detector collimation and slice thickness

The collimation describes the number and individual width of the detectors. Most 64-slice scanners have either 64 or 32 detector rows with double z-sampling (including dual-source CT). For coronary imaging the thinnest collimation, i.e. the smallest selectable detector width (0.5–0.6 mm) is usually selected to achieve maximum longitudinal spatial resolution. In case of noisy images (obese patients or insufficient dose), image noise can to a certain extent be averaged out by reconstruction of thicker slices at the expense of the spatial resolution (Figure 1.31).

Expansion of the number of detector rows has resulted in shorter scan times and more comfortable breath hold. The number of detector rows does not affect the spatial resolution.

Table advancement and pitch

The pitch is the table advancement (increment) per rotation relative to the width of the collimated detectors (where n is the number of detectors):

$$\text{Pitch} = \frac{\text{table advancement per rotation}}{n \times \text{individual detector width}}$$

To scan non-moving body sections the table advancement should be as high as possible while ensuring sufficient data acquisition. For non-gated scan protocols, the pitch usually varies between one and two. While a pitch of one results in optimal image quality, a higher pitch will shorten the scan time and reduce the radiation and contrast medium dose, but increase the effective slice thickness. For cardiac scanning, each z-position needs to be sampled during one entire heart cycle; therefore, the pitch is lower, significantly less than the width of the collimated detectors (Figure 1.32). Ideally, ECG-gated reconstruction results in consecutive slabs of isophasic images covering the entire object without gaps or overlap (Figure 1.33). At a fixed table speed the amount of z-axis overlap between slabs acquired during consecutive heart cycles depends on the heart rate. During very slow heart rates gaps are created, during fast heart rates excessive overlap will occur. Unless multisegmental reconstruction is anticipated, this

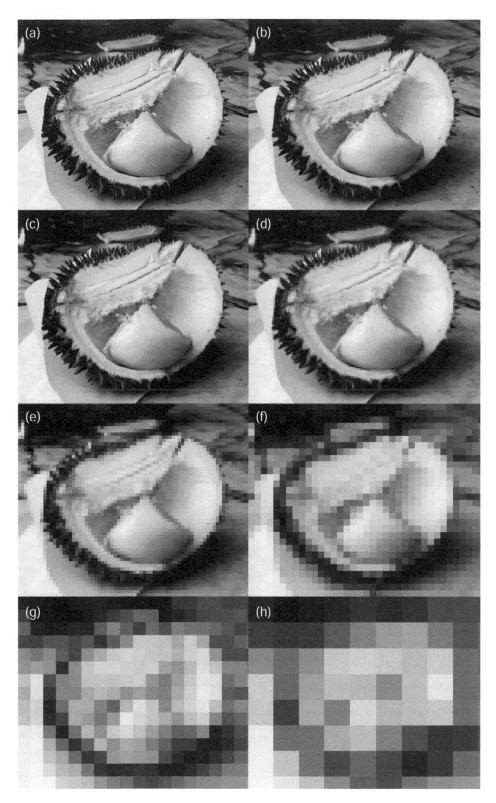

Figure 1 . 2 Decreasing spatial resolution results in partial voluming, i.e. averaging of the signal contributing to the density of the image element, and loss of detail.

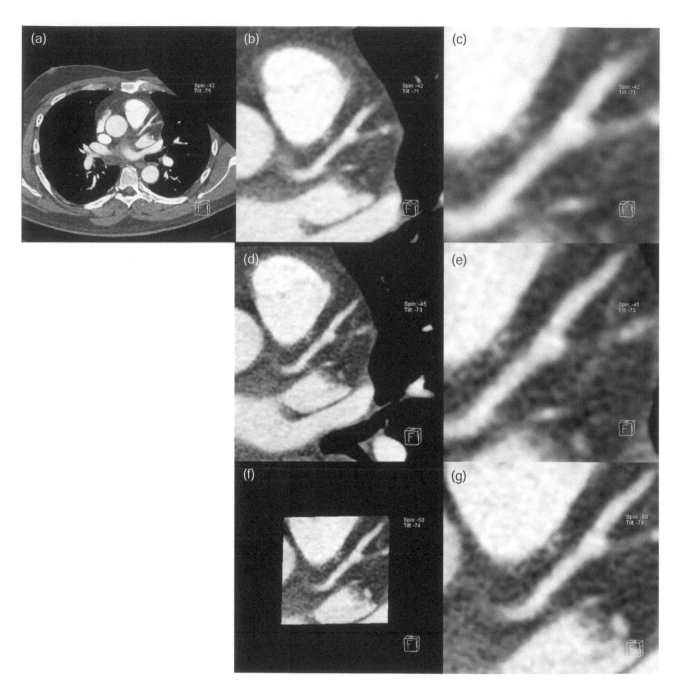

Figure 1 .03 By decreasing the field of view, and zooming in on the structure of interest, the spatial resolution will increase at a fixed matrix size. In the first series the entire thorax is reconstructed and a section of the left anterior descending coronar y artery is magnified (a)Đ(c). In the second series a section of approximately 10 × 10 cm is reconstructed and magnified (d) and (e). In the third series only the proximal left anterior descending artery is reconstructed (f) and magnified (g). When the pixel size becomes smaller than the fundamental spatial resolution, no improvement of spatial resolution can be expected.

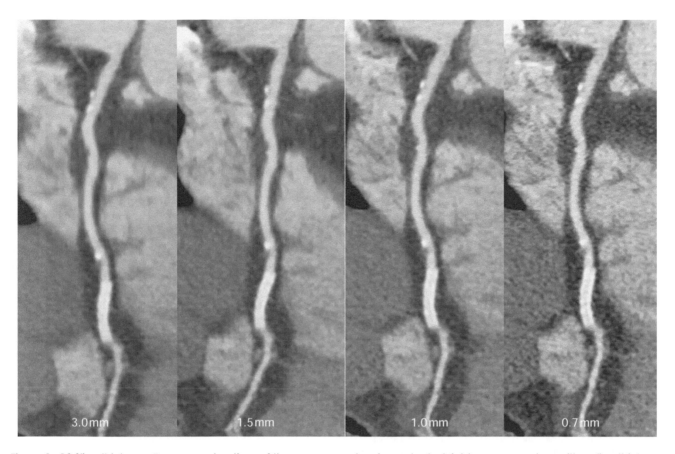

Figure 1.13 Slice thickness. Four reconstructions of the same scan showing a stented right coronary artery with a slice thickness of 3.0, 1.5, 1.0, and 0.7 mm, each with a reconstruction overlap of approximately 50%.

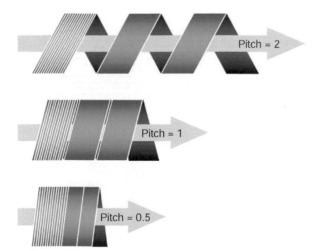

Figure 1.32 Pitch. Using a high pitch the table advancement per gantry rotation is large and extended sections can be scanned in a short period of time. Decreasing the pitch improves the image quality but results in a longer scan time. For cardiac imaging an even smaller pitch of less than one is required, which results in multiple acquisitions of each position to guarantee availability of data during the entire car diac cycle and allows for multiphasic reconstruction.

slab overlap results in unnecessary exposure to radiation. Therefore, some scanners are equipped with variable table speeds. A low table feed is selected in slow heart rates to allow complete coverage without gaps, a higher table speed is used to reduce the radiation dose and shorten the scan time.

Reconstruction increment

Axial images can be reconstructed at an increment that is smaller than the thickness of the slice. Overlapping images improve the through-plane continuity and to some extent (and at least subjectively) the longitudinal spatial resolution (Figure 1.34). The high number of overlapping slices improves the smoothness of three-dimensional reconstructions. For coronary angiography an overlap of between 30% and 50% is recommended.

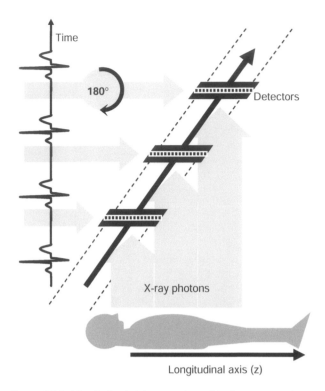

Optimally, the spatial resolution of current CT scanners is around 0.4 mm in three dimensions. However, in clinical practice such high resolution is unlikely to be realized on a routine basis. When a voxel contains more than one type of tissue the attenuation value of that image element will be a weighted average of both tissue types (Figure 1.35). Therefore, CT is more accurate in the larger proximal coronary arteries compared with the smaller side branches. While the spatial resolution determines the smallest detail that can be differentiated by CT, the minimal size of the image elements can be considerably smaller. By choosing a very small field of view and reconstructing images with a large overlap, voxels as small as 0.1 mm³ can be created. Reconstruction of voxels smaller than the spatial resolution of the scanner can be compared to the 'digital zoom' of a camera, the images are blown up using interpolation without added detail (Table 1.2).

Figure 1.33 Ideally the table speed would allow no overlap or gaps (in the longitudinal direction) between the isophasic data acquired during the consecutive heart cycles. In this case heart rate acceleration would result in overlapping acquisition, while heart rate deceleration would result in gaps.

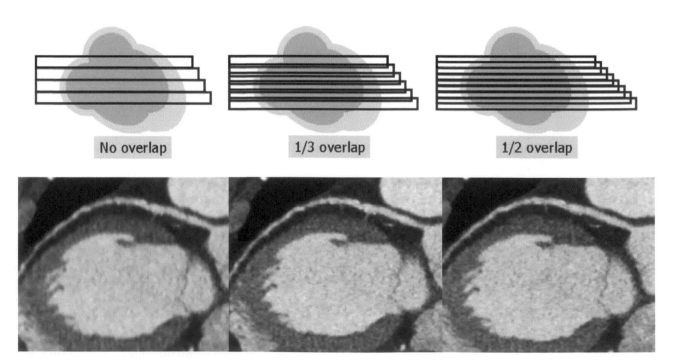

Figure 1 .43 Reconstruction increment. Comparison of the longitudinal or through-plane image quality after reconstruction of slices with no, one-third, or one-half overlap.

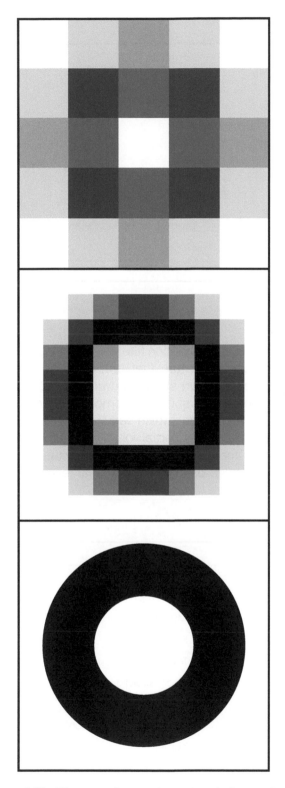

Figure 1.35 When one image element, a pixel or voxel, contains more than one type of tissue, the density value of the image element will represent a weighted average of both. When a black ring on a white background is digitized, the image consists of various shades of gray depending on the amount of black and white that is sampled within the pixel.

Contrast resolution and tissue differentiation (Table 1.3)

The degree of contrast and the ability to differentiate between tissues is called the contrast resolution. Differentiation of tissues is based on the variation of attenuation of the respective tissues and can be divided in to a limited number of groups: air/lung, fat tissue, soft tissue, and bone/metal. A contrast medium can be helpful to further differentiate tissue, for example blood and vessel wall as used in CT coronary angiography, or infarcted myocardium from normally perfused myocardium. The ability to recognize detailed variation of attenuation and tissue composition depends on the spatial resolution and image noise, and is influenced by numerous factors mentioned in the previous sections. Additionally, the perception of tissue contrast is affected by the window display settings, the display size, and the distance of the radiographer from the screen.

The roentgen attenuation by a given object varies depending on the energy of the photons. At lower energy levels (lower kV) photons are more easily dispersed (Compton effect), particularly when the tissue contains atoms with a high mass. Therefore, contrast between contrast-enhanced blood (containing iodine with a high atomic mass) and soft tissues may be improved using a lower tube current. Additionally, the variance of the contrast between tissues at different photon energy levels could be used to differentiate tissues. Dual-source CT allows acquisition of two data sets using different tube voltages during a single scan. The advantages of this technique for cardiac applications, such as differentiation of coronary calcium, delayed myocardial enhancement, still need to be further explored.

Image noise

Image noise is the fluctuation of the measurement compared with the nominal noise. It is responsible for the grainy appearance of CT scans or other imaging modalities. Image noise negatively affects the detailed evaluation of morphology and differentiation of tissues that are so important in coronary imaging. The amount of noise is influenced by the number of measurements per image element (voxel). If fewer

T ble 1 . 2 Spatial resolution and voxel size

	Spatial resolution	Voxel size
In-plane (xy)	Focal spot size	Field of view
	Tube– detector distance	Matrix size
	Detector size	
	Projections per rotation	
	Field of view	
	Matrix size	
	Filtering	
Through-plane (z)	Detector width	Reconstruction increment
	Pitch	
	Reconstructed slice thickness	

photons are collected per detector element per measurement, as a result of lower tube output, smaller detectors, faster rotation, or obese patients, image noise will increase. The increased noise level by use of thinner detectors, faster tube rotation, and scanning of obese patients is often compensated by increasing the tube current. Alternatively, or additionally, convolution filters or kernels can be used to modify the noise in the images.

Kernel

The kernel or convolution filter is a modifiable image reconstruction feature that enhances or smooths the edges between structures with varying attenuation properties. A soft kernel smooths intensity variation in the image, which reduces the amount of noise but increases partial voluming. Sharper kernels enhance the interface between structures, which improves edge definition and spatial resolution, but

T ble 1 . 3 Image quality parameters

Image quality parameters	Predefined factors	Modifiable factors
Temporal resolution and motion artifacts	Rotation speed	Heart rate
	Reconstruction algorithm	ECG synchronization
	Heart rate	Multisegmental reconstruction
Spatial resolution and image detail	Detector element size	Field of view
	Focal spot size	Table speed
	Projections per rotation	Reconstruction increment
Tissue contrast and lumen differentiation	X-ray tube peak power	Tube voltage
	X-ray attenuation	Contrast enhancement
		Kernel
Image noise	X-ray tube peak power	Tube current and voltage
	Patient size	
Inter-slab continuity	Number of detectors	Patient cooperation
	Arrhythmia	Arrhythmia
		ECG editing

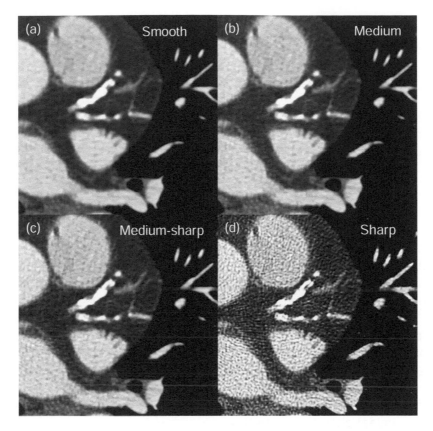

Figure 1 . 3 Reconstruction kernels. Filtering of data before reconstruction can either smooth (a) or sharpen (d) an image (showing an axial slice with a severely calcified left coronary artery).

also increases the image noise (Figure 1.36). Harder kernels can improve the image interpretability of stented or calcified vessels.

Scan time

The duration of the scan can be calculated as follows:

$$\text{Scan time} = \frac{\text{scan volume} \times \text{rotation time}}{\text{pitch} \times n \times \text{detector width}}$$

More and larger detectors (where n is the number of detectors), a faster rotation, and a higher pitch reduce the scan time of a given scan range. Because all data are preferably acquired in a single scan, which should be performed while the patient holds his breath and remains completely motionless, the total scan time needs to be as short as possible. Compared with non-cardiac protocols, ECG-synchronized protocols require a substantially longer scan time. Using four-slice MSCT, with a 500-ms rotation time and four 1-mm detector rows the heart can be covered in 35–40 s, which is a considerable period to hold one's breath. In addition to voluntary and involuntary patient movement, the long breath-hold time causes acceleration of the heart rate. Using 16-slice technology, with a less then 400 ms rotation time and 16 × 0.75-mm detector rows the scan time is less than 20 s. For comparison, the entire abdominal aorta and femoral run-offs can be scanned using a non-gated protocol and 1.5-mm slices in the same amount of time. The cardiac scan time of 64-slice CT and dual-source CT varies between 5 and 12 s, resulting in a comfortable breath-hold period for most patients.

REFERENCES

1. Nieman K, Rensing BJ, van Geuns RJ et al. Non-invasive coronary angiography with multislice spiral computed tomography: impact of heart rate. Heart 2002; 88: 470–4.

CHAPTER 2

Image post-processing

Image post-processing is defined as the process of using imaging techniques to modify the initial axial images (the source images) to make them more useful to the observer[1,2]. Post-processing is useful because it allows clinically relevant information to be extracted from the enormous amount of data of more than 300–800 axial images that are generated by a multislice CT (MSCT) acquisition from a single thoracic examination. The use of these post-processing techniques allows the investigators to better understand the complex coronary artery anatomy and related coronary abnormalities, which can be extremely difficult to ascertain from the large number of axial images. The usefulness and quality of image post-processing is highly related to the in-plane and through-plane resolution of MSCT. The data that form the CT slice are sectioned into elements, the width indicated on the x-axis and the height on the y-axis (Figure 2.1a) to create a two-dimensional square indicated as a pixel (picture element). However, there is a third component, the thickness of the slice, which is indicated on the z-axis. Taking the thickness into account turns the square (pixel) into a cube which is referred to as a voxel (volume element) (Figure 2.1b). The thickness of the slice is important, because the X-ray beam passes only through the selected slice thickness, thereby eliminating superimposition and radiation scatter of adjacent structures which creates high quality images. In computerized imaging, pictures are composed of pixels. The region of interest is mathematically divided into voxels. In each voxel the signals are averaged and turned into a number, which eventually represents a certain level on the gray scale. These numbers are used to create a picture consisting of pixels. The pixels are arranged in an image matrix, which is a grid consisting of rows (x-axis) and columns (y-axis). The matrix size used for CT is generally 512 x 512 pixels. The field of view (FOV) is the diameter of the area being imaged. The pixel size is determined by the ratio of the FOV and matrix or:

$$\text{Pixel size} = \frac{\text{FOV}}{\text{Matrix size}}$$

The smaller the pixel (or voxel) the higher is the resolution.

The voxel is the fundamental unit of the volume. Adding up all the voxels of the volume and applying a post-processing algorithm such as volume rendering will result in the anatomical representation of the data set. In terms of image quality, the smaller the voxel the better is the spatial resolution of the image (Figure 2.1c). It is important to note that the shape of voxels may differ and, depending on the slice thickness, the voxel may be constructed as an isotropic voxel, i.e. x-y-z measurements are identical, or as an anisotropic voxel, i.e. x-y are similar but z is usually larger.

Isotropic imaging is preferred because post-processing from isotropic voxels creates sharp images while anisotropic voxels may create less distinct images. Spiral CT creates two-dimensional images oriented in an axial plane. The resolution is high and image reconstruction is almost isotropic, which is optimized by selecting a reconstruction increment of 50% of the slice thickness, which increases the spatial resolution in the z-axis. The parameters for image reconstruction in CT coronary angiography typically are slice

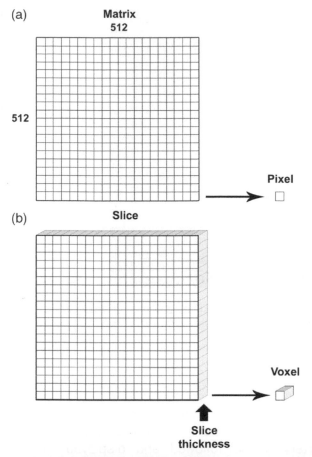

(a) Matrix 512

512

Pixel

(b) Slice

Voxel

Slice thickness

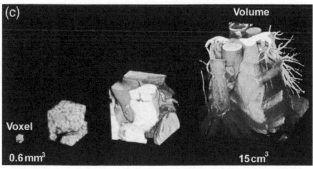

(c) Volume

Voxel

0.6 mm³

15 cm³

Figure 2 . 1 The matrix of the image represents the number of pixels that are by convention used for the reconstruction (a). In all current CT images the matrix is 512 x 512 pixels (262.144 pixels). The matrix is constant and is not affected by the size of the field of view. The field of view can be varied and in cardiac CT imaging it usually ranges around 150 mm. The size of the field of view affects the size of the pixel. For instance, for a field of view of 150 mm, the pixel in the matrix will be 0.3mm². When a slice is reconstructed, a third dimension is added to the matrix. This dimension corresponds to the slice thickness and d epends mainly on the collimati   on (b). Ideally, the slice thickness should be in the range of the size of the pixel in the matrix (i.e. 0.3 mm² for a field of view of 150 mm). When this requirement is met, the   voxel is called isotropic. (C) Voxel and volume.

thickness of 1mm (ideally less) reconstruction increment 0.5 mm (or less), and FOV 150 mm. Post-processing imaging is performed from a three-dimensional data set that is reconstructed from the obtained axial images which should always be considered as the source information of CT imaging (Figure 2.2). The three-dimensional data set can be reformatted according to the needs of the investigator using several types of post-processing algorithms (Table 2.1).

POST-PROCESSING TECHNIQUES

Axial image scrolling

The axial images are considered to be the source images providing the basic information in CT. Scrolling through these images in the cranio–caudal direction allows interpretation of the cardiac structures including the coronary arteries (Figure 2.3). However, because of the complex course of the coronary arteries interpretation of the axial images may be difficult and better insight may be obtained from multiplanar reconstructions.

Multiplanar reconstruction

Multiplanar reconstructions (MPR) can be generated from the volume data set which is reconstructed from a stack of axial images (Figure 2.4)[3]. In principle, any plane can be generated from the volume data set, but by convention the most often used relevant planes in radiological routine are the axial, sagittal, and coronal planes (Figure 2.4), while oblique planes may also be useful. Planes that are oriented parallel or orthogonal to the interventricular or atrioventricular grooves are very useful in coronary MPR reconstructions. The slice thickness can be modified to create a 'thick slab' which may be useful to visualize (a part of) a tortuous coronary artery. The advantages of MPR are: (1) first that it is a relatively simple algorithm which can be rendered quickly and accurately on any image-processing workstations without the need of segmentation of overlapping structures; (2) distance measurements

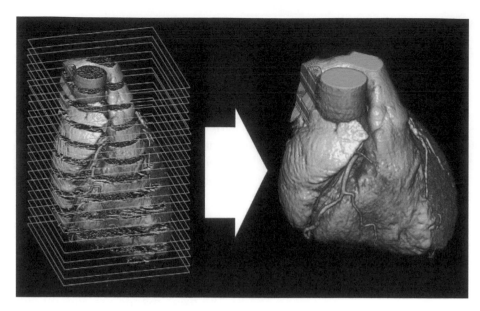

Figure 2 . 2 The source information of CT are the axial images. The axial images are reconstructed with a defined x-y-z-resolution. This stack of images is reconstructed to for m a volume. Post-processing is per formed on this volume data set.

in MPR are accurate and not subject to fore-shortening; (3) different structures in MPR are accurate and do not overlap; and (4) 100% of the available data is represented in the images (no loss of voxel value information due to thresholding). A disadvantage of MPR is that the image quality is highly dependent on the resolution and isotropy of data volume set.

Curved multiplanar reconstruction imaging

Curved MPR is defined as a plane that is reformatted along a curved plane. Curved MPRs are useful for visualization of coronary arteries where

T ble 2 . 1 Post-processing techniques

Axial image scrolling

Multiplanar reconstructions (MPR)

Curved multiplanar reconstructions (cMPR)

Maximum intensity projections (MIP)

Shaded surface display (SSD)

Three-dimensional volume rendering (VR)

Virtual endoscopy (VE)

Vessel analysis (VA) and vessel tracking (VT)

---

a curved MPR is reconstructed along the curved course of the coronary artery of interest (Figure 2.5). This enables the entire coronary artery to be followed and displayed in one reconstruction. The curved MPR planes tend to distort the actual configuration of the anatomical structures that are represented in the volume. It is recommended that at least two images in orthogonal planes are reconstructed to prevent under- or overestimation of the severity of coronary lesions.

Maximum intensity projection

Maximum intensity projection (MIP) is a projectional technique. Imaging rays are cast through the three-dimensional data volume from the viewpoint of the user and only the highest intensity voxels encountered by each ray are used to reconstruct the two-dimensional projection image (Figure 2.6)[3,4]. It resembles the principle of conventional angiography because the result is a projection of the highest attenuation values on the image. MIP vascular imaging allows differentiation between enhanced vascular structures and non-vascular structures and, because most

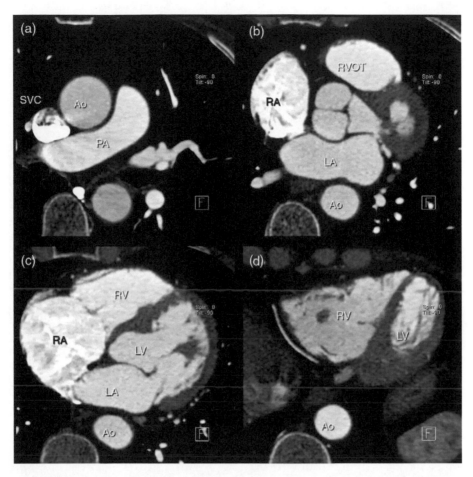

Figure 2 . 3 Axial images. The axial images are the basic infor mation of the CT scanner. Scrolling through them in the cranial to caudal direction will show the structures of interest in the axial plane. Usually a cardiac CT scan starts at the level of the main stem of the pulmonary artery (PA) where the ascending aorta (Ao) and superior vena cava (SVC) run orthogonal to the scan plane (a). At the level of the aortic valve both atria are visualized as well as the outflow tract of the right ventricle (RVOT) (b). More inferior, the four cardiac chambers are displayed (c). Finally, the inferior side of the heart is shown with the dist al right coronary artery and the inferior walls of the right and left ventricle (LV) (d). The aorta descendens is visualized in (b), (c) and (d). RA, right atrium; LA, left atrium; RV, right ventricle.

of the volume data are discarded, it requires a relatively short reconstruction time. A potential problem with MIP is that superimposed higher density structures obscure the lower density structures of interest, which is the case when calcium is present along the imaginary ray from the observer point of view. This problem can be avoided by using a limited stack of images (e.g. a 'slab') with a thickness adjusted to the size and course of the coronary arteries (Figure 2.6). Another problem is that MIP images lack 'depth' information, which fortunately does not play a significant role in coronary artery imaging.

Shaded surface display

Shaded surface display (SSD) is a three-dimensional technique that creates a surface of an object using contour information based on a selected threshold of the voxel within the volume data set (Figure 2.7). All the voxels above or below the preselected threshold form a solid surface. To improve the three-dimensional impression, a simulated light source is added to provide shading effects.

SSD provides no density information, implying that calcifications or contrast-enhanced coronary lumen are presented in the same way[4,5].

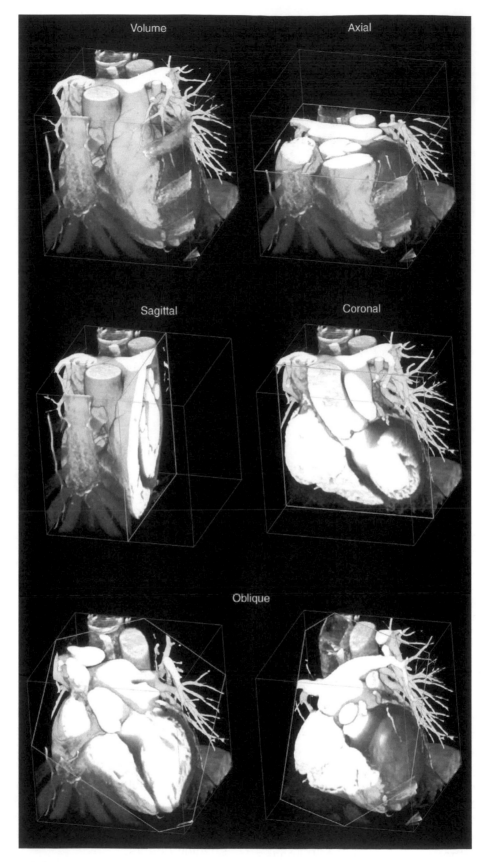

Figure 2.4 Multiplanar reconstructions are generated from the interpolation of the stack of axial images into a volume of data (Volume). The conventional planes that are used for visualization are the axial plane (Axial), the sagittal plane (Sagittal), and the coronal plane (Coronal). These planes should be imagined as slices that cut the volume with a defined spatial orientation. The cut planes can be arbitrarily tilted in any orientation to create orthogonal or parallel planes through the structures of interest(Oblique).

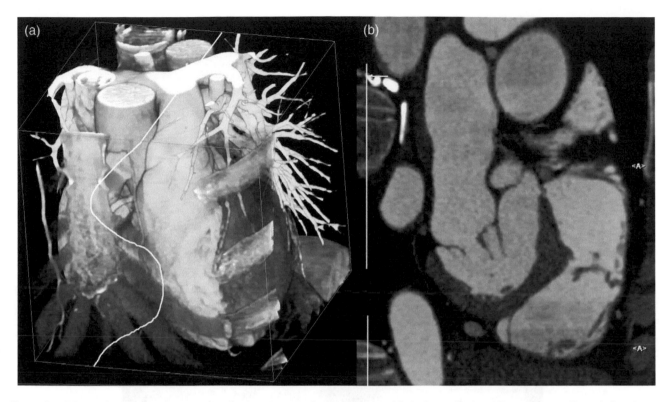

Figure 2 . 5 Curved multiplanar reconstructions are generated by means of flat planes that cut the volume with a defined spatial orientation. When the cut plane is not flat but instead is curved, the result is a curved multiplanar reconstruction (a). The main difference with conventional multiplanar reconstructions is that the resulting image is a flattened representation of the curve d plane (b). In this image the geometric relationships are less consistent.

Typically, SSD uses only 10% of the available volume data and is now replaced by three-dimensional volume rendering which uses 100% of the available volume data.

Three-dimensional volume rendering

Three-dimensional volume rendering uses all the voxels of the volume data to create a three-dimensional image based on the density of each voxel[1,3,6]. Volume rendering requires pre-processing tissue types contained in each voxel. The voxels are classified according to the density value in major tissues: air, fat, soft tissue, and bone. Air has a density of −1000 HU, fat approximately −100 HU, soft tissue +50 HU, and bone +1000 HU (Figure 2.8). Volume rendering assigns a certain opacity to each voxel density value to make some structures opaque and others transparent. Lowering the opacity of the voxel values which are not of interest causes the corresponding voxels to become transparent, while increasing the opacity causes these structures to become more opaque. The settings of the opacity function can be fully adapted to meet the requirements of the observer (Figure 2.9). In addition, a color can be assigned to the classified voxels, representing different tissues (Figure 2.10). The default setting for bone is yellowish white and for soft tissue is reddish brown. The default opacity setting is high for bone, medium to low for soft tissue, and fat and air are fully transparent. When processing the opacity value is set high for the tissues of interest and low for other tissues. It is of note that different settings may affect the appearance of a structure, and may have an effect on the size of the (in particular smaller) coronary vessels (Figure 2.11).

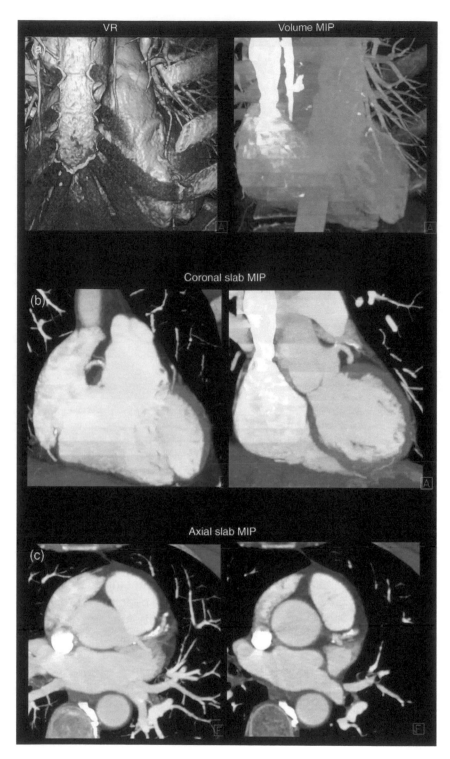

Figure 2 . 6 Maximum intensity projections (MIPs) are projectional images that visualize only the voxel with the highest attenuation along the observation line. The perception of depth is completely lost when MIPs are applied to a volume of data, especially if compared to volume rendering (a). MIP reconstructions are more effective and informative when applied to thick slabs of images (b) and (c).

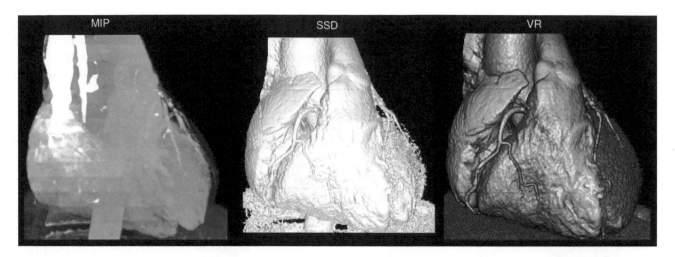

Figure 2 . 7 Shaded surface display (SSD) is the oldest of the three-dimensional techniques. The technique shows a sur face of an object based on the selection of a threshold. It gives more depth infomation when compared to volumetric maximum intensity projections (MIPs), but is very limited when compared to volume rendering (VR).

Virtual endoscopy

The concept of virtual endoscopy was first introduced in the context of the visualization of the inner surface of hollow organs. The main applications are in the colon (Figure 2.12), the airways (Figure 2.13), stomach, and the bladder. In virtual endoscopy the air within the colon is made transparent to create a virtual space within the colon. The surrounding tissues have a different attenuation (e.g. higher or lower) and are made opaque. Thus, a surface of the walls of the colon is created with the point of view of the observer positioned inside the colon. Virtual bronchoscopy uses the same technique (Figure 2.13). This concept applied to vascular imaging produces a virtual angioscopic visualization (Figure 2.14) of the arteries. The very dense contrast material inside the vessel is made transparent and the walls of the vessels are made opaque.

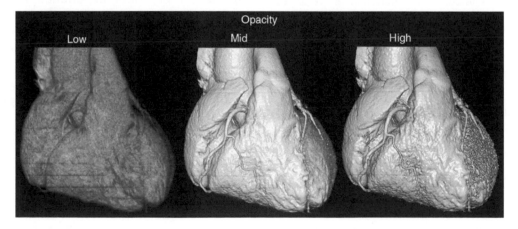

Figure 2 . 8 Volume rendering: opacity. The opacity (or transparency) is assigned to a voxel in order to allow the observer to see through it or to make it completely opaque. In the figure a volume of data is displayed with increasing opacity level from left to right.

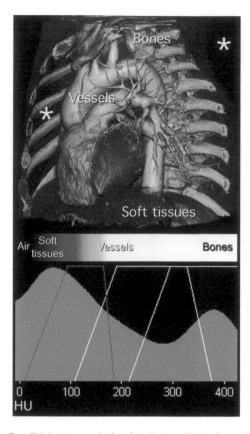

Figure 2 . 9 Volume rendering is a three-dimensional technique that displays the voxels of the volume based on the density. In addition, a value of opacity can be assigned to each voxel in order to let the observer look through defined ranges of attenuation. The opacity settings can be arbitrarily selected according to the requirements of the observer . In this example, the range of attenuation below 0 (fat, lung parenchyma, and air) are transparent (asterisk). The soft tissues with a range of attenuation between 0 HU and 180 HU (subcutaneous tissue, liver parenchyma, and myocar dium) are assigned to the color red. The tissues with a range of attenuation between 110 and 370 HU (vessels) are assigned a yellow color. The tissues with attenuation above 220 HU (bones) are assigned to the color white. The color stripe in the middle of the image shows the progressive change of color along the scale of attenuation.

This technique produces spectacular images but, so far, its clinical use is limited.

Vessel analysis and vessel tracking

Segmentation involves the simplification of an image by dividing it into its basic component elements or objects. Segmentation can be done in several ways such as vessel tracking, contouring, region growing, etc. Segmentation of the vessels by vessel tracking is a fast semi-automated or even fully automated software algorithm which significantly reduces the often time-consuming task of post-processing[7].

Segmentation of vessels is based on density, spatial geometry, and homogeneity of the vessel structure within the volume data set[6,8,9]. Vessel segmentation is a required step preceding quantitative vessel lumen analysis using contour-detection algorithms. With vessel tracking software a central lumen line can be generated simply by positioning a beginning and endpoint in the vessel region of interest. The lumen contours of the vessel are determined by contour-detection algorithms taking the central lumen line as the starting point. Thus, a cross-sectional contour of the vessel is generated, which allows quantification of the vessel lumen (Figure 2.15). Various software packages are available, but it is extremely difficult to produce an accurate and reliable algorithm for the coronary arteries which are small, have a tortuous course, and the image quality obtained by CT is not always optimal for automated construction of a central lumen line and lumen contour detection.

Post-processing techniques in clinical practice

Which, when, and how to use the various available post-processing techniques remains a matter of personal experience and may differ amongst various operators. In Table 2.2 we present the advantages and disadvantages of the available techniques. Table 2.3 is a summary of our experience using the various post-processing techniques in clinical practice. The techniques were scored according to a range of variables:

(1) Availability. The availability of post-processing techniques is inversely proportional to their computational complexity. All DICOM (Digital Imaging and Communication in Medicine) viewing software allows axial images to be scrolled, while for increasingly complex tasks, such as MPR, MIP and VR, more sophisticated software and computer power are required.

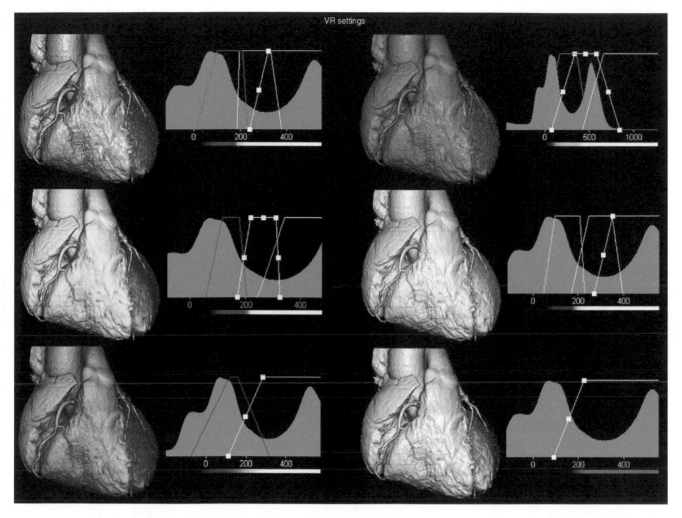

Figure 2 . 1 0 Volume rendering: color attribution. In volume rendering the parameters attributed to an image are arbitrary. Therefore, the appearance will change when the operator changes the colors of the algorithm.

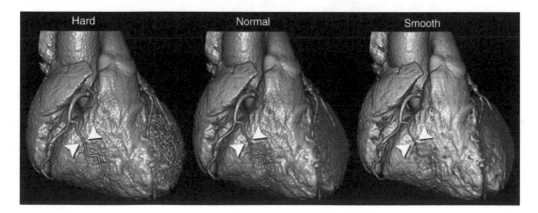

Figure 2 . 1 1 Volume rendering (VR) and vessel diameter. VR is based on arbitrary settings and modification of these settings may affect the size of the vessels. This is particularly evident for small vessels such as coronary arteries. The image shows how the diameter of a marginal branch of the right coronary artery (arrowheads) can be modified by the application of progressively smoother VR settings.

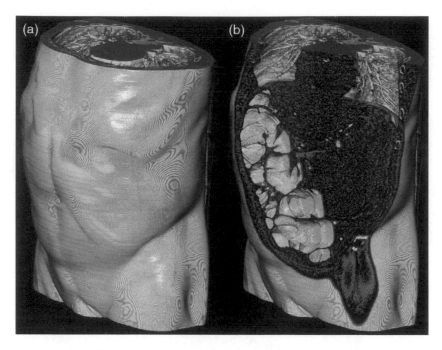

Figure 2 . 1 2 Virtual colonoscopy is based on the visualization of the colon as a hollow organ after the inflation of air The volume of data is made opaque (a) and the air is made transparent (b) and the walls of the colon are also made opaque. A surface is generated and the abnormalities of the surface, such as polyps, can be easily detected.

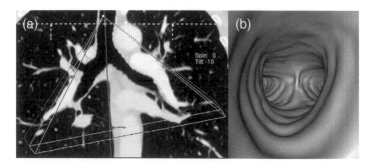

Figure 2 . 1 3 Virtual bronchoscopy is based on the same principles as virtual colonoscopy. The air inside the airways is made transparent while the walls of the trachea are opaque. A point of view inside the trachea is chosen (a) and the surface of the airways can be displayed as with fiberoptic bronchoscopy (b). The main applications of this technique are to detect upper airway abnormalities, e.g. carcinoma.

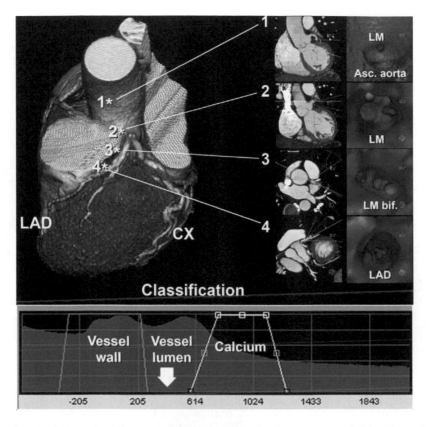

Figure 2 .41 Virtual angioscopy is based on the same principle as virtual colonoscopy and virtual bronchoscopy. The contrast material inside the vessel lumen is made transparent and the vessel wall is made orange and the calcium is made white (see the lower part of the figure). Virtual angioscopy is applied from the ascending (Asc.) aorta and the coronary arteries. The point of view of the observer is within the vessel and is progressing from the ascending aorta (1), to the ostium of the left main coronary artery (LM) (2), the bifurcation of left main (LM bif.) (3), to the left anterior descending (LAD) (4). LCX, left circumflex.

(2) Reliability. The reliability of the technique represents how the information displayed reflects the original data after the algorithm is applied.

(3) Experience. The experience required to use these techniques is dependent on the type of training. Radiologists are used to interaction with cross-sectional images and will feel comfortable using the technique, while a cardiologist, not by training familiar with the technique, might require additional education. Even though the techniques that show three-dimensional anatomical configuration, such as VR, provide information that is easier to understand, some experience is required to handle the data properly.

(4) Time. The time needed to obtain relevant images is also dependent on the training of the operator and on the complexity of the technique and, even more, on whether the output is qualitative (e.g. images) or quantitative (e.g. stenosis assessment).

(5) Diagnosis. The impact of each post-processing technique is different. For the assessment of stenoses and plaques the techniques that show the original data in planes favorable to coronary anatomy (e.g. axial scrolling, MPR, cMPR, and MIP) are preferred. With these images the real densitometric information can be evaluated. VR is used in coronary artery bypass graft evaluation to better understand the anatomical configuration of the grafts.

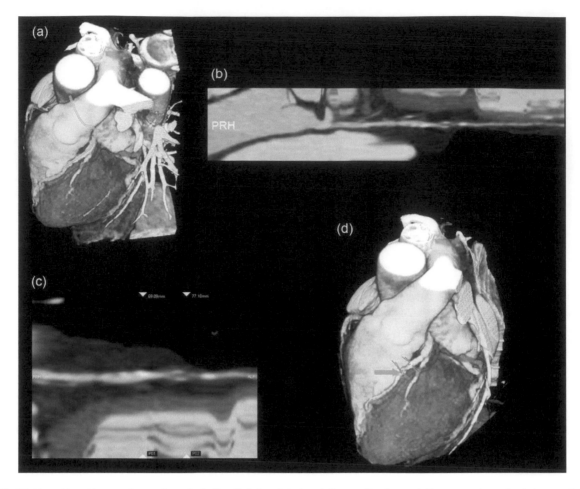

Figure 2.51 Vessel tracking and vessel analysis. The first step is to track the path of vessel. The operator selects two points: one at the beginning and one at the end of the vessel, which allows the software to identify the path of the vessel (a). The software then creates a stretched curved multiplanar reconstruction along the central lumen line (b). This longitudinal view can be rotated around its axis to evaluate the position of the branches and the location and longitudinal extent of plaques (c). In the longitudinal view automated lumen measurements can be performed and their position is easily indicated on the three-dimensional volume rendering (d).

In other non-coronary applications the diagnostic information should be evaluated on axial and multiplanar images.

(6) Presentation and communication. For presentation and communication purposes the axial and multiplanar images are less informative because they presuppose interaction with the volume which is difficult to display in a still frame.

Post-processing protocol

At the beginning of each evaluation an overview of the data set should be performed to detect gross abnormalities, artifacts, and the presence of extracoronary and myocardial abnormalities. To analyze coronary arteries a systematic approach should be followed. It is recommended that the coronary segments are evaluated in a

Table 2 . 2 Comparison of post-processing techniques

Technique	Advantages	Disadvantages
Axial scrolling	True data Artifacts easily recognized Anatomical overview	No three-dimensional perception
MPR	True data Artifacts easily recognized Anatomical overview Vessel area measurement	Poor three-dimensional perception
cMPR	Complete overview of the vessel of interest	Highly operator-dependent No anatomical overview Time-consuming Requires two or more orthogonal projections
MIP	Partial overview of the vessel of interest	Over-projection of calcium and stents No visualization of vessel wall Requires at least two orthogonal projections
SSD	Overview and orientation	User-dependent No visualization of vessel wall Poor evaluation of stents and calcium
VR	Three-dimensional perception Complete anatomical overview Relation to myocardium	User-dependent No visualization of vessel wall Poor evaluation of stents and calcium Time-consuming
VE	None	User-dependent No visualization of vessel wall No anatomical overview

MPR, multiplanar reconstructions; cMPR, curved multiplanar reconstructions; MIP, maximum intensity projections; SSD, shaded surface display; VR, volume rendering; VE, virtual endoscopy; VA, vessel analysis; VT, vessel tracking.

sequential order from segment 1 to segment 15 following the standard report of the American Heart Association.

Protocol

Axial images should always be reviewed first (Figure 2.16). Scrolling axial images up and down will allow all the non-coronary information that might be present within the data set to be reviewed. At the same time the location of cardiac structures (e.g. great vessels of the thorax, cardiac valves, atria, ventricles), including coronary arteries, can be screened for gross morphological abnormalities. After scrolling of axial images the observer should shift to MPR (Figure 2.17). With this technique dedicated planes can be generated better to represent coronary segments or entire coronary vessels.

There are two main planes (Figure 2.18) that are useful for the evaluation of coronary arteries:

(1) The plane for the right coronary artery and the left circumflex artery is parallel to the atrioventricular groove and can be defined as a paracoronal plane. Scrolling the plane on this axis the observer can follow the path of the right coronary artery and the left circumflex. Sometimes the ideal plane for the right coronary artery is slightly different to the one for the left circumflex.

Table 2.3 Post-processing techniques: impact and role in cardiac CT

Technique	Availability	Reliability	Experience	Time	Diagnosis			Presentation	Communication
					Stenosis plaques	CABG	Others*		
Axial scrolling	High	High	Low	Low	Low	Low	High	Low	Low
MPR	High	High	Low	Low	High	High	High	Low	Low
cMPR	Mid	High	Mid	Low	High	High	Mid	Mid	High
MIP	Mid	Mid	Mid	Low	Mid	High	High	Mid	High
SSD	Mid	Low	Mid	Mid	Low	Low	Low	Low	Low
VR	Mid	Low	High	Mid	Low	High	Mid	High	High
VE	Low	Low	High	High	Low	Low	Low	Mid	Low
VA and VT	Low	?	High	High	High?	High?	?	High	?

*Others relates to cardiac CT performed for non-coronary purposes. The question marks in the VA and VT are due to the still limited experience and validation of automatic or semiautomatic tools for vessel tracking and evaluation.

MPR, multiplanar reconstructions; cMPR, curved multiplanar reconstructions; MIP, maximum intensity projections; SSD, shaded surface display; VR, volume rendering; VE, virtual endoscopy; VA, vessel analysis; VT, vessel tracking.

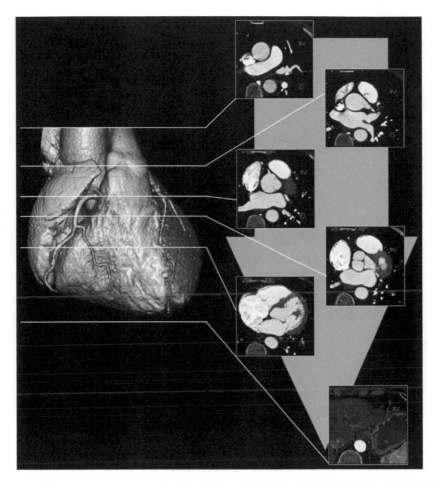

Figure 2 . 1 6crolling of axial images provides a quick view of the data set to crudely assess the main features of the coronary anatomy. When scrolling the images the observer should create in his mind a quick roadmap of the main features of the patient's vessels.

(2)   The plane for the left anterior descending artery is parallel to the interventricular septum and can be defined as a parasagittal plane. The vessel can be followed easily by scrolling these planes back and forth. When calcifications are not too prominent the application of a slab MIP, 3–5 mm thick, allows the entire vessel or most of it to be projected in the same image (Figure 2.19). Following the vessel throughout the optimal plane and manually or automatically tracing the central-lumen line will result in a single image representing the entire vessel (Figure 2.20). In order to obtain the orthogonal projection of this image, the tracing of the central-lumen line should be performed on a plane orthogonal to the one previously described, or, when automatic, the vessel should be rotated 360° around its axis. When lesions or suspected lesions are detected, the segment of interest should be magnified and a plane orthogonal to the path of the vessel should be used for the evaluation (Figure 2.21). Scrolling back and forth along the axis of the lumen the observer will be able to evaluate the patency of the vessel looking first at the proximal non-diseased region and then focusing the image on the diseased region. At the end of the evaluation a VR can be

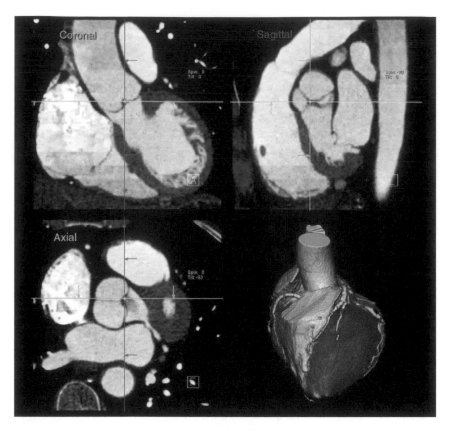

Figure 2 . 1 Scrolling multiplanar reconstructions. After scrolling the axial images the observer should use multiplanar reconstructions to better orientate the planes of visualization to the geometric orientation of the coronary structures. The starting planes, as previously described, are the axial, coronal, and sagittal planes (see Figure 2.4).

performed to give an anatomical picture of the coronary arteries and to create images useful for the report (Figure 2.22).

REPORTING

A report for coronary CT angiography (CTA) should be similar to that of a conventional coronary angiography report (Figure 2.23). A report should be based on a visual approach with clear reference to the segment with disease. Particular attention should be given to calcification and motion artifacts that may impair the visualization of the vessels.

CONCLUSION

Coronary artery bypass graft evaluation

VR should be used prior to other post-processing techniques to give an overview of the entire anatomy which is often helpful to understand the anatomy of the grafts (Figure 2.24).

Non-coronary studies

Axial and MPR images are recommended to detect non-coronary abnormalities.

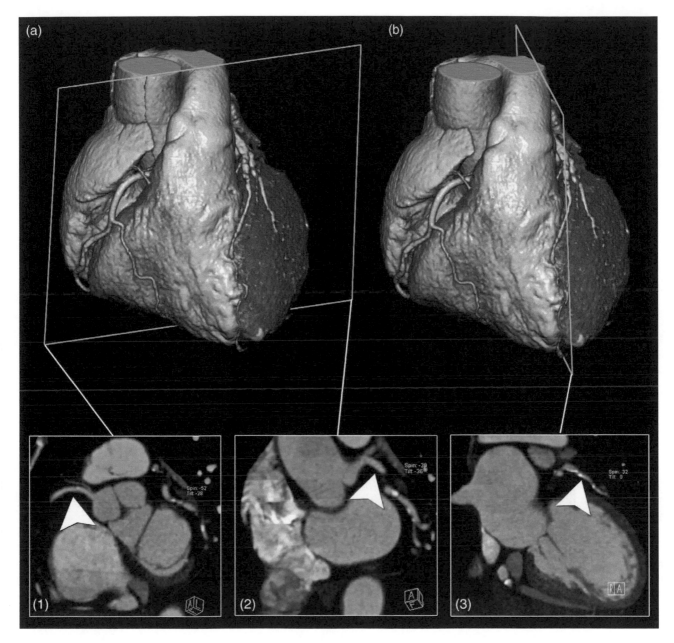

Figure 2 . 1 8 Multiplanar reconstruction planes for the coronary arteries. The planes that can help to visualize better the coronary arteries are a plane parallel to the atrioventricular groove (a) and a plane parallel to the interventricular groove (b). The first plane shows the right coronary artery (1) and the left circumflex (2). The second plane shows the left anterior descending artery (3). The tortuous anatomy of the left coronary artery most of the time it does not allow representation of the entire vessel in one single image.

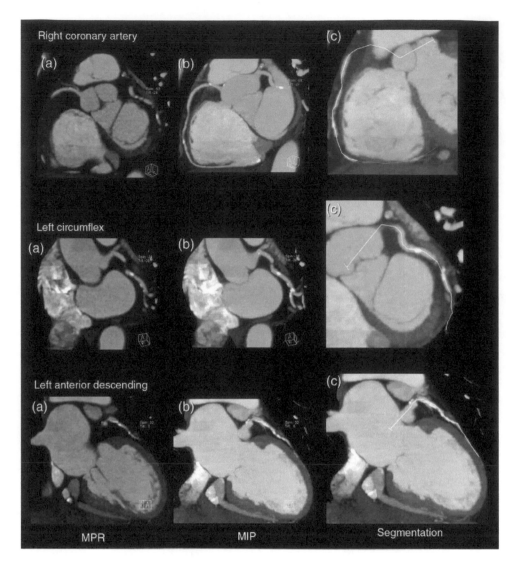

Figure 2 . 1 Maximum intensity projections (MIP) for the coronary arteries. Multiplanar reconstructions (MPR) can be used to set the cut planes in an orientation that matches one of the main coronary arteries. Nevertheless, the tortuous anatomy of coronary vessels does not allow the complete visualization of the vessel in many cases (a). The use of MIP can increase the overview for each vessel (b). Using MIPs it is also easier to track the path of the vessel when per forming curved MPR (c).

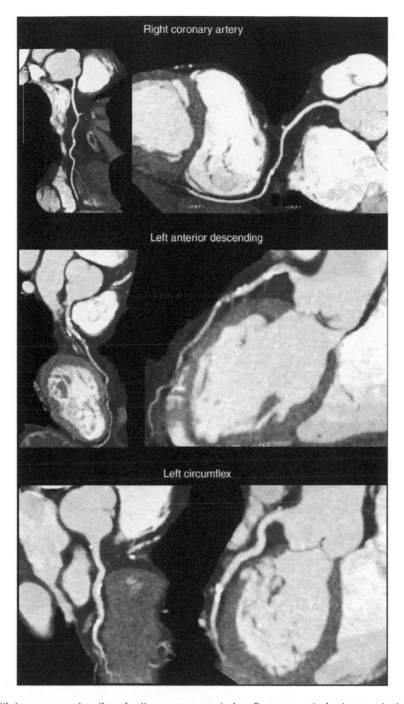

Figure 2 .02 Curved multiplanar reconstructions for the coronary arteries. Coronary arteries have a tortuous anatomy; therefore, it can be difficult to show the entire vessel in one image. An easy way to do this is by means of curved multiplanar reconstructions. The vessel is segmented using multiplanar planes with or without maximum intensity projections (see Figure 2.19). Then the resulting image is projected into one plane. From two orthogonal planes the observer can have a quick overview of the vessel anatomy and abnormalities.

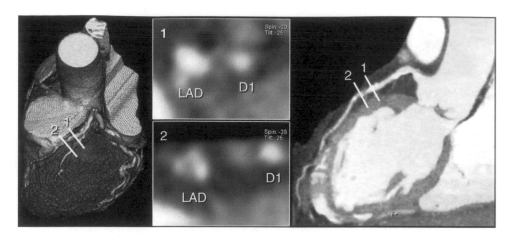

Figure 2 .12 Orthogonal views for the coronary arteries. When abnormalities are detected in the lumen or in the wall of coronary arteries, the observer can always create a plane orthogonal to the direction of the vessel. This view, which is commonly used in intravascular ultrasound, allows the configuration of the disease along the vessel to be seen. In the figure, two orthogonal views (1 and 2) are performed at the level of segment 7 (mid-left anterior descending) immediately after the bifurcation of the first diagonal. The first view (1) is performed at the level of normal lumen, while the second view (2) is performed at the level of a significant (>50%) lumen reduction in the left anterior descending (LAD). D1, first diagonal.

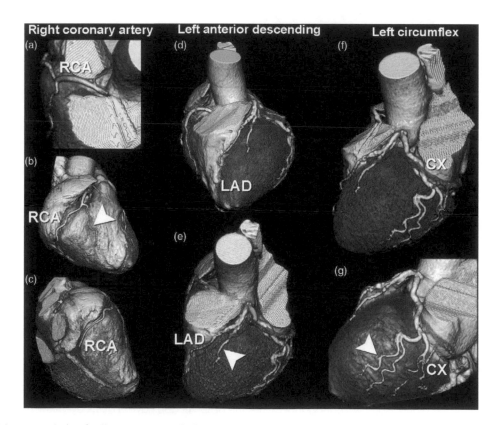

Figure 2 .22 Volume rendering for the coronary arteries. Volume rendering allows an easy overview of coronary artery anatomy. It does not allow quantitative or semi-quantitative evaluations regarding the patency of the lumen of the arteries to be performed. Nevertheless, it assists significantly in understanding the topography of coronary vessels and the position of the lesions in the coronary tree. Dedicated projections for each one of the three main vessels are performed. The proximal segment of the right coronary artery (RCA) is visualized in a cranial view (a). The mid-segment of the right coronary artery (b) is visualized in a view from the right side in which a marginal branch is clearly shown (arrowhead). The distal segment of the right coronary artery is visualized in a right caudal view (c). The left anterior descending (LAD) is visualized in a left anterior view (d) and in cranial left view (e) where the first diagonal branch is visualized (arrowhead). The left circumflex artery (CX) is visualized in left cranial view (f) and in a left view (g) where several marginal branches are clearly displayed (arrowhead).

Cardiac MSCT

Name:	Contrast typ.: mgl/ml	mAs:
Birth:	Contrast vol.: ml	kV:
ID:	Contrast rate: ml/s	Coll:
Date:	Metoprolol: mg	Slices:
	HR: bpm	Rot. Time:

Referring physician: ....

History: ....
....

Clinical question: ....

Coronary angiography

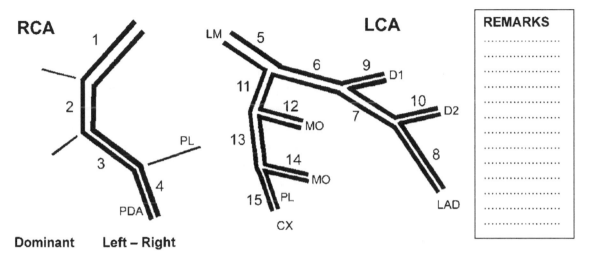

RCA   **LCA**   **REMARKS**

Dominant   **Left – Right**

Seg.	Vessel	Patent	Stenosis	Conf$^\alpha$	Small	Qual$^\beta$	Stent	Calcium
01	RCA	Y – N	0 / <50 / ±50 / >50 / NA	1-2-3	...	1-2-3	...	0 / + / ++
02	RCA	Y – N	0 / <50 / ±50 / >50 / NA	1-2-3	...	1-2-3	...	0 / + / ++
03	RCA	Y – N	0 / <50 / ±50 / >50 / NA	1-2-3	...	1-2-3	...	0 / + / ++
04	PDA	Y – N	0 / <50 / ±50 / >50 / NA	1-2-3	...	1-2-3	...	0 / + / ++
05	LM	Y – N	0 / <50 / ±50 / >50 / NA	1-2-3	...	1-2-3	...	0 / + / ++
06	LAD	Y – N	0 / <50 / ±50 / >50 / NA	1-2-3	...	1-2-3	...	0 / + / ++
07	LAD	Y – N	0 / <50 / ±50 / >50 / NA	1-2-3	...	1-2-3	...	0 / + / ++
08	LAD	Y – N	0 / <50 / ±50 / >50 / NA	1-2-3	...	1-2-3	...	0 / + / ++
09	D1	Y – N	0 / <50 / ±50 / >50 / NA	1-2-3	...	1-2-3	...	0 / + / ++
10	D10	Y – N	0 / <50 / ±50 / >50 / NA	1-2-3	...	1-2-3	...	0 / + / ++
11	CX	Y – N	0 / <50 / ±50 / >50 / NA	1-2-3	...	1-2-3	...	0 / + / ++
12	MO	Y – N	0 / <50 / ±50 / >50 / NA	1-2-3	...	1-2-3	...	0 / + / ++
13	CX	Y – N	0 / <50 / ±50 / >50 / NA	1-2-3	...	1-2-3	...	0 / + / ++
14	MO	Y – N	0 / <50 / ±50 / >50 / NA	1-2-3	...	1-2-3	...	0 / + / ++
15	PL	Y – N	0 / <50 / ±50 / >50 / NA	1-2-3	...	1-2-3	...	0 / + / ++

$^\alpha$ 1= non-reliable; 2= moderately reliable; 3= reliable
$^\beta$ 1= poor; 2= adequate, 3= good

Figure 2.32 Example of a reporting form for cardiac CT. The general CT report should assess coronary angiography, coronary calcium score, and overview of the heart. (a) Coronary angiography: coronary arteries are evaluated following the standard segmental classification of the American Heart Association. Each segment should be scored normal, <50% obstruction, >50% obstruction, or total occlusion. Sometimes the segment is not assessable (NA) for several reasons: too small, too calcified, or motion artifact. Additionally, a confidence level is assigned to the assessment as well as the quality of the image. The presence of stents should be noted and a visual score for calcium (absent = 0; nodules = +; bulk = ++) should be performed.

(Continued)

(b)

Coronary calcium score

Calcium score

	RCA	LM	LAD	CX	Total
Agatston	....	....	....	....	....
Volume (mm^3)	....	....	....	....	....
Mass (mg)	....	....	....	....	....

CALCIUM SCORE										
Gender	Perc.	Age (years)								
		<40	40–44	45–49	50–54	55–59	60–64	65–69	70–74	>74
Men	25th	0	0	0	1	4	13	32	64	166
	50th	1	1	3	15	48	113	180	310	473
	75th	3	9	36	103	215	410	566	892	1071
	90th	14	59	154	332	554	994	1299	1774	1982
	n	3504	4238	4940	4825	3472	2288	1209	540	235
Women	25th	0	0	0	0	0	0	1	3	9
	50th	0	0	0	0	1	3	24	52	75
	75th	1	1	2	5	23	57	145	210	241
	90th	3	4	22	55	121	193	410	631	709
	n	641	1024	1634	2184	1835	1334	731	438	174

Reproduced from Hoff JA et al. JACC 2003; 41: 1008–12.

General Guidelines for Interpretation of Calcium Score			
Calcium score*	Atherosclerotic plaque burden	Probability of significant CAD	Implications for CV risk
0	No detectable plaque	Very low (<5%)	Very Low
1–10	Minimal detectable plaque burden	Very unlikely (<10%)	Low
11–100	Mild atherosclerotic plaque burden	Mild or minimal	Moderate
101–400	Moderate atherosclerotic plaque burden	High likelihood of non-obstructive CAD Possibility of obstructive disease	Moderately High
>400	Extensive atherosclerotic plaque burden	High likelihood of one or more "significant" obstructive lesions (>90%)	High

Modified from Rumberger JA et al. Mayo Clin Proc 1999; 74: 243–52.
*Values in the Table should be age/gender adjusted.

REMARKS

....
....
....
....
....

Figure 2.23 Cont'd   (b) Coronary calcium: the calcium score is given as the Agatston, volume, and mass score. The calcium score (in quartiles) is presented for age and gender and general guidelines are given for interpretation of the calcium score.

(c)

Left ventricle

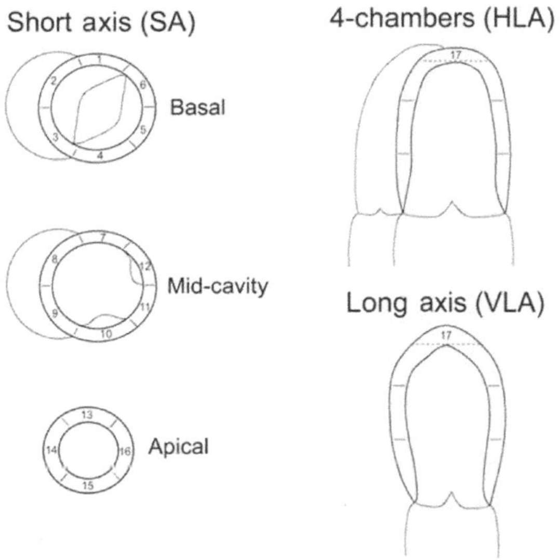

Short axis (SA)

Basal

Mid-cavity

Apical

4-chambers (HLA)

Long axis (VLA)

WALL MOTION	
Segment	Score
01	....
02	....
03	....
04	....
05	....
06	....
07	....
08	....
09	....
10	....
11	....
12	....
13	....
14	....
15	....
16	....
17	....

SCORE
1 = Normal
2 = Hypo
3 = Akin
4 = Dyskin

LVF		
EDV		ml
ESV		ml
SV		ml
EF		%
Mass		g

REMARKS
....
....
....
....
....

Valves	Visible	Calc	Thick
MV	....	....	....
PV	....	....	....
AoV	....	....	....
PV	....	....	....

COLLATERAL FINDINGS
....
....
....
....
....

CONCLUSION
....
....
....
....
....
....
....

Reporting physicians

Radiologist ....

Cardiologist ....

Figure 2.23 Cont'd   (c) Left ventricle: evaluation of left ventricular function and motion abnormalities. The presence of additional cardiac and non-cardiac abnormalities should be noted.

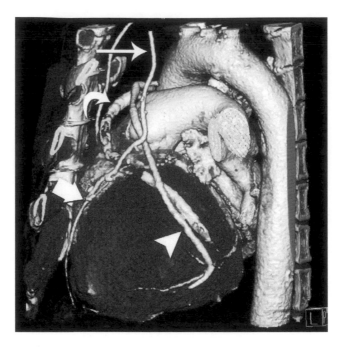

Figure 2 .42 Example of coronary artery bypass graft. The anatomical configuration of coronary artery bypass graft can be better evaluated with three-dimensional volume rendering. In the case of coronary artery bypass grafts, the native coronary arteries (left anterior descending, thick arrow) are crossed by other vessels such as the left internal mammary artery (thin arrow), the saphenous vein grafts, one of which is patent (arrowhead), the other is occluded (curved arrow).

REFERENCES

1. Calhoun PS, Kuszyk BS, Heath DG et al. Three-dimensional volume rendering of spiral CT data: theory and method. Radiographics 1999; 19: 745–64.
2. Fishman EK, Magid D, Ney DR et al. Three-dimensional imaging. Radiology 1991; 181: 321–37.
3. Lichtenbelt B, Crane R, Naqvi S. Introduction to volume rendering. Hewlett-Packard Professional Books. Upper Saddle River, NJ: Prentice Hall PTR, 1998.
4. Semba CP, Rubin GD, Dake MD. Three-dimensional spiral CT angiography of the abdomen. Semin Ultrasound CT MR 1994; 15: 133–8.
5. Sato Y, Shiraga N, Nakajima S et al. Local maximum intensity projection (LMIP): a new rendering method for vascular visualization. J Comput Assist Tomogr 1998; 22: 912–17.
6. Udupa JK. Three-dimensional visualization and analysis methodologies: a current perspective. Radiographics 1999; 19: 783–806.
7. Hohne KH, Hanson WA. Interactive 3D segmentation of MRI and CT volumes using morphological operations. J Comput Assist Tomogr 1992; 16: 285–94.
8. Masutani Y, MacMahon H, Doi K. Automated segmentation and visualization of the pulmonary vascular tree in spiral CT angiography: an anatomy-oriented approach based on three-dimensional image analysis. J Comput Assist Tomogr 2001; 25: 587–97.
9. Clarke LP, Velthuizen RP, Camacho MA et al. MRI segmentation: methods and applications. Magn Reson Imaging 1995; 13: 343–68.

CHAPTER 3

Radiation issues

INTRODUCTION

Multislice CT (MSCT) is a roentgen technique. The examination cannot be performed without exposure of the patient to (potentially) harmful radiation. The biological effects of ionizing radiation can be divided into deterministic and stochastic effects. Deterministic effects, in which loss of cells causes dysfunction of tissues, are dose dependent but only occur above a certain threshold. Because of the equal distribution of radiation these effects (skin erythema) are rare following CT. Stochastic effects are the result of cell modification and may result in cancer or genetic effects. These effects are dose related without a minimal threshold, and therefore most relevant in cardiac CT.

RADIATION DOSE PARAMETERS

To quantify the amount of radiation of a CT examination several related parameters can be measured and calculated (Table 3.1)[1]. The principal parameter of the absorbed dose, i.e. the amount of energy absorbed per unit mass, is the CT dose index (CTDI or $CTDI_{100}$). The CTDI is the integrated radiation dose (in milliGray) measured by an ionization chamber along the z-axis during a single tube rotation (Figure 3.1). To account for the non-homogeneous distribution of the CTDI within the body, i.e. the highest dose is absorbed around the edges of the object, the weighted CTDI ($CTDI_w$) can be calculated using a specific Perspex phantom: $\frac{2}{3}CTDI_{edge} + \frac{1}{3}CTDI_{center}$. Most CT examinations, including CT coronary

angiography, involve many scanner rotations at a variable longitudinal distance. Therefore, the total dose at a given position is increased by consecutive acquisitions at adjacent locations. In spiral CT the $CTDI_{vol}$ is determined by the $CTDI_w$ and the table speed (pitch): $CTDI_{vol} = CTDI_w/pitch$ (Figure 3.2). The $CTDI_{vol}$ is independent of the total volume that is being interrogated. To determine the radiation dose of an entire volume that is being scanned the $CTDI_{vol}$ is multiplied by the scan length, which results in the dose-length product (DLP, mGy × cm).

The damage or risk of a CT scan depends on the susceptibility of the organs or body region exposed to the X-ray. To account for the sensitivity of the body region that is being scanned, the effective dose (E, mSv) can be calculated. This value better reflects the risk of harm of the examination. To determine the effective dose the $CTDI_{vol}$ can be multiplied by a k value that is specific for the scanned body region. In case of thoracic CT the effective dose can be calculated as E (mSv) = 0.017 × DLP.

WHY IS THE RADIATION DOSE HIGH IN CARDIAC CT?

The amount of radiation that the patient is subjected to during CT coronary angiography depends on the scanner type, the scan protocol, and patient characteristics (Table 3.2). ECG-gated spiral CT requires overlapped scanning, with multiple sampling of tissues to ensure the availability of data from each position during the entire heart cycle. Therefore, the dose

Table 3.1 Radiation parameters in spiral CT

Parameter	Unit	Explanation
CT dose index (CTDI$_{100}$)	mGy	Measured radiation dose of a single slice (over 100 mm)
Weighted CTDI (CTDI$_w$ = $\frac{2}{3}$CTDI$_{edge}$ + $\frac{1}{3}$CTDI$_{center}$)	mGy	Correction for inhomogeneous attenuation
Volume CTDI (CTDI$_{vol}$ = CTDI$_w$/pitch)	mGy	Slice dose of a volumetric acquisition
Dose-length product (DLP = CTDI$_{vol}$ 8 × range)	mGy × cm	Dose of the scanned volume
Effective dose (E = k × DLP or E$_{chest}$ = 0.017 × DLP)	mSv	Tissue or body region dependent biological effect of an examination

is higher than comparable non-gated thoracic protocols. Also, electron-beam CT, which acquires consecutive axial slices, with only short exposures, involves significantly less radiation exposure. Because imaging of the coronary arteries requires high spatial resolution the thinnest available collimation is recommended. Thinner detectors result in increased noise levels when the same tube current is maintained. In addition, faster tube rotation will also reduce the number of photons that reach the detectors per rotation, which can also be compensated for by increasing the tube current. For these reasons we have witnessed a gradual increase of the radiation dose during the development of cardiac CT.

MEASURES TO REDUCE DOSE

With increased concerns about the potential consequences of radiation exposure, the cardiac CT community has taken efforts to reduce the radiation dose and also to define appropriate use of the technique. From a technical perspective several measures can be taken to reduce dose without compromising on image quality.

Effective use of the transmitted radiation depends on the scanner design. Filtering and tight collimation of the X-ray beam is important to remove X-rays that do not contribute to the generation of images. Detector technology is important in maximizing the imaging information derived from the emitted X-rays.

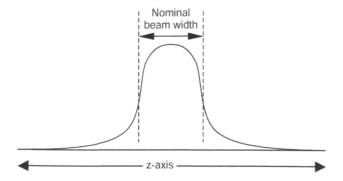

Figure 3.1 Radiation dose profile. From the measured radiation along a 100 mm ionization chamber, the CT dose Index (CTDI$_{100}$) can be calculated by integrating the area under the curve of the radiation dose profile.

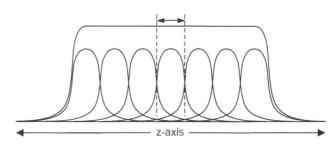

Figure 3.2 The volume CTDI (CTDI$_{vol}$) takes into account the added radiation from adjacent acquisitions. The CTDI$_{vol}$ increases when the spacing between the acquisitions decreases, in case of slow table speed or pitch.

Table 3.2 Radiation and influencing factors

Scanner variables	Influence
Roentgen beam filtration	Filtering of low-energy radiation
Roentgen beam collimation	Narrowing of the roentgen beam (cone)
Detector efficiency	Photons needed to create a signal
Detector size	Increased noise compensated for by higher tube current
Rotation speed	Fewer photons per rotation compensated for by higher tube current
Scan protocol	
Tube current and voltage	
Table speed	Oversampling at low pitch
Scan length	
Tube modulation	Based on anatomy and heart rhythm
Patient characteristics	
Weight and gender	Amount of absorption and susceptibility
Heart rate	Efficiency ECG-tube modulation and/or pitch

Anatomic tube current modulation

The amount of radiation needed for a CT examination depends on the roentgen absorption as the beam trasverses through the object. A large and tissue-dense body region such as the abdomen requires a higher tube current compared with a limb. By reducing the tube current when there is less absorption the radiation dose can be reduced without sacrificing image quality. For chest CT more radiation is needed around the shoulders and at the level of the diaphragm compared with the midsection which contains the lungs. Longitudinal tube current modulation adjusts the tube current to maintain a constant flux of photons to the detectors while consecutive body regions with a varying roentgen absorption rate are being scanned (Figure 3.3)[2]. Angular tube modulation operates in a similar fashion. Because roentgen absorption of the chest is lower in an anteroposterior direction compared with a lateral direction, the tube current can be lowered in the anteroposterior direction, while maintaining a constant flux of photons to the detector (Figure 3.3). The regional absorption can be estimated using the overview scan. Using automatic exposure control the tube current is adjusted during the data acquisition depending on the intensity of the transmitted amount of X-ray radiation that reaches the detectors.

ECG-gated tube modulation

Most of the time late-diastolic CT data are used to reconstruct and assess the coronary arteries. In this case data acquired outside this period are of little diagnostic value. Using ECG-gated tube modulation the tube current can be varied during the cardiac cycle (Figure 3.4). Nominal tube output is delivered during the motion-sparse diastolic phase, while the tube current is decreased during the systolic phase. The tube is not turned off completely, thus allowing reconstruction low-quality images to be produced during the systolic phase. ECG-triggered tube modulation can reduce the radiation dose by 30–40%[3]. Because the period of nominal output is usually fixed, dose savings are most substantial in patients with a low heart rate and a long R-to-R interval. The high-output period is generally sufficiently long to vary the position of the reconstruction window within the diastolic phase. In patients with a faster heart rate reconstructions during end-systole may be needed. In these patients the pulsing interval must include both end-diastole and end-systole, which is another reason why ECG-triggered tube modulation is less useful in the patient with a fast heart rate. Timing of the high tube current is established by prospective ECG triggering. Based on the previous heart cycles the timing of the diastolic phase is predicted. Therefore, arrhythmia may result in inappropriate tube variation and may cause insufficient signal during the diastolic phase. By narrowing the window of nominal output and lowering the systolic tube current further dose saving can be achieved (Figure 3.4).

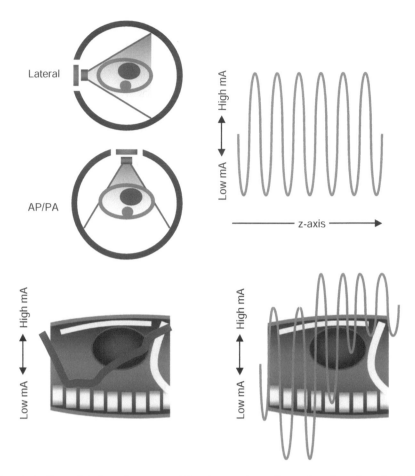

Figure 3 . **3**Angular tube current modulation. Because of the lower absorption rate when the chest is scanned in an antero-posterior (AP) direction, the tube current can be decreased without significant sacrifice to the image noise in the final image s. PA, posteroanterior.

Sequential CT scanning

Sequential scanning can be considered the ultimate tube modulation algorithm. Using ECG triggering, emission of X-ray radiation is limited to a single acquisition of one set of axial slices. Although image quality of sequential CT is regarded as inferior to spiral CT (non-overlapping slices, vulnerability to arrhythmia, single phase-reconstruction, etc., sequential CT angiography protocols are available on some 64-slice CT scanners in an effort to further reduce dose.

Adaptable pitch

At a fixed table speed, which accommodates a wide range of heart rates, substantial over-sampling will occur in patients with a fast heart rate. Acquisition of data during more than one cardiac cycle can be advantageous to decrease the effective temporal resolution (multi-segmental reconstruction algorithms). Alternatively, by increasing the pitch the total radiation dose (DLP) can be reduced substantially.

Dose reduction by the imager

Perhaps the most efficient way of reducing the dose is avoiding unnecessary examinations. If the indication for the scan is unsound (Chapter 7), the risk is particularly high (young women) or insufficient image quality is expected (non-cooperative, very fast heart rate, arrhythmia), one should consider an alternative diagnostic approach.

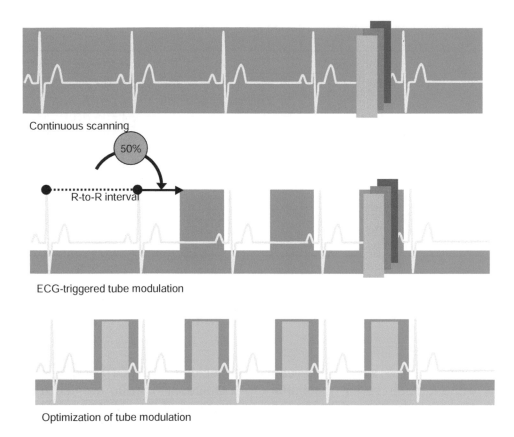

Continuous scanning

50%

R-to-R interval

ECG-triggered tube modulation

Optimization of tube modulation

Figure 3 . 4ECG-triggered tube modulation. Prospectively triggered modulation of the roentgen tube allows lowering of the tube current during the systolic phase, while maintaining optimal image quality during the motion-sparse diastolic phase.

If the indication is appropriate there are multiple means to acquire diagnostic images while minimizing radiation exposure (Table 3.3). Image quality can be maximized without consideration for radiation dose. However, an image does not need to be esthetically perfect to be diagnostic. According to the ALARA (as low as reasonably possible) one should strive for maximum diagnostic accuracy with minimal radiation dose.

In addition to the tube modulation applications described above, the imager has several other options to reduce dose without sacrificing image quality. Smaller patients require a smaller tube current to obtain comparable image quality with that in larger patients[2]. Use of lower tube voltage (100 kV) results in increased image noise but improved contrast. Hausleiter et al showed that comparable contrast-to-noise and image quality can be achieved while reducing the radiation exposure of 64-slice CT by nearly 50%[3]. The shorter scan time of 16- and 64-slice CT

scanners has resulted in easier breath holds. Without the restriction of the breath hold time longer ranges can be scanned without the risk of missing anything. The tendency of excessively wide scan ranges results in a dramatic increase of dose. It is important to practice a reproducible breath hold (also during the scout acquisition) with the patient and base the range on anatomical landmarks. Images acquired before the CT angiogram, such as the test bolus acquisition or the calcium scan, can be used to optimize the scan range.

REPORTED DOSE MEASUREMENTS AND ESTIMATIONS

As mentioned above the radiation dose by cardiac CT has increased with the development of more powerful CT equipment. While the reported radiation dose of 4-slice CT varies around 9–10 mSv,[4]

T ble 3 . 3 Dose measurements and estimations in CT coronary angiography

	MSCT	Method	Radiation dose (mSv)
Hunold et al [4]	4-CT	Phantom	6.7– 10.9 (men); 8.1– 13.0 (women)
Hausleiter et al [3]	16-CT	Estimation	10.6 ± 1.2 (120 kV) 6.4 ± 0.9 (120 kV, tube modulation) 5.0 ± 0.3 (100 kV, tube modulation)
	64-CT	Estimation	14.8 ± 1.8 (120 kV) 9.4 ± 1.0 (120 kV, tube modulation) 5.4 ± 1.1 (100 kV, tube modulation)
Leber et al[5]	64-CT	Estimation	10– 14
Mollet et al[6]	64-CT	Estimation	15.2 (men), 21.4 (women)
Ropers et al[7]	64-CT	Estimation	7.5 (men), 10.2 (women)

64-slice CT involves a dose varying between 8 and 20 mSv, without dose saving measures (Table 3.3)[3,5–7]. However, applying dose saving measures results in significant reduction of the radiation dose. Hausleiter et al showed that ECG-triggered tube current modulation reduced the radiation dose by 36%, while decreasing the tube voltage to 100 kV resulted in another 43% decrease in dose[3]. In comparison, the dose of a non-gated thoracic CT scan varies between 5 and 7 mSv. The radiation dose of a myocardial perfusion scan using technetium is somewhat less than that of a 64-slice CT scan, while using thallium the radiation dose is much higher[8]. Radiation exposure during conventional angiography varies between 3 and 10 mSv depending on the indication for the examination, the equipment used, and the angiographer. The yearly radiation exposure from natural sources is 1.9 mSv in The Netherlands and 3.6 mSv in the USA.

Whether the radiation dose of cardiac CT, or any other medical examination involving radiation, is justified will depend on a combination of factors including the indication, the diagnostic performance of CT, the availability of alternative tests, and patient preferences. The radiation dose may be acceptable if another test that involves a comparable X-ray dose (single photon emission CT (SPECT)) or different risks (catheter angiography) can be avoided. Particularly at the other end of the spectrum, i.e. screening of non-symptomatic individuals, the (current) radiation dose of CT angiography is much more of a concern. Based on data from the atom bomb victims of Hiroshima, the International Commission on Radiation Protection has estimated the risk of radiation-induced lethal cancer as 1 in 20 000 per mSv, based on 40–60-year-old adults[9]. Based on these models the estimated risk of cancer from a single coronary CT scan was recently published for different age groups and gender (Figure 3.5)[10]. Although the potential harm of radiation should not be underestimated, the

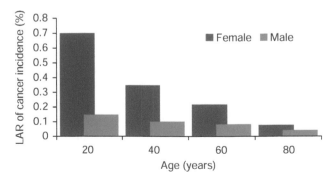

Figure 3 . 5 Lifetime attributable risk of (LAR) cancer from a single 64-slice cardiac CT scan[10].

effect of medical radiation on the incidence of cancer remains controversial[11]. Increased risk due to high background radiation or increased occupational exposure has not been demonstrated[12,13]. Additionally, patients undergoing CT coronary angiography are generally older. Nevertheless, it remains the responsibility of the cardiologists and radiologists to use cardiac CT appropriately, apply radiation-saving methods, and optimize scan protocols to achieve diagnostic image quality without excessively exposing the patient to radiation.

REFERENCES

1. Morin RL, Gerber TC, McCollough CH. Radiation dose in computed tomography of the heart. Circulation 2003; 107: 917–22.
2. McCollough C, Bruesewitz M, Kofler J. CT dose reduction and dose management tools: overview of available options. RadioGraphics 2006; 26: 503–12.
3. Hausleiter J, Meyer T, Hadamitzky M et al. Radiation dose estimates from cardiac multislice computed tomography in daily practice. Circulation 2005; 113: 1305–10.
4. Hunold P, Vogt FM, Schmermund A et al. Radiation exposure during cardiac CT: effective doses at multi-detector row CT and electron-beam CT. Radiology 2003; 226: 145–52.
5. Leber AW, Knez A, Von Ziegler F et al. Quantification of obstructive and nonobstructive coronary lesions by 64-slice computed tomography. J Am Coll Cardiol 2005; 46: 147–54.
6. Mollet NR, Cademartiri F, van Mieghem C et al. High-resolution spiral computed tomography coronary angiography in patients referred for diagnostic conventional coronary angiography. Circulation 2005; 112: 2318–23.
7. Ropers D, Rixe J, Anders K et al. Usefulness of multidetector row spiral computed tomography with 64- × 0.6-mm collimation and 330-ms rotation for the noninvasive detection of significant coronary artery stenoses. Am J Cardiol 2006; 97: 343–48.
8. Picano E. Sustainability of medical imaging. BMJ 2004; 328: 578–80.
9. International Commission on Radiological Protection. 1990. Recommendations of the International Commission on Radiological Protection. ICRP Publication 60. Ann ICRP 1991; 21: 1–3.
10. Einstein AJ, Henzlova MJ, Rajagopalan S. Estimating risk of cancer associated with radiation exposure from 64-slice computed tomography coronary angiography. JAMA 2007; 298: 317–23.
11. Zanzonico P, Rothenberg LN, Strauss HW. Radiation exposure of computed tomography and direct intracoronary angiography: risk has its reward. J Am Coll Cardiol 2006; 47: 1846–9.
12. Pukkala E, Aspholm R, Auvinen A et al. Incidence of cancer among Nordic airline pilots over five decades occupational cohort study. BMJ 2002; 325: 567–72.
13. Langner I, Blettner M, Gundestrup M et al. Cosmic radiation and cancer mortality among airline pilots: results from a European cohort study (ESCAPE) Radiat Environ Biophys 2004; 42: 247–56.

CHAPTER 4

Coronary imaging: normal coronary anatomy

Volume-rendered CT cardiac images resemble the gross anatomy of the heart and provide a precise anatomic presentation of the presence and course of the right and left coronary arteries in relation to the surrounding cardiac structures. The coronary arteries are presented in a three-dimensional fashion, and as cross-sectional images. Superimposed structures, such as the atria and appendages, the pulmonary trunk, and cardiac veins can obscure the view and are preferably removed.

CORONARY ANATOMY

The left main coronary artery arises from the left posterior aortic sinus. It varies in length, but is usually 1–2 cm (Figure 4.1). In a small proportion of cases the left main coronary artery is very short and bifurcates almost immediately. In 0.41% of cases the left main coronary is not developed, and the left anterior descending and circumflex artery each individually arise from in the left coronary sinus. The main left coronary artery bifurcates, beneath the left atrial appendix, into the left anterior descending (LAD) and the circumflex arteries (Figure 4.2). The LAD artery passes to the left of the pulmonary trunk and turns forwards to run downwards in the anterior interventricular groove (Figure 4.2). The LAD artery provides two main groups of branches: first, the septal branches, which supply the anterior two-thirds of the septum; and, second, the diagonal branches which lie on the lateral aspect of the left ventricle. The circumflex artery turns backwards shortly beyond its origin to run downwards in the left atrioventricular groove. It, too, gives rise to a variable number of marginal

branches, which run on and supply the lateral aspect of the left ventricle. In the atrioventricular groove the circumflex artery is often covered by the auricle of the left atrium, which obstructs

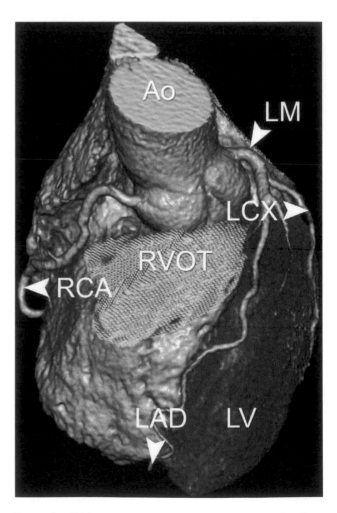

Figure 4 . 1 Volume-rendered image: superior anterior view of left and right coronary arteries. Ao, aorta; LM, left main coronary artery; LCX, left cir cumflex artery; RCA, right coronary artery; RVOT, right ventricular outflow tract; D1; first diagonal branch.

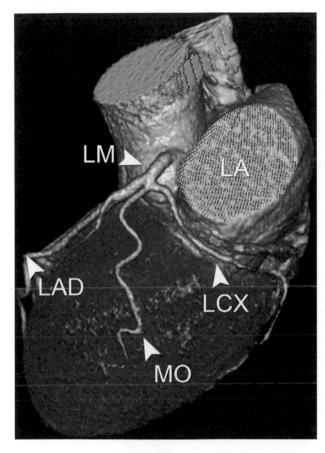

Figure 4 . 2 Volume-rendered image: lateral left view of left coronary artery. LM, left main coronary artery; LAD, left anterior descending artery; MO, marginal obtuse branch; LCX, left circumflex artery; LA, left atrium.

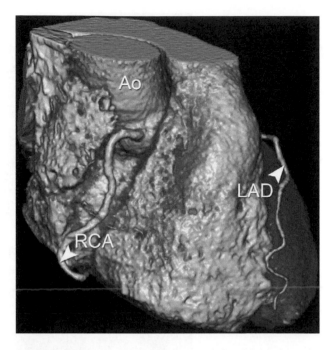

Figure 4 . 3 Volume-rendered image: lateral right view of right coronary artery (RCA). Ao, aorta; LAD, left anterior descending.

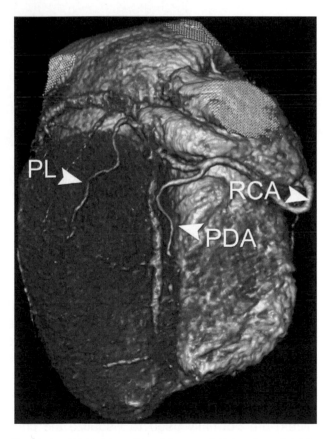

Figure 4 . 4 Volume-rendered image: inferior view of right coronary artery (RCA). PL, posterolateral branch; PDA, posterior descending artery.

visualization and therefore has to be removed from the data set. In one-third of subjects the left main coronary artery trifurcates into the LAD, left circumflex, and an intermediate artery, which follows a course between the circumflex and LAD arteries over the anterolateral wall of the left ventricle.

The right coronary artery (RCA) arises from the anterior aortic sinus, passes forwards and then downwards, in the right atrioventricular groove and continues around the margin of the heart towards the crux, a point where the atrioventricular groove and the posterior interventricular groove meet (Figures 4.3 and 4.4). In the majority (80%) of individuals the RCA is the dominant vessel and continues forwards from the crux along the posterior interventricular groove to become the posterior descending artery (PDA) (Figures 4.5 and 4.6). The posterolateral branch

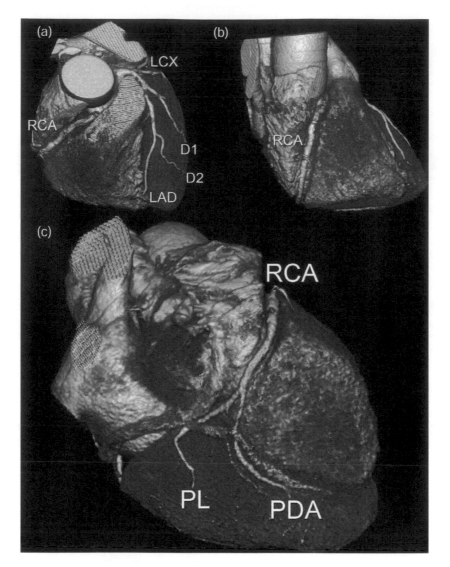

Figure 4 . 5(a) Volume-rendered image: superior view of right and left coronary arteries. Left anterior descending (LAD) give rise to two large diagonal branches. (b) Volume-rendered image of right coronary artery (RCA). (c) Volume-rendered image: inferior view of right dominant coronary artery. D1 first diagonal; D2 second diagonal; PL, posterolateral branch; PDA, posterior descending artery.

supplying the posteroinferior aspect of the left ventricle also arises from the RCA close to the crux. Left coronary dominance exists when the PDA arises from the circumflex artery (Figures 4.7 and 4.8). A balanced situation exists when the RCA and left circumflex (LCX) are of similar size.

The tomographic axial slices (the source slices) are normally used to visualize the coronary arteries. The course of the coronary arteries on the axial slices in relation to other cardiac structures is presented at different levels of the heart shown in Figure 4.9 and Figure 4.10.

CONCLUSION

The coronary anatomy can easily be assessed from the volume-rendered CT cardiac images. Knowledge of the gross anatomy of the coronary arteries is essential for accurate CT image interpretation.

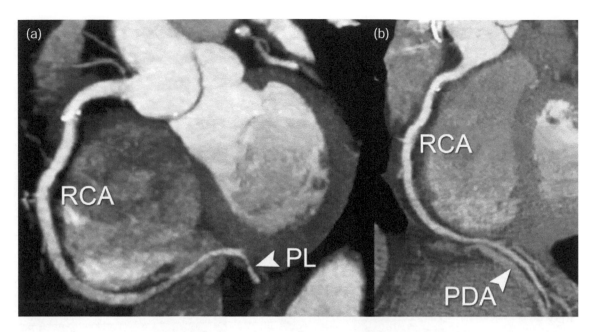

Figure 4 6 (a) Maximum intensity projection of right coronary artery (RCA) and posterolateral branch (PL). (b) Curved multiplanar reconstruction of RCA and posterior descending artery (PDA). Same patient as in Figure 4.5.

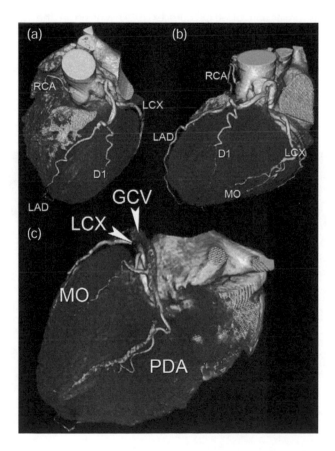

Figure 4 . 7 (a) Volume-rendered image: superior anterior view of left circumflex (LCX). (b) Volume-rendered image: lateral left view of LCX. (c) Volume-rendered image: inferior view of dominant LCX. Note: great cardiac vein (GCV) obscures the course of LCX. RCA, right coronary artery; LAD, left anterior descending; D1, first diagonal branch; MO, marginal obtuse branch; PDA, posterior descending artery.

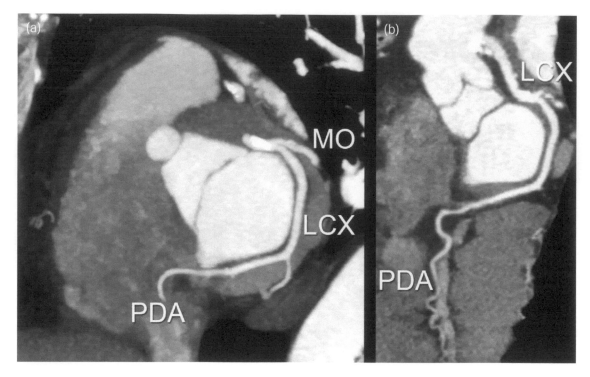

Figure 4 . 8(a) Maximum intensity projection of left cir cumflex (LCX) running in the atrioventricular groove. (b) Curved multiplanar reconstruction of the LCX. MO, marginal obtuse branch; PDA, posterior descending artery.

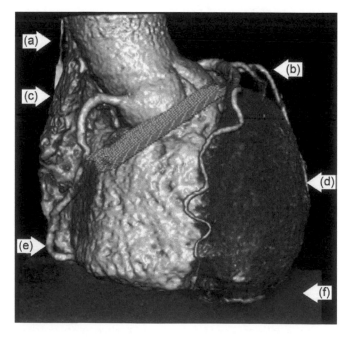

Figure 4 . 9 Volume-rendered image of coronary arteries. The arrows indicate the levels of the heart where axial images of the coronary arteries are chosen and shown in Figure 4.10.

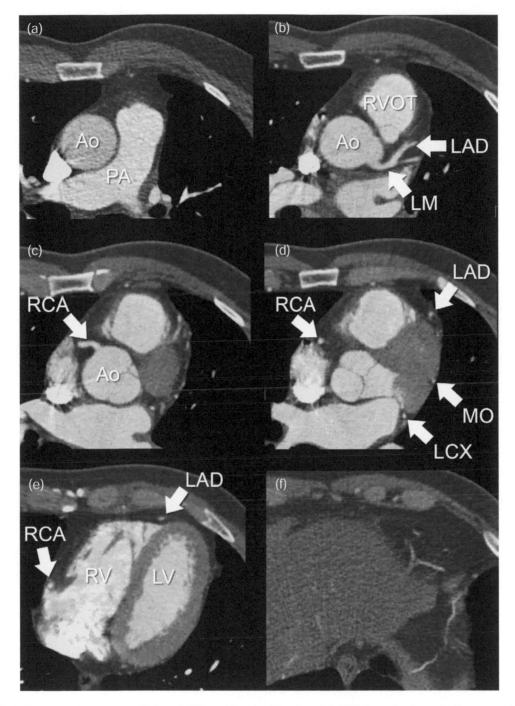

Figure 4 . 1 0 Axial images of coronary arteries at different levels of the heart. (a)–(f) From the base to the apex of the heart. (a) Level at aortic root and common pulmonary artery (PA). (b) Level at origin of left coronary artery. (c) Level at origin of right coronary artery (RCA) (d) Level of RCA and left cir cumflex (LCX) at atrioventricular groove. (e) Mid-ventricular level: RCA. (f) Dome of the diaphragm. Ao, aorta; RVOT, right ventricular outflow track; LM, left main; LAD, left anterior descending; MO, marginal obtuse branch; RV, right ventricle; LV, left ventricle.

SUGGESTED READING

James T. Anatomy of the coronary arteries in health and disease. Circulation 1965; 32: 1020–33.

Yamanaka O, Hobbs R. Coronary artery anomalies in 126 595 patients undergoing coronary angiography. Cathet Cardiovasc Diagn 1990; 21: 28–40.

Levin DC, Harrington DP, Bettmann MA et al. Anatomic variations of the coronary arteries supplying the anterolateral aspect of the left ventricle; possible explanation for the 'unexplained' anterior aneurysms. Invest Radiol 1982; 17: 458–62.

Braunwald E. Heart Disease. A Textbook of Cardiovascular Medicine, 4th edn. Philadelphia: WD Saunders Company, 1992.

CHAPTER 5

Coronary angiogram evaluation

INTRODUCTION

There is more than one way to assess a CT coronary angiogram. Depending on the indication, scanning equipment, image quality, and available post-processing software, as well as personal experience and preferences, various approaches can be taken. This chapter describes the evaluation process as it is performed in Rotterdam as well as alternative approaches. It functions as an initial guide for those new to coronary CT angiography.

PRIOR TO THE EVALUATION

Optimized image quality is key to accurate and confident assessment of the data. Before starting an evaluation, the reader needs to be assured that the most optimal reconstructions have been prepared. It is important to take note of the overall image quality. Is there patient motion or coronary blurring due to a high heart rate? Is contrast enhancement sufficient? Is the image noise level acceptable? Does the reconstructed field of view contain the entire heart, and was there sufficient longitudinal coverage? In case of motion artifacts additional phases may be reconstructed, cases with excessive image noise may benefit from reconstruction of thicker slices, while cases with stents or calcification may be better interpreted using thinner slices and sharper filters.

Screening the image quality of the data set also allows the gross cardiac and coronary anatomy to be interpreted. A general idea about the size and shape of the cardiac cavities, the dominance of the respective coronary arteries, and the presence and extent of coronary calcification and stents, etc. can be gained.

DETECTION OF CORONARY STENOSIS

Assessment of the coronary lumen, to detect or exclude significant coronary stenosis, is often the primary indication for a coronary CT scan (Table 5.1). Several tools and applications are available to assist in the assessment, each with their own advantages and pitfalls. It is important to realize the finite spatial resolution of the CT images, as

Table 5. 1Assessment of the coronary CT angiogram

Image quality
Artifacts
Motion
Noise
Contrast enhancement
Coronary artery disease
Anomalies
Plaque burden
Coronary stenosis (severity)
Cardiac morphology
Dimensions
Myocardium
Valves
Pericardium
Left ventricular function
Global function
(Wall motion abnormalities)
Intrathoracic pathology
Great vessels
Pulmonary disease
Mediastinum
Chest wall and spine

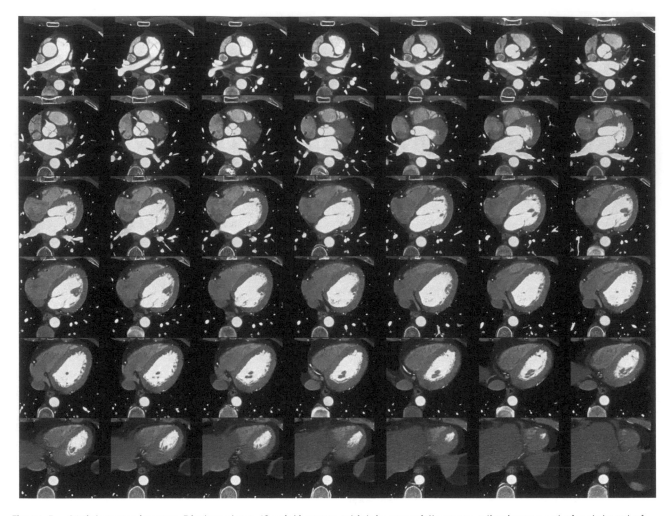

Figure 5 . 1 Axial source images. Displayed are 42 axial images, which is every sixth consecutive image out of a data set of approximately 250. Rather than looking at all the images at once (on a printed sheet), one can scroll back and forward through the images to track and assess each individual coronary branch.

well as the influence of filtering and image interpolation to improve the (subjective) image quality. Under clinical conditions the spatial resolution will be at best 0.5–0.7 mm in three dimensions, not accounting for residual motion artifacts or suboptimal contrast enhancement.

Despite the availability of sophisticated postprocessing applications, many scans can be assessed by merely scrolling through the axial source images (Figure 5.1). Particularly in cases with little or no coronary calcification or apparent plaque, stenotic disease in the larger branches is virtually excluded in a very short time. Smaller branches may be better assessed using maximum intensity projection (MIP), which displays

the vessel over a longer trajectory in a single plane (Figure 5.2). Because the MIP only shows the highest intensity within the slab it should be used with caution in calcified vessels (because of the risk of disease overestimation), and is rarely useful in the presence of stents. When the vessel runs perpendicular to the MIP plane, noncalcified tissue may not be noticed and luminal narrowing could be overlooked. Identification of atherosclerotic plaque or suspected narrowing is followed by closer examination to assess stenosis severity. Orthogonal and (double-)oblique cross-sectional planes (MPR, multiplanar reformation) can be placed in any position or angle within the three-dimensional data. By aligning

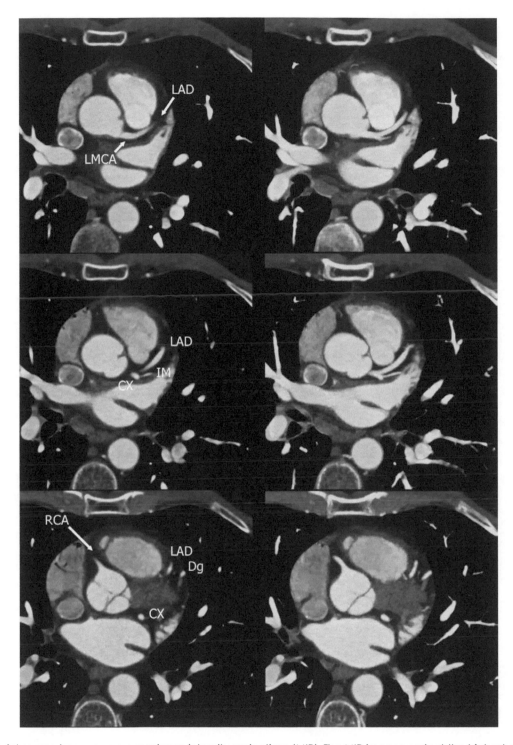

Figure 5 . 2 Axial source images versus maximum intensity projections (MIP). The MIP images project the highest densities within a selected slab. The images are usually less noisy and quite useful for the assessment of longer segments of tortuous vessels and smaller branches. Axial sour ce images (left column) and maximum intensity projections (MIP) images (right column) at corresponding levels show the difference in appearance. LAD, left anterior descending; LMCA, left main coronary artery; CX, circumflex; IM, intermediate branch; RCA, right coronary artery; Dg, diagonal branch; Mg, marginal branch.

(Continued)

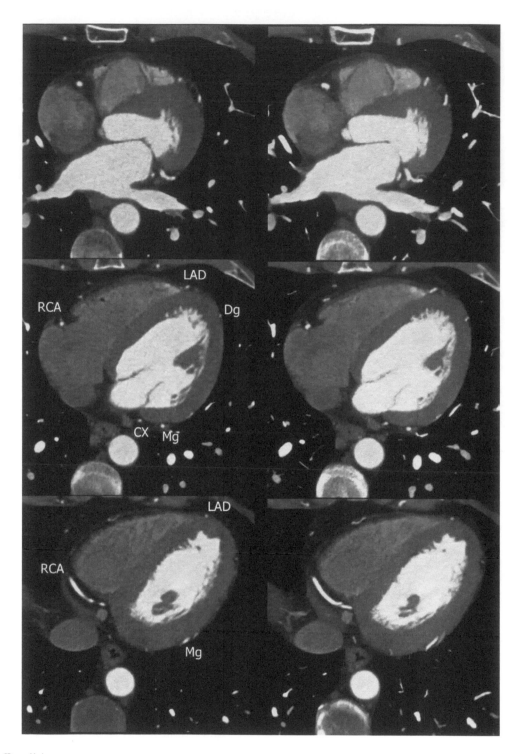

Figure 5 .—Cont'd

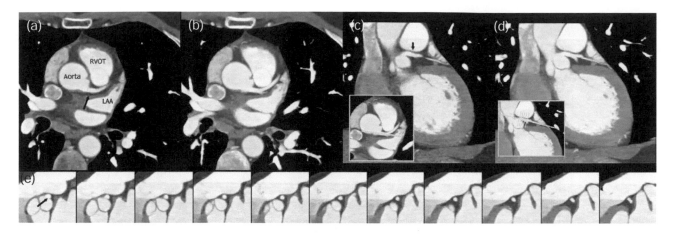

Figure 5 . 3 Assessment of the left main coronary artery (LMCA). The LMCA can be found on the axial slices (a) and MIP images (b) arising from the left coronary sinus between the right ventricular outflow tract (RVOT) and the left atrial appendage (LAA). By angulating an MPR plane around the vessel, perpendicular to the axial slice (as indicated by the line in the insert), a second view of the vessel can be obtained (MPR (c), MIP (d)), which better shows the initial cranial take-off of the LMCA. A cross-sectional view of the vessel can be obtained by positioning another MPR plane   perpendicular to the LMCA in the previous image. A detailed view of the vessel and vessel wall can be obtained by scrolling through the cross-sectional images along the LM (from the origin towards the bifurcation (e)), In this case no plaque or luminal narrowing was observed.

these cross-sectional planes along a certain vessel the diameter of a suspected lesion can be assessed and compared with other (non-diseased) vessel segments. These angulated planes may be converted to MIP images to demonstrate a longer segment of the vessel. Alternatively, in case of diffuse disease short-axis cross-sectional images of the vessel may be created. If it is necessary to display a longer segment of the vessel, or the entire vessel, curved MPR or MIP can be helpful.

ASSESSMENT OF THE CORONARY BRANCHES

Left main coronary artery

The left main coronary artery (LMCA) can be assessed in the vast majority of cases, as it has the largest diameter of all coronary branches. Nevertheless, it is usually assessed closely because of the importance of the vessel and the lower threshold for it to be classified as significantly diseased. In addition to the axial source images, short-axis cross-sectional images are useful to exclude ostial or bifurcation disease (Figure 5.3).

Left anterior descending coronary artery and diagonal branches

The left anterior descending coronary artery (LAD) can be found in the anterior interventricular groove of the heart, usually continuing in the same direction as the distal LMCA. When athero-sclerotic plaque is present axial slices may be difficult to interpret. The proximal and mid-segments of the LAD are fairly straight and can often be caught in one or even two perpendicular planes using the double-oblique MPR function (Figure 5.4). The angulated image plane can be moved back and forth. Alternatively, MIP conversion may be useful in the absence of extensive calcifications. If still unsuccessful, running a short-axis cross-section through the segment may be attempted if the image quality allows (Figure 5.5). The distal LAD is smaller and generally contains little calcification, and can often be assessed using MIP. Moderate-sized diagonal

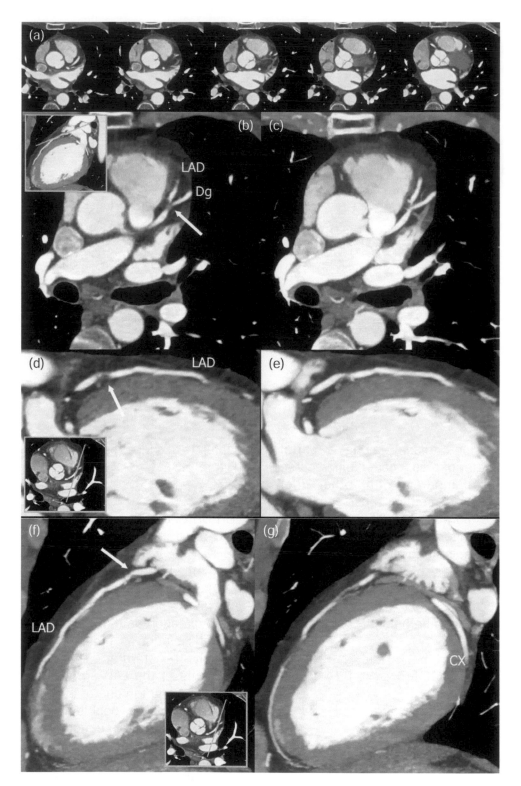

Figure 5 . 4 Assessment of the left anterior descending coronary artery (LAD). The first series are a selected number of axial slices in which coronary disease may be difficult to recognize (a). Using MPR a slightly oblique cross-section brings the proximal and mid-LAD in-plane (b), and reveals a severe lesion at the level of the bifurcation of the diagonal branch (Dg) (arrow). MIP conversion makes the lesion even more obvious (c). A second orthogonal view is created using MPR (d) and MIP (e). For the smaller and tortuous distal LAD MIP imaging is applied (f). When the vessel cannot be contained within a single (thin) slab, interpretation of the vessel may require adjacent images to be scrolled through (f) and (g).

(continued)

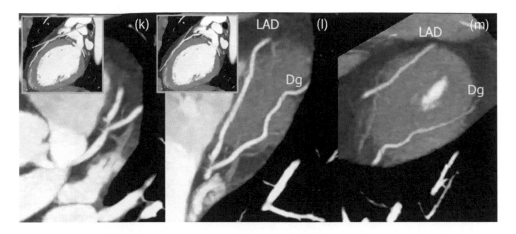

Figure 5.—C ont'd The smaller diagonal branches can be followed by rolling an MIP plane along the suface of the anterior wall (k)Đ(m).

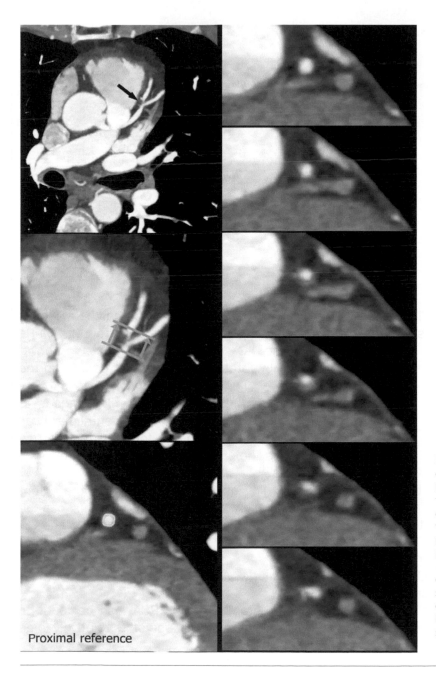

Proximal reference

Figure 5.5 Short-axis views of the left anterior descending (LAD). A short-axis view may be helpful to assess a vessel segment, for instance the mid-LAD (a). The MPR function is used to create two orthogonal planes along the vessel of interest. The thir d plane is then positioned perpendicular to these longitudinal planes to create a short-axis view of the LAD (c). This plane can be scrolled back and forth along the vessel (right column). Views that show lumen narrowing can be selected to compare with reference sites. The lumen can be traced manually to assess the stenosis severity.

(Continued)

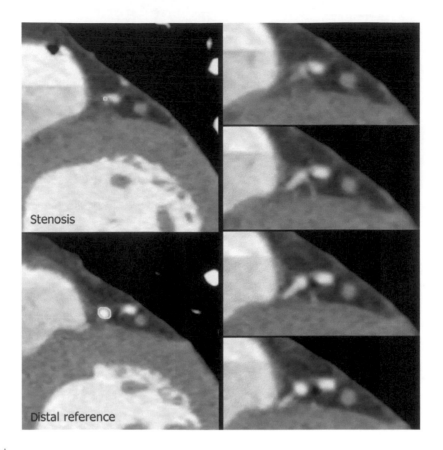

Figure 5.—Cont'd

branches may be evaluated using MIP. The ostium may require closer examination using (short-axis) MPR, particularly in the presence of extensive plaque in the LAD.

Left circumflex coronary artery and side branches

The left circumflex coronary artery (LCX) has the most varying anatomy of all coronary branches. Assessment may be complicated by the presence of the great cardiac vein adjacent to the LCX in the left atrioventricular (AV) groove. The proximal part of the LCX can be observed in a single view by rotating a plane around the LMCA–LAD axis (Figure 5.6). In case of a substantial LCX, the atrioventricular course can often be caught in a single plane by MPR or MIP, which allows a good overview of the vessel. This view can be achieved by positioning the rotation point of the MPRs within the LCX half-way along the AV groove, followed by rotation of the planes parallel to the AV groove. For assessment of the marginal branches of the LCX an image plane needs to be positioned parallel to the ventricular wall where the side branch was found. Often the use of MIP is helpful to interpret these tortuous branches.

Depending on the vessel size and the extent of calcification, the ramus intermedius can be evaluated using angulated MPR or MIP planes.

Right coronary artery

The right coronary artery (RCA) can be found in the right AV groove. Because of its relatively large

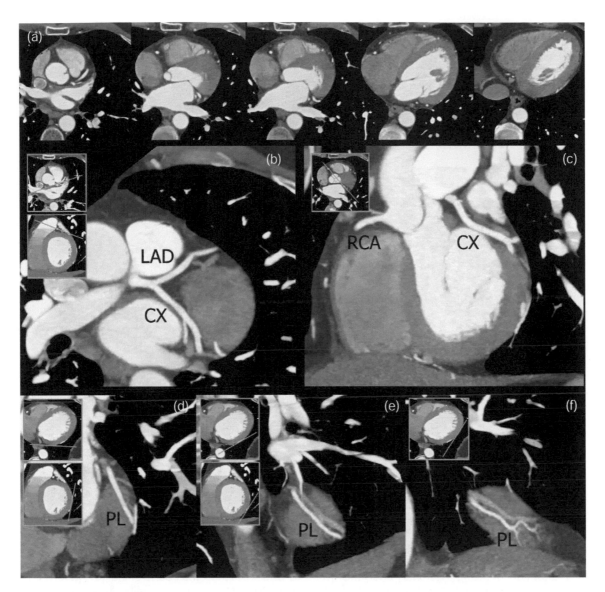

Figure 5 . 6 Assessment of the left circumflex coronary artery (CX). The first series shows selected axial slices of the CX, and the course, size, and anatomy of the vessel and side branches (a). From an axial image at the level of the left main coronary artery (LMCA) bifurcation it is often possible to capture the proximal CX in a single image using MPR with the origin of the CX as the rotational point of the MPR planes (b) and (c). The marginal or posterolateral branches (PL) can be evaluated by rolling an MIP plane along the lateral surface of the left ventricle.

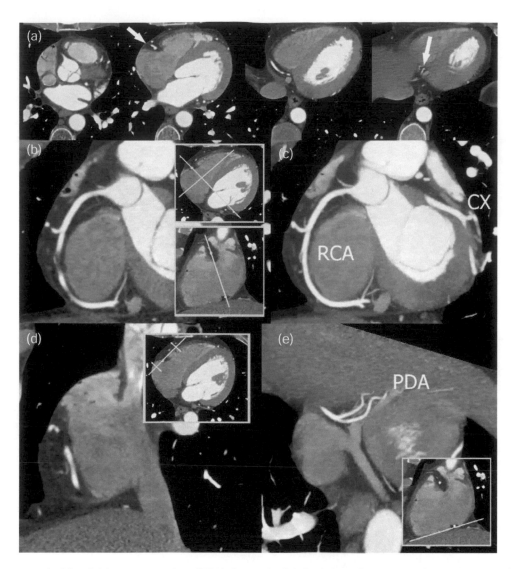

Figure 5 . 7 Assessment of the right coronary artery (RCA). Several axial slices show the course of the RCA (arrow) from the right sinus of Valsalva through the right atrioventricular (AV) groove, terminating into two branches within the posterior interventricular groove (a). To bring the RCA into a single plane, an axial plane at mid-ventricular level is selected. One MPR plane is positioned along the base of the heart (through the right and left AV groove). A second plane is positioned perpendicularly to the previous plane, through the right ventricle. This second plane is used to rotate the plane through the AV groove to intersect with both the proximal and distal RCA. The resulting plane will show the RCA within the A V groove (b). Particularly if the RCA has a more tortuous course, MIP conversion can bring the entire course of the RCA into view (c). The proximal and distal RCA are usually well visualized in the axial slices. An alternative (longitudinal) view of the mid-segment can be created by placing a plane along the right border of the heart (d). The smaller branches, such as the posterior descending branch (PDA) are often better assessed using (oblique) MIP (e).

size it can often be evaluated well on the axial images. It is also possible to view the vessel in a single plane positioned parallel to the AV groove (Figure 5.7), creating a view similar to the left-anterior oblique projection on conventional angiography. The smaller side branches, such as the marginal, posterior descending, and posterior lateral branches, are better evaluated using MIPs positioned parallel to the respective branches.

CHAPTER 6

Coronary pathology relevant to coronary imaging

A thorough review of the pathogenesis of coronary atherosclerosis is beyond the scope of this book; however, we believe it is worthwhile to provide a simple framework of the pathogenesis of coronary atherosclerosis to facilitate better understanding and interpretation of coronary plaque images.

The natural history of lumen atherosclerotic disease from the initial, only microscopically visible, lipid filled macrophages to advanced lesions that cause symptoms is represented in the morphological classification scheme for lesions proposed by the American Heart Association (AHA)[1,2] (Table 6.1).

This classification scheme has been widely accepted as the framework of our current understanding of progression of atherosclerosis. However, this scheme emphasizes mainly the histological features of plaque progression. From a clinical point of view, one might be more interested in a classification of coronary plaques that are associated with pathogenetic mechanisms associated with intracoronary thrombus formation and the subsequent occurrence of acute coronary syndromes or sudden cardiac death.

Davies et al demonstrated that rupture of the fibrous cap of an advanced atherosclerotic plaque exposes thrombogenic plaque components, in particular, tissue factor, to circulating

Table 6.1 Current American Heart Association classification[1,2]

Type	Histological classification	Gross classification	Lesion	MSCT detection
I	Isolated macrophage foam cells	Fatty dot, fatty streak	Early lesion, minimal lesion	No
II	Multiple foam cell layers	Fatty dot, fatty streak	Early lesion, minimal lesion	No
III	Preatheroma, intermediate lesion	Visually assessed	Chronological annotation	No
IV	Atheroma	Fibrolipid plaque	Advanced	Yes
V	Fibroatheroma	Fibrous plaque, plaque	Advanced	Yes
VI	Fissured, ulcerated, hemorrhagic, thrombotic lesion	Complicated lesion	Advanced	Yes
VII	Calcific lesion	Calcified lesion	Advanced	Yes
VIII	Fibrotic lesion	Visually assessed	Advanced	Yes

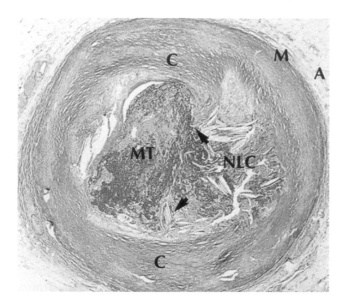

Figure 6 . 1 Advanced complicated plaque with fibrous cap rupture. MT, mural thrombus; NLC, necrotic lipid core; C, collagen; M, media; A, adventitia; arrow, rupture fibrous cap. From reference 6, with permission.

blood thereby initiating platelet aggregation and intracoronary thrombus formation[3,4,5]. The fibrous cap is the region of the plaque that separates the necrotic core from the lumen, and when the thickness of the cap is less than 65 μm it may be vulnerable to rupture. Typically, ruptured lesions have a large necrotic lipid core with a disrupted fibrous cap infiltrated by macrophages and lymphocytes, and the number of smooth muscle cells is low (Figure 6.1). Plaque rupture is the most common cause of acute coronary thrombosis formation and occurs in approximately 65–70% of cases. However, another cause of coronary thrombosis is plaque erosion[7,8]. Erosion occurs much less frequently in approximately 25–30% of cases, and in these lesions, typically, the endothelium is absent at the erosion site. These lesions usually do not have a necrotic core, but if present it is small; they have a thick fibrous cap, and smooth muscle cells and proteglycans are abundant while the eroded site contains minimal inflammation[7,8] (Figure 6.2). The majority of plaque erosions are eccentric and occur most frequently in young men and women under 50 years of age, often associated with smoking.

Finally, a calcified nodule, albeit infrequent (2–5%), may be the cause of a thrombotic occlusion. Calcific nodules are plaques with luminal thrombi showing a calcific nodule protruding into the lumen through a disrupted thin fibrous cap[8] (Figure 6.2b). This plaque is associated with a large underlying calcific plaque. The lesion is usually seen in elderly male patients with heavily calcified and tortuous arteries.

Based upon our recent knowledge that intracoronary thrombosis formation is caused by plaque

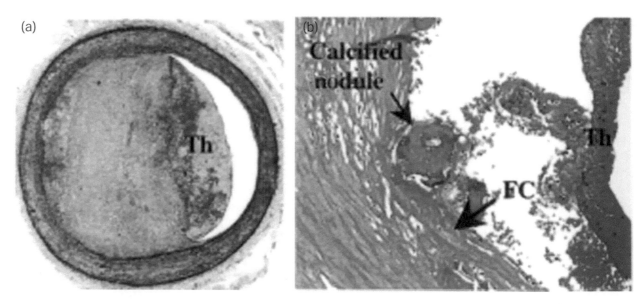

Figure 6 . 2 Plaque erosion/calcific nodule. (a) Plaque erosion with thrombus (Th). (b) Calcific nodule with Th FC, fibrous cap. From reference 8, with permission.

Table 6.2 Modified American Heart Association classification based on morphological description of progressive atherosclerotic lesions. From reference 8, with permission

Figure	Fibrous cap atheroma	Necrotic core with overlying fibrous cap
6.1	Thin fibrous cap atheroma	Thin fibrous cap, infiltrated by macrophages and lymphocytes with rare smooth muscle cells and an underlying necrotic core
6.2b	Calcified nodule	Rupture of nodular calcification with underlying fibrocalcific plaque
6.3	Fibrocalcific plaque	Collagen-rich plaque with significant stenosis usually contains large areas of calcification with few inflammatory cells
6.1 and 6.2a	Intracoronary thrombosis	Erosion or rupture causing non-occlusive or occlusive thrombus

rupture, plaque erosion, and calcific nodule, which are associated with certain types of coronary plaques, Virmani et al proposed a modified AHA lesion classification (Table 6.2). This modified AHA lesion classification describes the progression of atherosclerotic lesions from early stages through advanced thrombosis-prone plaques. It forms an important link between histology, intracoronary thrombus formation, and clinical presentation of coronary artery disease. The classification may further guide evolving research into the identification of a high-risk (vulnerable) plaque.

For the purpose of multislice CT (MSCT) plaque imaging we have adapted and simplified this modified AHA classification (Table 6.2 and Figures 6.1–6.3)[8].

IN VIVO MULTISLICE CT CORONARY PLAQUE IMAGING

The current resolution of MSCT scanners does not permit the initial phases of coronary atherosclerosis to be identified, and it cannot distinguish between plaque rupture and erosion as the cause of intracoronary thrombosis. Furthermore, the more subtle features of a plaque, such as fibrous cap thickness, disruption, or signs of inflammation, cannot be identified. Because of its limited resolution non-invasive MSCT only allows the depiction of advanced lesions according to the AHA classifications or progressive atherosclerotic lesions according to the modified AHA classification. Advanced plaques may or may not be associated with luminal narrowing depending on the presence of compensatory vessel wall remodeling that tends to preserve the lumen size in the earlier stages of plaque progression. CT coronary plaque imaging allows plaques to be classified into obstructive and non-obstructive. However, so far, precise quantification of the size of plaques is not possible due to either over- or underestimation and lack of quantification algorithms. In general, the size of low-density plaques tends to be underestimated and the size of calcific plaques tends to be overestimated. The precise composition of tissues within the plaque cannot be accurately assessed. MSCT can easily discriminate between a low-density and high-density plaque. Low-density plaques represent lipid core, necrotic, or fibrous tissue and high-density plaques represent calcium, whereas in the setting of an acute coronary syndrome a very low-density lesion of the culprit artery may be assumed to be a thrombotic lesion.

Current MSCT scanners cannot reliably discriminate between lipid accumulation in the plaque and fibrous tissue, and, to date, cannot reliably identify a plaque prone to rupture. Higher resolution scanners may resolve this problem.

CONCLUSION

MSCT plaque imaging allows, albeit rather crudely, discrimination between different types of advanced coronary plaques (Table 6.3 and Figures 6.4–6.9).

T ble 6 . 3MSCT features helpful to identify plaques

Figure	MSCT features	Density (HU)	Advanced plaques (AHA)	Progressive atherosclerotic lesion (modified AHA)
6.4	High density	>150	—	Calcific nodule
6.5	High density	>150	Calcific plaque	Ñ
6.6	High–low density		Ñ	Fibrocalcific plaque
6.7	Intermediate density	50–100	Fibrous plaque	Fibrous cap atheroma
6.8	Low density	20–50	(Fibro)atheroma	Thin fibrous cap atheroma
6.9	Very low density	< 20	Complicated plaque	Thrombus

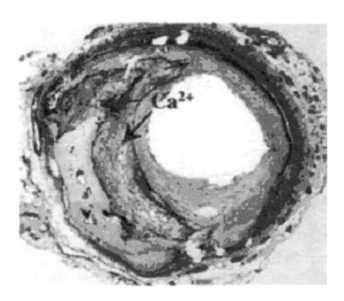

Figure 6.3 Fibrocalcific plaque. Ca^{2+}, calcium. From reference 8, with permission.

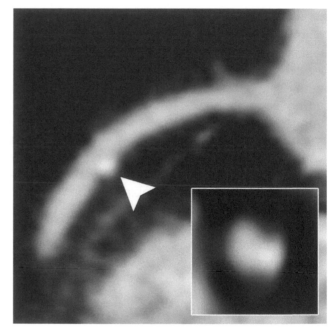

Figure 6 . 4 Axial and cross-sectional image of small calcific plaque (arrowhead: small high-density plaque (375 HU)).

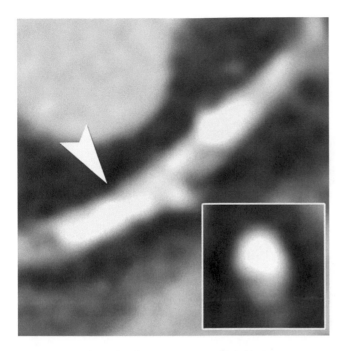

Figure 6.5 Axial and cross-sectional image of calcific plaque (arrowhead: high-density plaque (480 HU)).

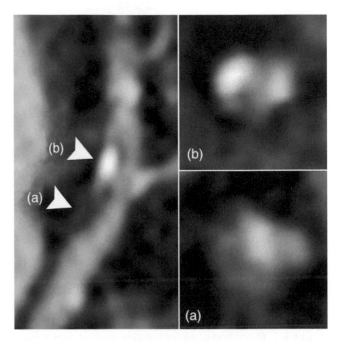

Figure 6.6 Axial and cross-sectional images of fibrocalcific plaque. (Arrowhead (a): low density (40 HU) and arrowhead (b): high density (350 HU).)

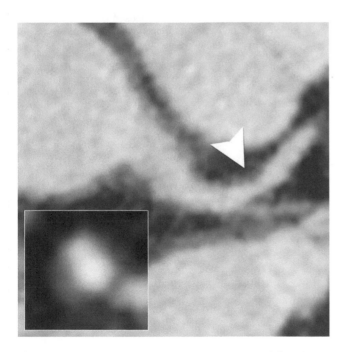

Figure 6.7 Axial and cross-sectional images of fibrotic plaque. (Arrowhead: intermediate-density plaque (95 HU).)

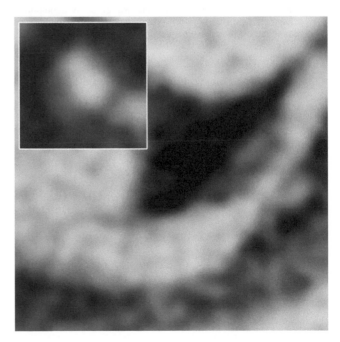

Figure 6.8 Axial and cross-sectional images of (fibro) lipid plaque. (Arrowhead: low density plaque (35 HU).)

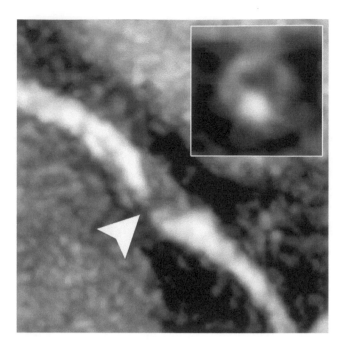

Figure 6 . 9 Axial and cross-sectional images of thrombotic occlusion. (Arrowhead: very low-density plaque (10 HU).)

REFERENCES

1. Stary HC, Chandler AB, Glagov S et al. A definition of initial, fatty streak, and intermediate lesions of atherosclerosis. A report from the Committee on Vascular Lesions of the Council on Arteriosclerosis, American Heart Association. Arterioscler Thromb 1994; 14: 840–56.
2. Stary HC, Chandler AB, Dinsmore RE et al. A definition of advanced types of atherosclerotic lesions and a histological classification of atherosclerosis. A report from the Committee on Vascular Lesions of the Council on Arteriosclerosis, American Heart Association. Arterioscler Thromb Vasc Biol 1995; 15: 1512–31.
3. Davies MJ, Thomas AC. Plaque fissuring – the cause of acute myocardial infarction, sudden ischaemic death, and crescendo angina. Br Heart J 1985; 53: 363–73.
4. Davies MJ. Anatomic features in victims of sudden coronary death. Coronary artery pathology. Circulation 1992; 85 (Suppl 1): 119–24.
5. Falk E. Plaque rupture with severe pre-existing stenosis precipitating coronary thrombosis. Characteristics of coronary atherosclerotic plaques underlying fatal occlusive thrombi. Br Heart J 1983; 50: 127–34.
6. Wilson PWF. Atlas of Atherosclerosis. Risk Factors and Treatment, 3rd edn. Part 1. Philadelphia: Current Medicine, Inc., 2001.
7. van der Wal AC, Becker AE, van der Loos CM, Das PK. Site of intimal rupture or erosion of thrombosed coronary atherosclerotic plaques is characterized by an inflammatory process irrespective of the dominant plaque morphology. Circulation 1994; 89: 36–44.
8. Virmani R, Kolodgie FD, Burke AP, Farb A, Schwartz SM. Lessons from sudden coronary death: a comprehensive morphological classification scheme for atherosclerotic lesions. Arterioscler Thromb Vasc Biol 2000; 20: 1262–75.

CHAPTER 7

Coronary stenosis: description and quantification

Coronary obstructions are generally described by location and severity. To describe the location of the lesion a standardized coronary segment classification is used (Figure 7.1 and Table 7.1), with further details of relevance (bifurcation lesion).

In clinical practice lesion severity is often visually estimated using the axial source images, (oblique) multiplanar reformations, and maximum intensity projections (Table 7.2). Despite the limitations of CT, in terms of the spatial resolution in relation to the small size of the coronary arteries, objective and reproducible stenosis quantification is possible with a certain degree of accuracy. The potential advantage of CT over catheter angiography is the ability to measure the cross-sectional vessel area. Particularly in cases of borderline lesions, manual tracing and measurement of the stenosis vessel in comparison to

Table 7.1 Coronary artery reporting system[1]

Number	Branch	Description
1	Proximal right coronary artery (RCA)	First half of the distance from the ostium to the acute margin of the heart
2	Mid-RCA	Second half of the distance from the ostium to the acute margin of the heart
3	Distal RCA	From the acute margin to the origin of the posterior descending branch
4	Posterior descending artery (PDA)	Branch groove in case of right dominance
5	Left main coronary artery (LMCA)	Including the bifurcation
6	Proximal left anterior descending (LAD)	From the origin to the first major septal branch
7	Mid-LAD	To the LAD angle. If unidentifiable, the first half until the apex of the left ventricle (often coinciding with the second diagonal branch)
8	Distal LAD	Terminal part of the LAD
9	First diagonal branch (D1)	Largest and usually first diagonal branch
10	Second diagonal branch (D2)	Second diagonal branch
11	Proximal circumflex artery (LCX)	From the origin to the bifurcation of the first marginal branch
12	Obtuse marginal branch (MO)	First marginal branch off the LCX
13	Distal LCX	Distal part running within or close to the left atrioventricular groove
14	Posterolateral branch (PL)	Branch along the posterolateral left ventricular wall
15	Posterior descending artery (PDA)	PDA from the LCX in case of left dominance
16	Intermediate branch (IM/AL)	Branch along the anterolateral wall between the LAD and LCX in case of a LM trifurcation

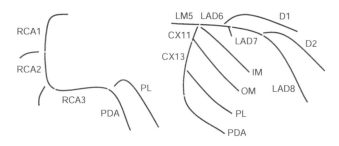

Figure 7.1 Classification of coronary artery segments. For abbreviations see Table 7.1.

Table 7.2 Semiquantitative stenosis severity scale

Semiquantitative scale	Diameter reduction(%)
Normal	0
Non-significant stenosis	< 50
Moderate stenosis	50–70
Severe stenosis	70–99
Occlusion	100

reference sites can be helpful to classify whether a lesion is significant or not. It is important to realize that (similar to catheter quantitative coronary angiography) measurements are affected by many variables including the projection angle, selection of the proximal and distal reference, and even the display settings (window level and width).

Contemporary vessel analysis software allows (semi-)automatic quantification of stenosis severity (Figure 7.2). Vessel recognition and lumen segmentation are affected by motion, slab misalignment noise, etc., and the results are most reliable in high-quality scans. Therefore, it is important to verify the results, check vessel contours, and exclude artifacts, before accepting the calculated stenosis severity.

CALCIFIED VESSELS

Calcified deposits, as part of atherosclerotic disease, cause beam hardening and blooming artifacts that increase the apparent size of these high-density structures and complicate assessment of the adjacent coronary lumen. To improve the interpretability of calcified vessels the first step is to optimize the acquisition. Because calcium-related artifacts are aggravated by motion, it is even more important to reduce the heart rate when the presence of advanced atherosclerotic disease is expected. Measures to minimize image noise should be taken.

When reconstructing the images, finding a motion-free phase is crucial. Improved edge-enhancement using sharper kernels may be helpful. In severely calcified vessels axial slices and multiplanar reconstructions (MPR) may not give a good (longitudinal) view of the vessel, while maximum intensity projections (MIP) will worsen the blooming effects. In these cases short-axis views can be helpful to identify the lumen, and confirm vessel patency.

In general calcium causes overestimation of the lesion severity. Despite the previously discussed measures, calcifications remain an important limitation of coronary CT angiography, and may render cases non-interpretable.

CORONARY PLAQUE

CT can detect atherosclerotic plaque in the coronary artery wall, which may or may not cause obstruction of the coronary artery lumen. Generally, coronary plaque identified by CT is classified as calcified, non-calcified, or mixed (Table 7.3). Prospective differentiation of fibrous (stable) and lipid-rich plaque (presumably unstable) is to date unreliable. The value of coronary calcium imaging by CT is well established. The significance and consequences of finding non-calcified plaque by CT remain unclear. Generally, we document the presence, localization (coronary segment), and composition (calcified or non-calcified) of coronary plaque.

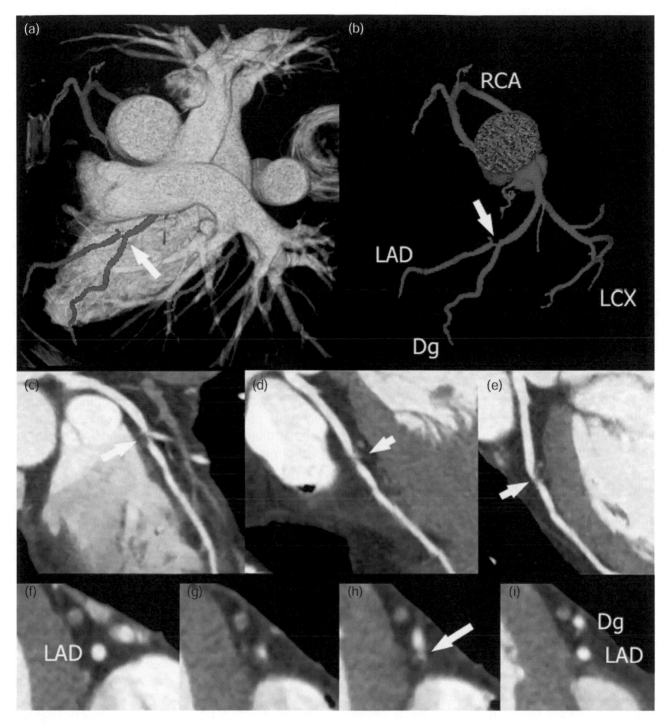

Figure 7.2 Vessel segmentation and stenosis quantification. Contemporary vessel analysis software allows automatic segmentation of the coronary arteries within the three-dimensional volume (a) and (b). In a selected vessel the center lumen line can be determined, after which multiple radial cross-sections can be reformatted (c)–(e). The residual lumen at the stenosis site (arrow) is automatically measured (h). Based on the proximal (f) and distal reference site (i) the stenosis severity can be calculated as percentages (0.9/7.4 mm^2, 90%) The residual lumen at the stenosis site (g) and (h) (arrow) is automatically measured. (Circulation‾, Siemens AG, Erlangen, Ger many). RCA, right coronary artery; LAD, left anterior descending; Dg, diagonal branch; LCX, left circumflex artery.

Table 7 . 3 Plaque classification

Plaque type	Criteria
Non-calcified	Attenuation (HU) of >90% of the plaque below enhanced coronary lumen
Calcified	Attenuation (HU) of >90% of the plaque above enhanced coronary lumen
Mixed	Both >10% calcified and non-calcified tissue. Particles with an attenuation value below enhanced lumen but above 130 HU are generally considered to be calcified tissue

PRESENTATION OF FINDINGS

Demonstration of findings on axial source images and MIPs and MPRs from arbitrary angles can be difficult to interpret by other healthcare professionals, i.e. referring physicians. Post-processing software provides an intuitive and attractive means by which to present CT findings. Despite the robustness and ease of use of contemporary post-processing applications, reliance on these tools for the primary coronary assessment is generally discouraged. A detailed description, as well as the drawbacks and pitfalls of these software tools can be found in other chapters.

To improve interpretability of source images, MIPs and MPRs, standardized angulations can be used, similar to catheter angiography projections. Additionally, labeling of side branches is important, particularly when non-standard views are presented.

Curved MPRs allow an entire coronary artery to be displayed in a single view (Figure 7.3). Similar to a world map, flattening a cross-section along a tortuous vessel will result in distortion of the vessel and, in particular, the surrounding structures. In cases with sufficient image quality automatic vessel tracking can create a center lumen line and display curved MPRs at an infinite number of rotational cross-sections around this center lumen line. The fidelity of the curved MPR depends on the accuracy of the traced or automatically defined center lumen line.

Three-dimensional volume-rendering allows attractive representation of angiographic findings in relation to the cardiac anatomy (Figure 7.4).

Different software enable (semi)automatic segmentation of the coronary arteries from the other cardiac cavities and surrounding tissues. Combined with detailed images of the local pathology three-dimensional images can be very useful for the transfer of CT results. Good three-dimensional images require high image quality. Reconstruction of thicker slices reduces image noise and improves the (subjective) quality of the three-dimensional reconstructions. When the image quality is suboptimal smaller branches may appear interrupted, suggesting obstructive disease. Obstructions in calcified vessels are difficult to demonstrate on three-dimensional rendered images.

CARDIAC ANATOMY AND FUNCTION

In addition to the coronary arteries, the remaining cardiac anatomy also needs to be reviewed. This includes the dimensions and morphology of the cardiac cavities, the ventricular wall, the integrity of the atrial and ventricular septum, the pericardium, the aortic root, and morphological abnormalities of the cardiac valves.

Reconstruction of several cardiac phases allows functional assessment of the left (and right) ventricle. Global left ventricular parameters, end-systolic volume, end-diastolic volume, stroke volume, and ejection fraction can be determined semiautomatically. Additionally, wall motion abnormalities can be visualized using a dynamic display of the consecutive phases. Dynamic assessment of the cardiac valves is currently being explored.

CLINICAL INDICATIONS FOR CORONARY CT ANGIOGRAPHY

The technical feasibility of CT coronary angiography compared with invasive coronary angiography has been validated extensively. Because of the high negative predictive value, CT is clinically used to rule out coronary artery disease. The quantitative accuracy of CT is inferior to invasive angiography and anatomical images are often not sufficient to establish the hemodynamic significance of a coronary stenosis. Therefore, cardiac

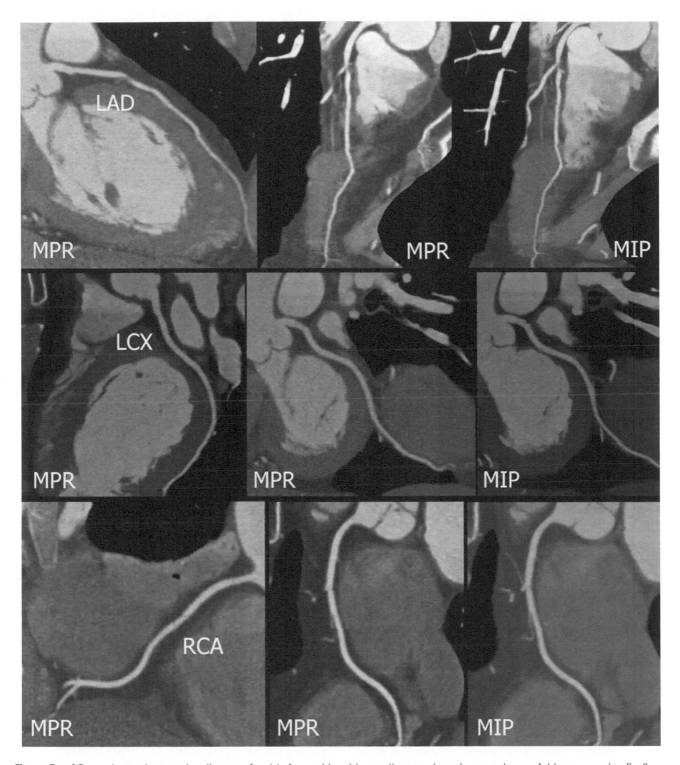

Figure 7 . 3 Curved vessel reconstruction, preferably from at least two orthogonal angles, can be useful to summarize findings. The three main branches, left anterior descending (LAD), left circumflex (CX, continuing as a large marginal branch), and right coronary artery (RCA), have been reconstructed as curved multiplanar reconstructions (MPRs) (left and middle columns) and a curved (MIP) maximum intensity projection (right column).

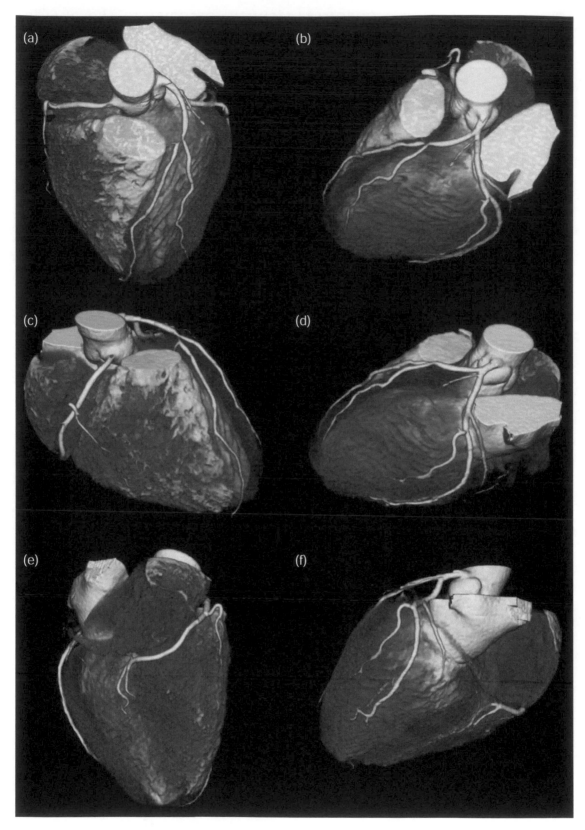

Figure 7 . 4 After segmentation and removal of the surrounding structures a three-dimensional volume-rendered CT coronary angiogram has been created. The lesion in the left anterior descending artery is clearly visible from an (extreme) cranial angle (a), a left lateral-cranial angle (b), and a right-anterior oblique angle (c). (c) Also shows the proximal right coronary artery (RCA). The distal RCA can be followed along the diaphragmatic sur face of the heart (e). The left cir cumflex coronary artery can be followed on the left-lateral views (b), (d), and (f).

Table 7.4 American Heart Association recommendations for the clinical use of coronary CT angiography. From reference 2, with permission

Indication	Class	Evidence
Assessment of obstructive coronary artery disease in symptomatic individuals (particularly in low–intermediate probability)	IIa	B
Screening of asymptomatic individuals	III	C
Follow-up after percutaneous intervention	III	C
Follow-up after coronary artery bypass graft	IIb	C
Anomalous coronary arteries	IIa	C
Non-calcified plaque	III	C

Class I, evidence or general agreement that the procedure is useful and effective; class II, conflicting evidence or divergence of opinion about the usefulness/efficacy of the procedure; class IIa, weight of evidence/opinion is in favor of usefulness/efficacy; class IIb, usefulness/efficacy is less well established by evidence/opinion; class III, evidence and/or general agreement that the procedure is not useful/effective and in some cases may be harmful. Weight of evidence A, high; B, intermediate; C, low.

CT is regarded to be most useful as a tool to rule out coronary artery disease in symptomatic patients and avoid conventional coronary angiography 2 (Table 7.4). Appropriateness criteria published in 2006 favor the use of CT in symptomatic patients at intermediate risk to rule out obstructive coronary artery disease, particularly when a functional test is not feasible or has produced non-interpretable or equivocal results 3 (Table 7.5). Furthermore, the use of CT to rule out coronary artery disease in patients with acute chest pain without ECG changes or elevated markers is considered appropriate. In general, the use of cardiac CT in asymptomatic individuals is discouraged. Also, in patients with new onset heart failure without evident ischemic heart disease, CT can be useful to rule out coronary artery disease as the causative etiology.

The ability to evaluate stented coronary arteries depends on the stent design, the stent material, and the diameter size of the stent. Because of the limited data, routine use of CT in patients who previously have undergone coronary intervention is not recommended. In selected patients, with larger stents (in the left main coronary artery

Table 7.5 Appropriateness criteria for contrast-enhanced cardiac CT in the detection of coronary artery disease (CAD). From reference 3, with permission

	Appropriateness criteria score
Evaluation chest pain syndrome	
Intermediate pretest probability of CAD ECG interpretable and able to exercise	5
Intermediate pretest probability of CAD ECG uninterpretable or unable to exercise	7
High pretest probability	2
Uninterpretable or equivocal stress test	8
Moderate to severe ischemia on stress test	2
Evaluation of intracardiac structures	
Suspected coronary anomalies	9
Acute chest pain	
Low pretest probability of CAD No ECG changes and cardiac markers negative	5
Intermediate pretest probability of CAD No ECG changes and cardiac markers negative	7
High pretest probability of CAD No ECG changes and cardiac markers negative	6
High pretest probability of CAD ST elevation or positive cardiac markers	1
Triple rule out	
Low pretest probability No ST elevation and cardiac markers negative	4
Asymptomatic	
Low CHD risk	1
Moderate CHD risk	2
High CHD risk	4
Prior to non-cardiac surgery	
Low-risk surgery	1
High-risk surgery	4
Post-CABG	
Symptomatic	6
Asymptomatic	2–3

(Continued)

Table 7.5 Appropriateness criteria for contrast-enhanced cardiac CT in the detection of coronary artery disease (CAD). From reference 3, with permission—Cont'd

	Appropriateness criteria score
Post-PCI	
Symptomatic	5
Asymptomatic	1
Complex congenital heart disease	
Coronary and non-coronary	7
New onset heart failure	
Coronary evaluation	7
LV function	
Following infarction or heart failure	3
Following infarction or heart failure	
Technically limited images echo	5
Native and prosthetic valves	
Technically limited images echo, MRI, TEE	5
Cardiac mass	
Technically limited images echo, MRI, TEE	8
Pericardial disease	
Technically limited images echo, MRI, TEE	8
Prior to invasive ablation therapy	
Pulmonary vein anatomy	8
Prior to biventricular pacemaker	
Coronary vein anatomy	8
Prior to repeat CABG	
Coronary anatomy	8

Score 7–9, generally acceptable and a reasonable approach; score 4–6, uncertain clinical scenario; score 1–3, not acceptable and not a reasonable approach.
CHD, coronary heart disease; CABG, coronary artery bypass graft; PCI, percutaneous coronary intervention; MRI, magnetic resonance imaging; TEE, transesophageal echocardiogram.

or grafts), contemporary stent designs with thin struts, or non-metalic stents, the use of CT as an alternative to conventional angiography can be considered.

CT is a very reliable tool to assess bypass grafts. However, for the complete evaluation of patients after bypass graft surgery, CT has a class IIb recommendation as a result of the more complicated assessment of the coronary arteries in these patients.

The appropriate or recommended role of coronary CT in clinical cardiology is still developing. Research into the usefulness of CT compared with established approaches, as well as its long-term prognostic value, is still ongoing. With ongoing technical innovation and improving diagnostic accuracy, lower radiation dose, and emerging clinical evidence, the (recommended) indications of coronary CT angiography are expected to expand in the future.

REFERENCES

1. Austen WG, Edwards JE, Frye RL et al. A reporting system on patients evaluted for coronary artery disease. Report of the Ad Hoc Committee for Grading of Coronary Artery Disease, Council on Cardiovascular Surgery, American Heart Association. Circulation 1975; 54 (Suppl 4): 5–40.
2. Budoff MJ, Achenbach S, Blumenthal RS et al. Assessment of coronary artery disease by cardiac computed tomography: a scientific statement from the American Heart Association Committee on Cardiovascular Imaging and Intervention, Council on Cardiovascular Radiology and Intervention, and Committee on Cardiac Imaging, Council on Clinical Cardiology. Circulation 2006; 114: 1761–91.
3. Hendel RC, Patel MR, Kramer CM et al. ACCF/ACR/SCCT/SCMR/ASNC/NASCI/ SCAI/SIR 2006 appropriateness criteria for cardiac computed tomography and cardiac magnetic resonance imaging. A report of the American College of Cardiology Foundation Quality Strategic Directions Committee Appropriateness Criteria Working Group. J Am Coll Cardiol 2006; 48: 1475–97.

CHAPTER 8

Coronary stenosis

Invasive X-ray coronary angiography using selective contrast enhancement of the lumen of the coronary arteries, is regarded as the reference standard for the detection of coronary obstructions in humans. High-resolution projections of only contrast-enhanced coronary arteries are acquired at a high frame rate throughout the cardiac cycle. This provides motion artifact-free high-quality images which allow precise quantification using contour detection algorithms. The high frame rate acquisition gives an impression of coronary flow and allows assessment of the collateral circulation. Catheter-based coronary angiography functions as a road map for intracoronary imaging techniques, including intracoronary ultrasound, virtual histology, palpography, optical coherence tomography or magnetic resonance imaging, and flow and pressure measurements to determine the functional severity of coronary obstructions or microcirculation. Thus, invasive coronary angiography plays an essential role in the diagnosis of coronary artery disease and it will be not easy, or may even seem unlikely for multislice CT (MSCT) coronary angiography to replace invasive coronary angiography although MSCT should provide sufficient diagnostic information regarding the coronary integrity to enable it to serve as a reliable alternative to invasive coronary angiography. The advantages of MSCT are its lower costs, reduced patient risk and discomfort, and higher throughput.

IMAGING CHARACTERISTICS

MSCT coronary angiograms are different from conventional angiograms. Conventional angiograms are projections of a vessel that has been enhanced with a high concentration of contrast material (Figure 8.1). During the injection of contrast, multiple images of this vessel are acquired throughout a number of cycles. For MSCT angiography the cross-sectional images of the coronary arteries are reconstructed during a single phase of a number of consecutive heart cycles (Figure 8.1). Because contrast is injected intravenously and scanning is performed during the plateau phase of the contrast enhancement, all blood-containing cavities are opacified. The intracoronary blood opacification in MSCT is of a relatively low magnitude and calcium or stents, having high densities, are much more visible, compared to conventional angiography (Figure 8.2). The technical boundaries of CT limit the spatial and temporal resolution, which are significantly lower than in catheter-based angiography (Table 8.1). This limits the applicability of stenosis severity quantification software, particularly in the smaller branches. On the other hand, because MSCT is a cross-sectional technique, it allows appreciation of the non-enhanced soft tissues in the proximity of the vessels and allows for three-dimensional reconstruction of the cardiac and coronary anatomy (Figure 8.3).

HISTORY OF CT CORONARY ANGIOGRAPHY

For the purpose of completeness and historical reasons, due to the rapid technological developments in CT, the diagnostic performance of electron beam CT (EBCT) and four- and eight-slice MSCT compared with coronary angiography are presented in Tables 8.2[1–10] and 8.3[11–20].

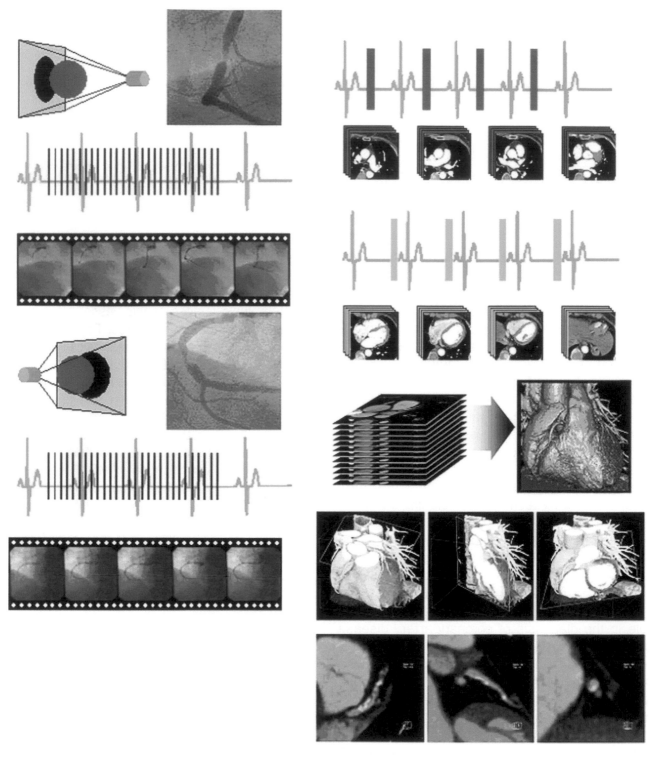

Figure 8.1 Coronary angiogram (CAG) versus multislice CT (MSCT) coronary imaging. While contrast is selectively injected into the coronary artery, more than 20 roentgen projections are acquired, showing the dynamic contrast enhancement of the vessel. Computer-assisted contour-detected quantification of a coronary stenosis (minimum lumen diameter) requires at least two perpendicular projections. The minimum luminal diameter is calculated as the average of the shortest diameters in the two perpendicular projections. MSCT requires intravenous injection of contrast and data are acquired during the steady state of contrast enhancement. During each cycle a consecutive and overlapping volume of the heart is scanned. Images are reconstructed during mid-diastolic phase in the heart cycle and reconstruction of an entire volume requires isocardiophasic data from a sequence of heart cycles. Different phases can be reconstructed depending on the position of the reconstruction window within the R-to-R interval. From these individual slices a three-dimensional data volume can be created that allows reconstruct ion of cross-sectional planes through the volume and display of the vessel or lesion of interest at any position or angle. If the s   patial resolution in relation to the vessel size permits, stenosis quantification can be performed by direct measurement of the vessel area.

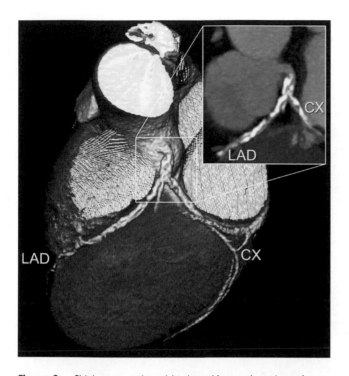

These early landmark studies were exciting and the sometimes spectacular coronary images stimulated cardiologists and radiologists to take part in further studies. The enormous potential of non-invasive coronary angiography, with its associated high number of cardiac patients who would need coronary angiography, was a powerful additional stimulus for the industry rapidly to further develop CT technology. Sixty-four-slice CT coronary angiography is now available, and newer developments such as dual-source CT or 256-slice CT are in the preclinical or early clinical test phase[21]. Although much has been achieved, CT technology is still evolving and CT coronary angiography is slowly entering the clinical arena.

DIAGNOSTIC PERFORMANCE OF 16-SLICE CT CORONARY ANGIOGRAPHY

The diagnostic accuracy of the 16-slice CT scanner to detect a significant coronary stenosis (≥50% luminal diameter) is presented in Table 8.4[22–35]. The weighted average of all published studies shows that the sensitivity is 87%,

Figure 8 . 2 Volume-rendered (colored image) and maximum intensity projection (insert) CT images readily highlight the presence of coronary calcifications (high-density structures displayed as white). CX, circumflex coronary artery; LAD, left anterior descending coronary artery.

T ble 8 . 1 Conventional versus MSCT coronary angiography

	Conventional angiography	MSCT angiography
Contrast injection	Intracoronary	Intravenous (peripheral)
Contrast enhancement	Selective coronary	Complete vascular
Image acquisition	Projection	Cross-section (3D)
Acquisition rate	≈20 projections per heart cycle	1 data set in ≈10 heart cycles
Radiation exposure	3–6 mSv	5–13 mSv
Examination time	³ 30 min	<15 min
In-hospital time	≤1 day	1– 2 h
Spatial resolution	$0.1 \times 0.1 \times \infty$ mm	$0.4 \times 0.4 \times 0.4$ mm
Temporal resolution	50 ms	83–200 ms
Additional advantages	Lesion quantification	Minimally invasive procedure
	Coronary flow	Cardiac anatomy
	Additional diagnostics (IVUS, pressure measurements, etc.)	Plaque imaging
	Intervention	
Additional disadvantages	Complications and discomfort related to the arterial puncture and coronary intubation	Sensitive to arrhythmia Calcified vessels

IVUS, intravascular ultrasound; ∞, infinity.

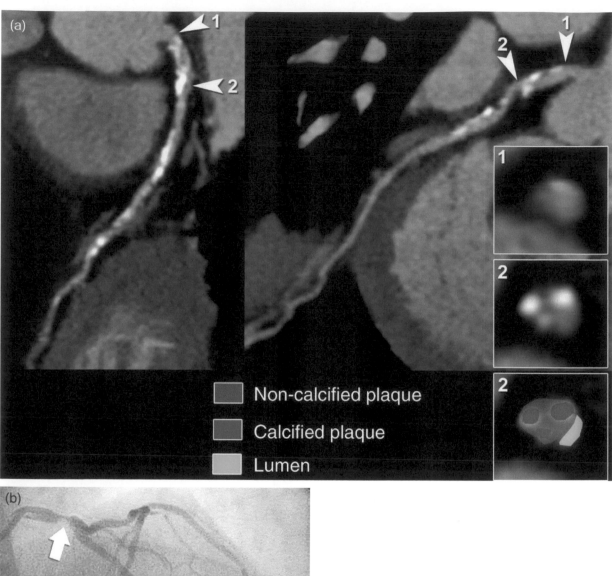

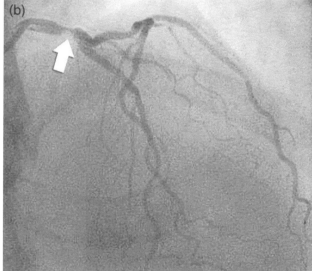

Figure 8.3 (a) Curved multiplanar reconstructed images of the left main and left anterior descending coronary arteries in two orthogonal directions (large images) showing a severely diseased left main coronary artery and the presence of both calcified and non-calcified tissue components. Cross-sectional images at different levels of the left main coronary artery (arrowheads) suggest significant narrowing of the coronary lumen. Arrowheads at site of cross-sectional images (1) and (2). At (2) narrow-lumen large mixed plaque and remodeling. (b) Invasive angiography confirming the presence of a significant stenosis in the left main coronary artery (arrow).

Table 8 . 2 Diagnostic performance of contrast-enhanced electron beam CT with conventional coronary angiography as the reference standard

	Patients	Sensitivity (%)	Specificity (%)	Excluded (%)
Moshage et al[1]	20	74	100	NR
Achenbach et al[2]	125	92	94	25
Rensing et al[3]	37	77	94	19
Reddy et al[4]	23	88	79	8
Schmermund et al[5]	28	83	91	12
Nakanishi et al[6]	37	74	94	12
Budoff et al[7]	52	78	91	11
Moshage et al[8]	118	90	82	24
Achenbach et al[9]	36	92	91	20
Lu et al[10]	107	91	93	7

NR, not reported

Table 8 . 3 Diagnostic performance of four- and eight-slice MSCT to detect coronary stenosis, with conventional angiography as the reference standard (four-slice CT)

	CT	Use of beta-blockers	n	Basis of assess-ment	Significant diameter reduction (%)	Previous disease per patient* (n)	Excluded segments or branches (%)	Sensitivity (%)	Specificity (%)	PPV (%)	NPV (%)	Sensitivity[†] (%)
Nieman et al[11]	4	–	31	Branch	50	0.9	27	81	97	81	97	68
Achenbach et al[12]	4	–	64	Branch	50	1.1	32	85	76	56	93	55
					70	0.9	32	91	84	59	98	58
Knez et al[13]	4	–	43	Segment	50	1.2	6	78	98	84	96	51
Vogl et al[14]	4	+	64	Segment	50	NR	28	75	99	92	98	NR
Nieman et al[15]	4	–	53	Segment	50	1.3	30	82	93	66	97	61
Kopp et al[à][16]	4	–	102	Segment	50	1.5	15	86	96	76	98	86
								93	97	81	99	93
Giesler et al**[17]	4	+	100	Branch	70	1.0	29	91	89	66	98	49
Nieman et al**[18]	4	–	78	Segment	50	0.9	32	84	95	67	98	63
Kuettner[19]	4	+	66	Segment	70	1.6	43	66	98	83	95	37
Maruyama et al[20]	8	–	25	Segment	50	1.5	14	90	99	93	99	73

*Number of diseased vessels or segments per patient; [†]overall sensitivity including missed lesions in non-assessable segments or branches; [à]results by two observers, without consensus reading; **studies that include patients from earlier publications; PPV, positive and NPV, negative predictive value with respect to the assessable segments and branches; NR, not reported.

Table 8 . 4 Diagnostic performance of 16-slice MSCT to detect significant coronary stenosis (more than of 50% of luminal diameter)

Author	n	Excluded segments (%)	Sensitivity (%)	Specificity (%)	PPV (%)	NPV (%)
Nieman et al[22]	58	0 (0/231)	95 (82/86)	86 (125/145)	80 (82/102)	97 (125/129)
Mollet et al[23]	127	7 (92/1384)	92 (216/234)	95 (1092/1150)	79 (216/274)	98 (1029/1110)
Martuscelli et al[24]	72	16 (116/729)	89 (83/93)	98 (450/459)	90 (83/92)	98 (450/460)
Kuettner et al[25]	58	21 (158/763)	72 (54/75)	97 (667/688)	72 (54/75)	97 (667/688)
Leta et al[26]	31	12 (55/474)	75 (62/83)	91 (341/375)	65 (62/96)	94 (341/362)
Hoffmann et al*[27]	33	17 (92/530)	63 (34/54)	96 (457/476)	64 (34/53)	96 (457/477)
Mollet et al[28]	51	0 (0/610)	95 (61/64)	98 (537/546)	87 (61/70)	99 (537/540)
Kuettner et al[29]	72	7 (62/936)	82 (96/117)	98 (742/757)	86 (96/111)	97 (742/763)
Cademartiri et al[30]	40	0 (0/428)	96 (88/92)	96 (322/336)	86 (88/102)	99 (322/326)
Schuijf et al[31]	45	6 (19/317)	98 (59/60)	97 (231/238)	89 (59/66)	99 (231/232)
Kefer et al[32]	52	0 (0/447)	82 (64/78)	79 (293/369)	46 (64/140)	95 (293/307)
Hoffmann et al[33]	103	6 (88/1384)	95 (149/157)	99 (1117/1125)	95 (149/157)	99 (1117/1127)
Kuettner et al[34]	120	7 (106/1560)	85 (304/359)	98 (1073/1095)	93 (304/326)	95 (1073/1128)
Achenbach et al[35]	50	4 (28/663)	94 (50/53)	96 (559/582)	68 (50/73)	99 (559/562)
Weighted	912	7.8 (816/10456)	87 (1402/1605)	96 (8006/8341)	81 (1402/1737)	97.5 (8006/8211)

*Stenosis >70%; PPV, positive predictive value; NPV, negative predictive value.

the specificity is 96%, the positive predictive value is 81%, and the negative predictive value is 97.5%. These results clearly indicate that a negative CT scan reliably rules out the presence of a significant coronary stenosis. However, a significant problem is the rather higher percentage (7.8%) of coronary segments that were excluded from analysis. This was mainly as a result of the presence of motion artifacts or severe calcifications, and the still limited spatial resolution of the 16-slice CT scanner prevented reliable assessment of the smaller parts of the coronary tree such as the distal segments and side branches.

DIAGNOSTIC PERFORMANCE OF 64-SLICE CT CORONARY ANGIOGRAPHY

Significant technical advances in CT technology have been introduced with almost unprecedented speed during the past few years, which has culminated in the production of a 64-slice CT scanner which is now available for clinical use and offered by various vendors (Siemens, Philips, General Electronic, and Toshiba). The 64-slice CT scanners from the various vendors differ slightly in design and configuration but all scanners feature a high temporal and spatial resolution, and rapid coverage of the entire heart with an acquisition time ranging from as low as 6 s to as high as 12 s. The diagnostic performance of the 64-slice CT scanner when compared with quantitative invasive coronary angiography, to detect (Figures 8.4–8.12) or rule out a significant coronary stenosis, is shown in Tables 8.05 and 8.6[36–47]. In Table 8.5 the per-segment analysis is performed, and it is of note that approximately 6% of the coronary segments were excluded from analysis (owing to poor image quality or severe calcification) which 'artificially' increased the diagnostic performance[36–47]. Inclusion of these segments would have resulted in a less favorable outcome.

In Table 8.6 the per-patient analysis is shown[36–47]. Again, exclusion of 3% of patients from the analysis suggests too favorable an outcome. The per-vessel analysis is demonstrated in Table 8.7. There were no significant differences in the outcome of the right coronary artery, left circumflex coronary artery, or the left anterior descending coronary artery. Stenoses in the left main stem were always detected. The 64-slice CT scanner is still not perfect but the high negative predictive value of 96% underscores the reliability of CT to exclude the presence of significant coronary stenosis. Unfortunately, the 64-slice CT scanner was still not always able to analyze all coronary segments, and around 6% of coronary segments were excluded from analysis.

DIAGNOSTIC PERFORMANCE OF DUAL-SOURCE 64-SLICE CT CORONARY ANGIOGRAPHY

The temporal resolution (165 ms) of 64-slice CT scanners remains too limited, which causes motion artifacts of fast moving coronary segments such as the right coronary artery. These motion artifacts occur most often during fast heart rates, i.e. more than 70 bpm. The dual-source CT scanner features a gantry composed of two X-ray tubes placed at an orthogonal angle, each tube having a fixed opposite detector row[48]. This new CT configuration has significantly improved the temporal resolution which is now 83 ms. This allows almost motion-free images to be obtained

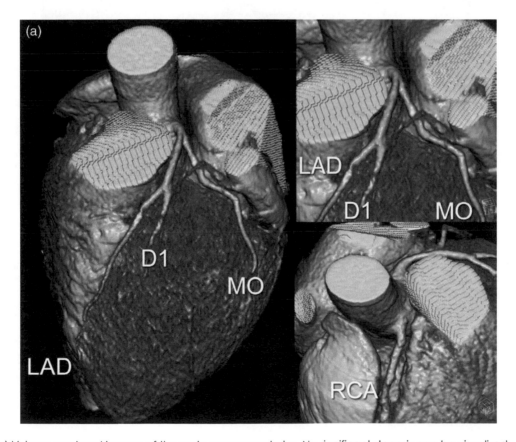

Figure 8 . 4(a) Volume-rendered images of the main coronary arteries. No significant stenosis can be visualized.

(Continued)

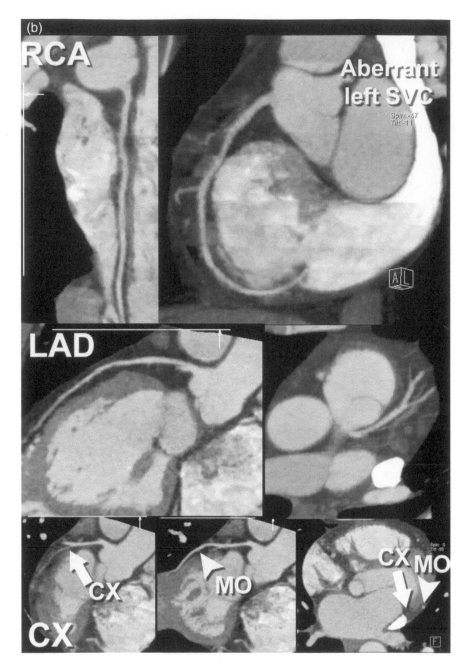

Figure 8.4 Cont'd (b) Curved multiplanar reconstructed and maximum intensity projected CT images of the same patient again do not show significant lumen narrowing of the main coronary arteries. An incidental finding is the presence of an aberrant left superior vena cava (SVC).

(Continued)

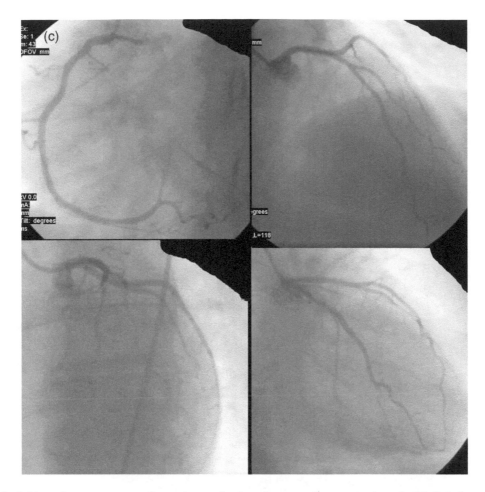

Figure 8.4 Cont'd (c) Invasive coronary angiography confirming absence of coronary stenosis. D1, first diagonal branch; LAD, left anterior descending coronary artery; MO, marginal obtuse branch; CX, circumflex coronary artery; RCA, right coronary artery.

during higher heart rates, thereby obviating the need for prior administration of beta-blockers if a CT scan is performed in patients with higher heart rates[48–51] (Figures 8.13–8.16). The initial results are excellent (Table 8.8) and have been obtained from analysis of the entire coronary tree without exclusion of coronary segments[52,53].

IMAGE INTERPRETABILITY (TABLE 8.09)

To determine whether a CT angiogram, or part of a CT angiogram, is evaluable or not depends on a number of factors, including observer experience and confidence. Using four-slice MSCT, the

number of segments with a subjectively adequate image quality varied between 6% and 43% in the different studies (Table 8.3). Studies with 16-slice technology and routine beta-receptor blocking report that approximately 8% of the coronary segments were excluded from analysis owing to poor image quality (Table 8.4)[21–35]. This was reduced to 5% with 64-slice CT technology (Table 8.5). The main reasons for reduced assessability are related to motion artifacts caused by residual cardiac motion, severe coronary calcification, fast heart rate, and voluntary patient movement. Fast heart rates (>65 bpm) are often associated with blurred images owing to the fact that during fast heart rates the

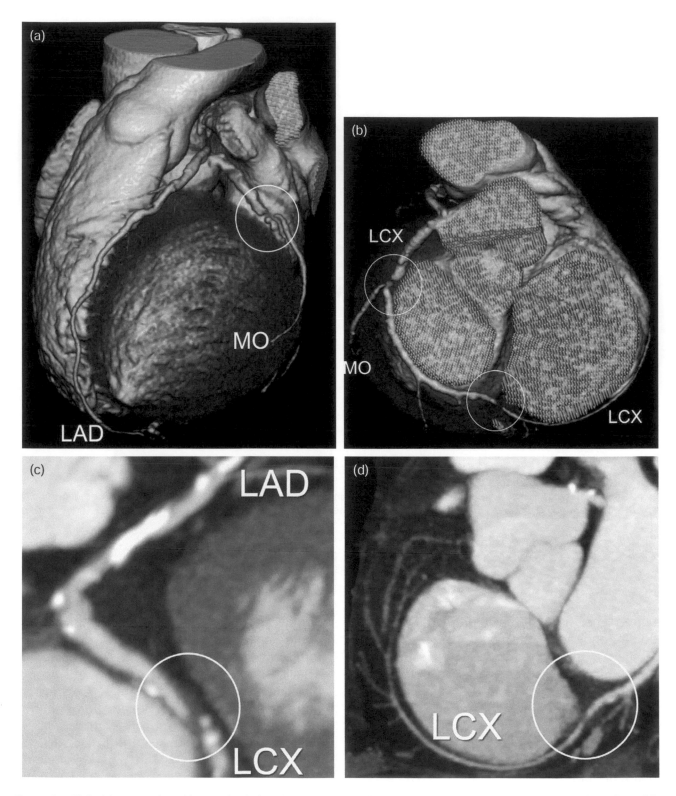

Figure 8 . 5(a) Volume-rendered image (anterior view) showing a significant lesion (circle) located at the bifurcation of the circumflex coronary artery (LCX) and the first marginal obtuse branch (MO). (b) Volume-rendered image (posterior view) after removing the left and right atrium showing two significant lesions (circles). The proximal lesion is located at the bifurcation of the LCX and the MO and the distal lesion in the posterolateral branch. Maximum intensity projections of the proximal (c) and the distal (d) coronary lesions.

(Continued)

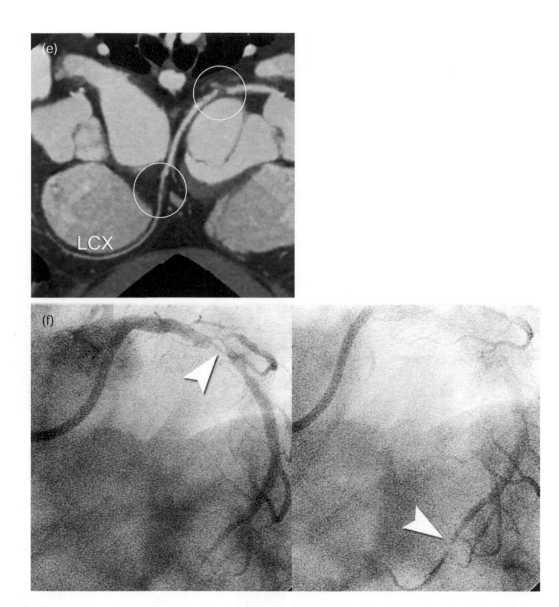

Figure 8.5 Cont'd   (e) Curved multiplanar reconstructed image of the LCX showing the proximal and the distal coronary lesions. (f) Invasive angiography confirming the presence of both significant obstructive coronary lesions located in the LCX (arrowheads). LAD, left anterior descending coronary artery.

motion-free diastolic cardiac phase is relatively short and thereby the likelihood of motion artifacts increases. Fast heart rates usually are reduced by administration of beta-blockers prior to the investigation to reduce the heart rate, ideally to less than 65 bpm. Other incidental causes for reduced interpretability are motion and beam hardening artifacts from the inflow of highly concentrated contrast medium into the superior caval vein or high-density artifacts from pacemaker wires. Patients with arrhythmia are generally unsuitable for MSCT coronary angiography because of the beat-to-beat end-diastolic volume variation. However, occasional premature contractions, which occur in many patients, can adversely affect the assessment, but this can be adequately managed by a post-processing editing algorithm. The contrast enhancement also influences the interpretability, and when stenosis detection of luminal narrowing is the objective, a high intracoronary concentration of contrast media is preferred. Finally, patient size adversely

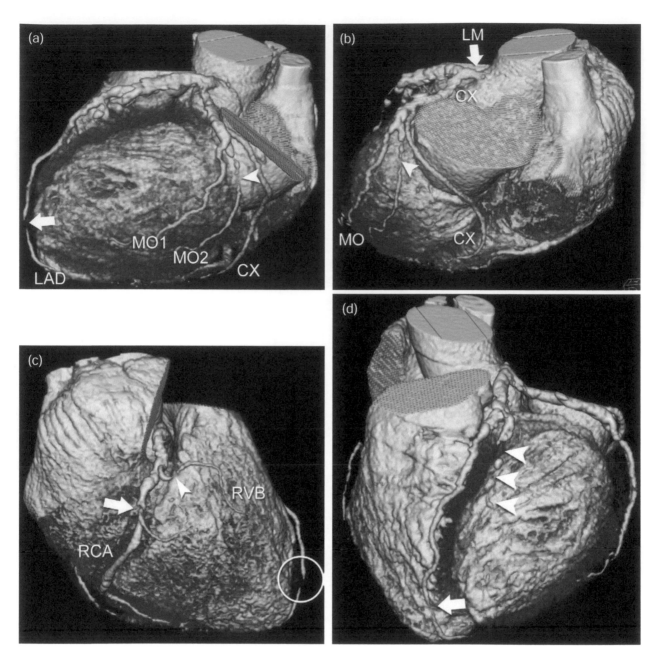

Figure 8.6 (a) Volume-rendered image (left lateral view) highlighting significant stenosis in the left anterior descending coronary artery (LAD, arrow) and second marginal obtuse branch (MO2, arrowhead). (b) Volume-rendered image (left posterolateral view) highlighting the significant stenosis in the second marginal obtuse branch (MO, arrowhead). (c) Volume-rendered image (right posterolateral view) highlighting significant stenosis in the right coronary artery (RCA, arrow), right ventricular branch (RVB, arrowhead), and left anterior descending coronary artery (circle). (d) Volume-rendered image (anterior view) highlighting a total occlusion of the first diagonal branch (arrowheads) and a significant stenosis in the LAD artery (arrow).

(Continued)

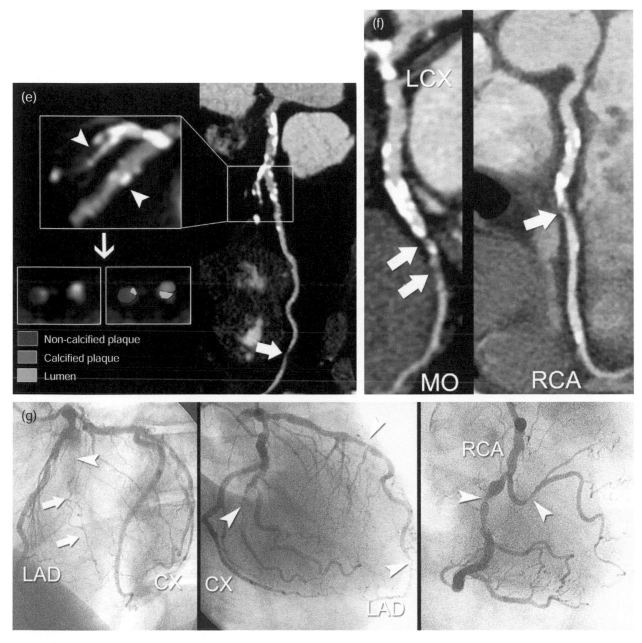

Figure 8.6 Cont'd (e) Curved multiplanar reconstructed image of the left main and LAD again showing the occluded first diagonal branch (box) and a significant lesion in the LAD (arrow). The maximum intensity projection (upper panel) and cross-sectional images (lower panels) visualize different plaque tissue components.(f) Curved multiplanar reconstructed images of the left circumflex (LCX, left panel) and right (RCA, right panel) coronary artery showing two significant lesions (arrows). (g) Invasive angiography confirming the presence of three-vessel disease (arrows, total occlusion of the first diagonal branch; arrowheads, significant stenoses). CX, circumflex coronary artery; MO1, first marginal obtuse branch; LM, left main coronary artery.

affects the quality of the scan. Factors influencing image interpretability are listed in Table 8.9.

CONSIDERATIONS AND LIMITATIONS

Despite significant technological progress and increasing experience with the evaluation of MSCT coronary angiography, a number of challenges remain (Table 8.10). Technical limitations in terms of spatial resolution, temporal resolution, and contrast-to-noise have been discussed in previous chapters. As a consequence, some patient characteristics are unfavorable and are more likely to result in non-interpretable examinations. Image quality is poorer in patients with a fast or irregular heart rate. Coronary arteries with diffuse and calcified atherosclerotic disease are more difficult to assess. A high body mass index results in more image noise and requires a higher roentgen dose. Contrast-enhanced MSCT is contraindicated in patients with impaired renal function or known intolerance to iodine-containing contrast media. The considerable radiation dose remains a matter of concern, limiting the application of this technique.

When coronary artery segments are regarded as evaluable, a number of misinterpretations continue to be made. Overestimation, and occasionally underestimation, of lesion severity can be caused by motion artifacts, or be related to the lack of objective quantification tools, lack of a representative reference diameter, and misuse of the window level and width settings (Figure 8.17). Other reasons for stenosis overestimation include cardiac arrhythmia, which results in discontinuity of vessels in the longitudinal direction, giving the impression of an obstruction with three-dimensional post-processing applications. Highly attenuating materials, such as stents or calcific plaques, cause blooming artifacts that create or exaggerate the apparent severity of

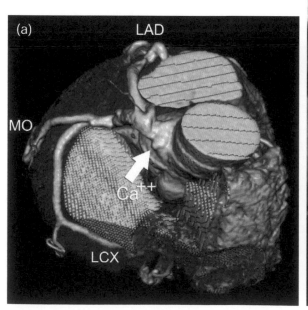

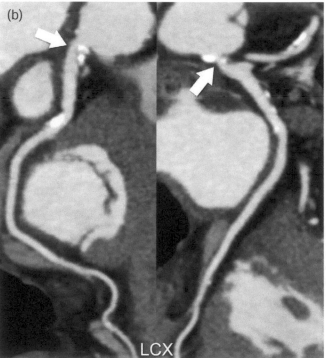

Figure 8 . 7(a) Volume-rendered image (left posterolateral view) showing severe calcification of the left main coronary artery (LM). The calcified plaque completely obscures the presence of a significant lumen narrowing of the LM. (b) Curved multiplanar reconstructions of the LM and left circumflex coronary artery (LCX) in two orthogonal directions show a significant stenosis of the LM (arrows). Ca++, calcium plaque; LAD, left anterior descending coronary artery; MO, marginal obtuse branch.

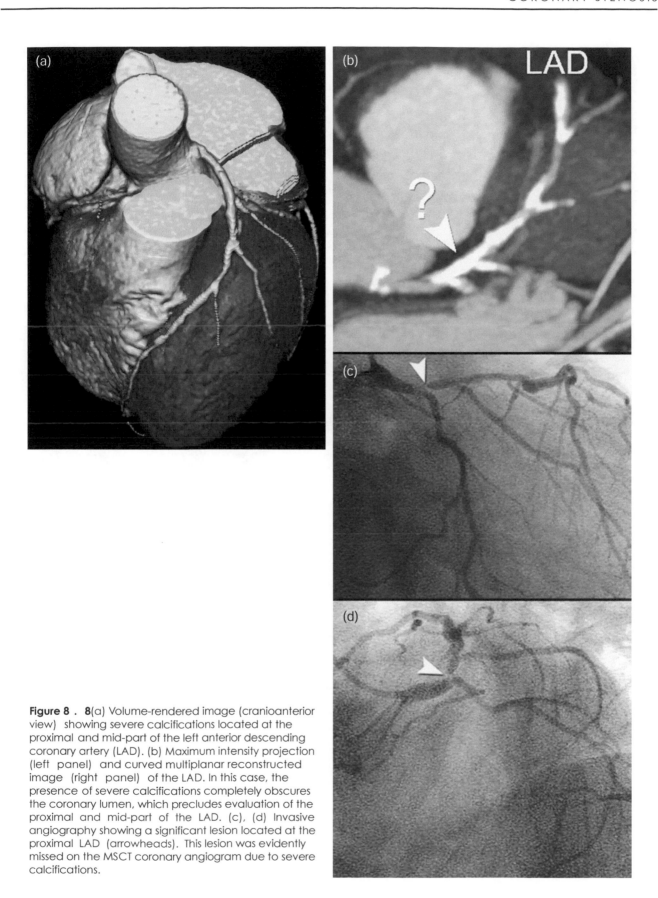

Figure 8 . 8(a) Volume-rendered image (cranioanterior view) showing severe calcifications located at the proximal and mid-part of the left anterior descending coronary artery (LAD). (b) Maximum intensity projection (left panel) and curved multiplanar reconstructed image (right panel) of the LAD. In this case, the presence of severe calcifications completely obscures the coronary lumen, which precludes evaluation of the proximal and mid-part of the LAD. (c), (d) Invasive angiography showing a significant lesion located at the proximal LAD (arrowheads). This lesion was evidently missed on the MSCT coronary angiogram due to severe calcifications.

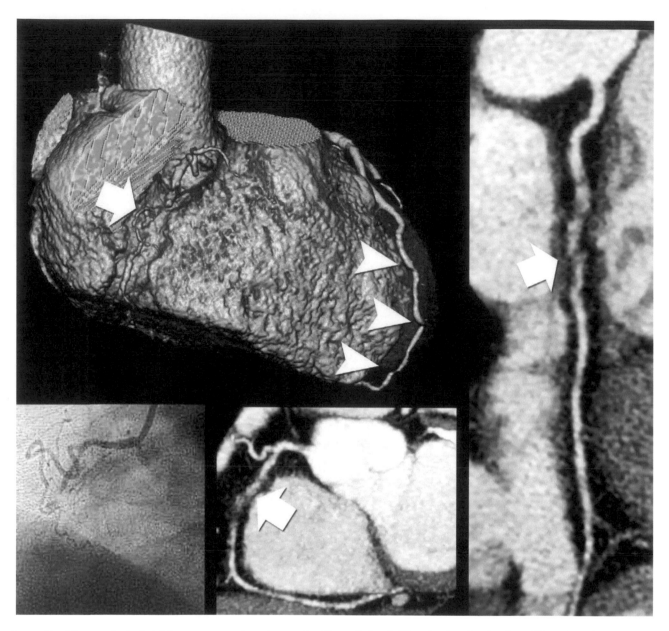

Figure 8 . 9 An occluded right coronary artery (arrows) with collateral filling is visualized using different post-processing techniques. This finding was confir med with invasive coronary angiography (left lower panel). However, image quality of the MSCT angiogram is severely reduced due to the motion artifacts. These motion artifacts did not only affect the evaluation of the right coronary artery, but also the evaluation of the left anterior descending coronary artery (arrowheads).

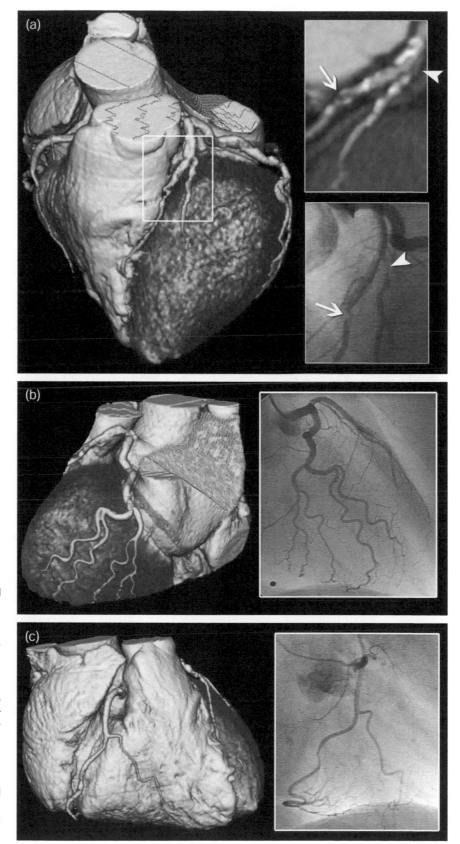

Figure 8.10 (a) Volume-rendered image (anterior view) providing an anatomical overview of the left coronary artery. Detail shows maximum intensity projection showing a significant lesion of the mid-part of the left anterior descending coronary artery and an ostial lesion of the first diagonal branch. Both lesions were confirmed on the conventional angiogram (right lower panel). (b) Volume-rendered image (left lateral view) and corresponding conventional angiogram of the circumflex coronary artery. No significant lesions are visualized. (c) Volume-rendered image (right lateral view) and corresponding invasive angiogram of the right coronary artery. No significant lesions are visualized.

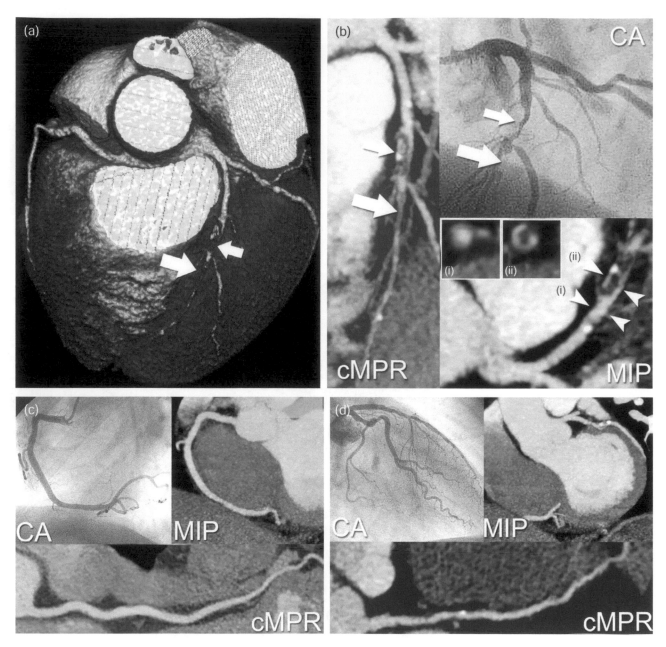

Figure 8 . 1 (a) Volume-rendered image (cranioanterior view) showing an anatomical overview of the proximal parts of the main coronary arteries. A significant lesion of the mid-part (small arrow) and a total occlusion of the distal part (large arrow) of the left anterior descending coronary artery are visualized. (b) Different post-processing techniques (curved multiplanar reconstruction (cMPR) and maximum intensity projection (MIP)) are used to visualiz ethe coronary lesions in more detail (arrows). Cross-sectional images (i) and (ii) at different locations (arrowheads) illustrate a high-grade stenosis of the mid-part of the left anterior descending coronary artery and calcified as well as non-calcified plaque tissue components. Both lesions were confirmed on the invasive coronary angiogram (CA). (c) MIP and cMPR CT images of the right coronary artery rule out the presence of significant lesions. These findings are confir med on the corresponding invasive coronary angiogram. (d) MIP and cMPR CT images of the cir cumflex coronary artery rule out the presence of significant lesions. These findings are confir med on the corresponding invasive coronary angiogram.

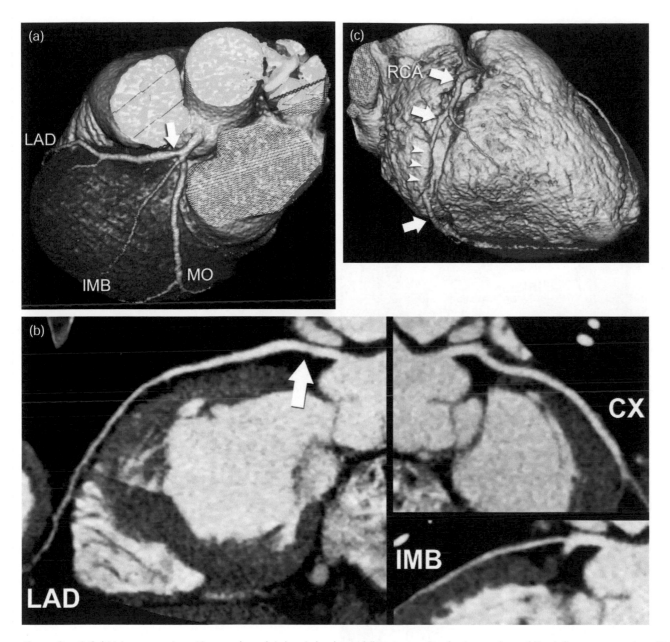

Figure 8 . 1 2 a) Volume-rendered image (craniolateral view) providing an anatomical overview of the left coronary artery. This image suggests a non-significant lesion (arrow) located at the proximal part of the left anterior descending coronary artery (LAD). (b) The presence of a non-significant lesion located at the proximal part of the LAD is also visualized on multiplanar reconstructed images. No significant lesions are visualized throughout the left coronary system. (c) Volume-rendered image (right lateral view) providing an anatomical overview of the right coronary artery (RCA). An incidental finding is the aberrant course of the RCA running within the right atrium (arrowheads).

(continued)

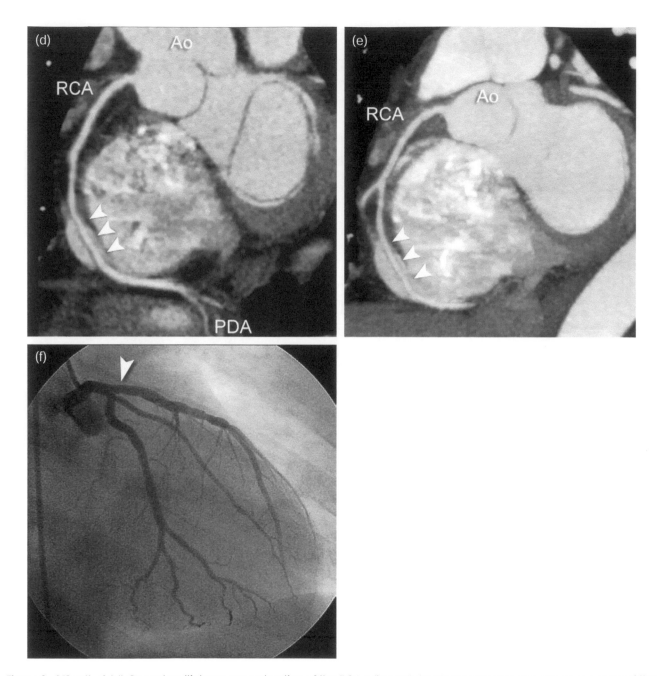

Figure 8 .2 Cont' d (d) Curved multiplanar reconstruction of the RCA ruling out significant stenoses. The aberrant course of the RCA is again visualized (arrowheads). (e) Maximum intensity projection confirming the findings of the other image processing techniques. Arrowheads indicate the aberrant course of the RCA. (f) Invasive angiography image confirming the presence of only a non-significant lesion (arrowhead) within the left coronary artery.   IMB, intermediate coronary branch; MO, marginal obtuse coronary branch; CX, circumflex coronary artery; Ao, aorta: PDA, posterior descending coronary artery.

Table 8.5 Diagnostic performance of 64-slice MSCT to detect significant coronary stenosis (more than 50% o⁼ luminal diameter). Segmental analysis

Author	Excluded patients	Year	Patients n	Excluded segments (%)	Sensitivity (%)	Specificity (%)	PPV (%)	NPV (%)
Leschka et al[36]	0	2005	67	0 (0/1005)	94 (165/176)	97 (805/829)	88 (165/189)	99 (805/816)
Leber et al[37]	4	2005	55	0 (0/732)	76 (57/75)	97 (638/657)	75 (57/76)	97 (638/656)
Raff et al[38]	0	2005	70	12 (130/1065)	86 (79/92)	95 (802/843)	66 (79/120)	98 (802/815)
Mollet et al[39]	1	2005	51	0 (0/725)	99 (93/94)	95 (601/631)	76 (93/123)	100 (601/602)
Ropers et al[40]	3	2006	81	4 (45/1128)	93 (39/42)	97 (1010/1041)	56 (39/70)	100 (1010/1013)
Schuijf et al[41]	1	2006	60	1 (12/854)	85 (62/73)	98 (755/769)	82 (62/76)	99 (755/766)
Ong et al[42]	2	2006	134	10 (143/1474)	82 (177/217)	96 (1067/1114)	83 (177/214)	96 (1067/1107)
Ehara et al[43]	2	2006	69	8 (72/956)	90 (275/304)	94 (545/580)	89 (275/310)	95 (545/574)
Nikolaou et al[44]	4	2006	72	11 (92/1015)	82 (97/118)	95 (762/805)	69 (97/140)	97 (762/783)
Herzog et al[45]	0	2007	55	8 (63/825)	82 (50/61)	97 (743/765)	70 (50/72)	99 (743/754)
Mühlenbruch et al[46]	0	2007	51	5 (39/765)	87 (91/105)	95 (530/560)	75 (91/121)	98 (530/544)
Oncel et al[47]	0	2007	80	0 (0/1200)	96 (155/161)	98 (1023/1039)	91 (155/171)	99 (1023/1029)
Total (weighted)	17		845	5.3 (617/11744)	89 (1340/1508)	96 (9281/9633)	80 (1340/1682)	98 (9281/9449)

PPV, positive predictive value; NPV, negative predictive value.

Table 8 . 6 Diagnostic performance of 64-slice MSCT to detect significant coronary stenosis (more than 50% of luminal diameter). Patient-based analysis

Author	Year	Patients (n)	Sensitivity (%)	Specificity (%)	PPV (%)	NPV (%)
Leschka et al[36]	2005	67	100 (47/47)	100 (20/20)	100 (47/47)	100 (20/20)
Leber et al[37]	2005	45	88 (22/25)	85 (17/20)	88 (22/25)	85 (17/20)
Raff et al[38]	2005	70	95 (38/40)	90 (27/30)	93 (38/41)	93 (27/29)
Mollet et al[39]	2005	51	100 (38/38)	92 (12/13)	97 (38/39)	100 (12/12)
Ropers et al[40]	2006	81	96 (25/26)	91 (50/55)	83 (25/30)	98 (50/51)
Schuijf et al[41]	2006	60	94 (29/31)	97 (28/29)	97 (29/30)	93 (27/29)
Ehara et al[43]	2006	67	98 (59/60)	86 (6/7)	98 (59/60)	86 (6/7)
Nikolaou et al[44]	2006	68	97 (38/39)	79 (23/29)	86 (38/44)	96 (23/24)
Herzog et al[45]	2007	55	100 (19/19)	84 (30/36)	79 (19/25)	100 (30/30)
Mühlenbruch et al[46]	2007	51	98 (44/45)	50 (3/6)	92 (44/48)	75 (3/4)
Oncel et al[47]	2007	80	100 (62/62)	100 (18/18)	100 (62/62)	100 (18/18)
Total (weighted)		695	97 (421/432)	89 (234/263)	93 (421/451)	96 (234/245)

PPV, positive predictive value; NPV, negative predictive value.

stenosis (Figure 8.18). When the coronary arteries show severe and diffuse calcified atherosclerosis, MSCT angiography interpretation is not suitable. It has been proposed that a non-enhanced calcium quantification scan should be performed first to exclude patients with an unfavorably high coronary calcium load, prior to contrast-enhanced CT angiography. In our opinion, motion artifacts related to fast heart rates are currently the most important limitation of 64-slice CT coronary angiography. They result in non-assessable investigations, and thereby reduce the clinical applicability of the technique. Two studies evaluated the diagnostic accuracy of MSCT in relation to the heart rate of the patient. Giesler et al divided 100 patients into four groups and showed that in patients with a heart rate below 60 bpm motion artifacts occurred in only 8% of the coronary arteries, compared with 18% at a heart rate between 61 and 70 bpm, 41% at between 71 and 80 bpm, and 22% at more than 80 bpm. The respective percentages

Table 8 . 7 Diagnostic performance of 64-slice CT coronary angiography (per-vessel analysis)

	Vessels (n)	Sensitivity (%)	Specificity (%)	PPV (%)	NPV (%)
Raff et al[38]	279	91	92	80	97
Schuijf et al[41]	239	87	96	82	96
Ropers et al[40]	321	95	93	64	99

PPV, positive predictive value; NPV, negative predictive value.

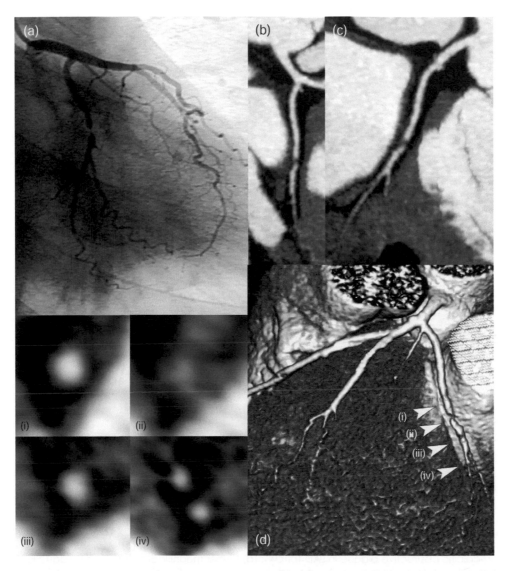

Figure 8 .31 (a) Invasive coronary angiography showing severe lesion of left cir cumflex coronary artery (LCX). (b) and (c) Multiplanar reconstructions showing LCX lesion. (d) Volume-rendered image showing LCX lesion (i–iv with corresponding cross-sections at i–iv).

of non-assessable vessels were 22%, 23%, 50%, and 24%, which resulted in a decreasing overall sensitivity to detect more than 70% coronary diameter narrowing in 67%, 55%, 35%, and 22%, for the respective heart rate groups[17]. In a study by Nieman et al, 78 patients were equally divided into three groups according to the average heart rate during MSCT coronary angiography[18]. In the low-heart rate group (56 ± 4 bpm), intermediate-heart rate group (67 ± 3 bpm), and high-heart rate group (82 ± 9 bpm), the number of assessable segments were 78%, 73%, and 54%, resulting in an overall sensitivity to detect more than 50% luminal stenosis of 82%, 61%, and 32%, respectively. The accuracy of MSCT to classify patients as having no, single, or multivessel disease, without exclusion of non-assessable segments, was 73%, 54%, and 42%, for each respective group[18]. Based on experiences like these, many centers now routinely use anti-chronotropical medication,

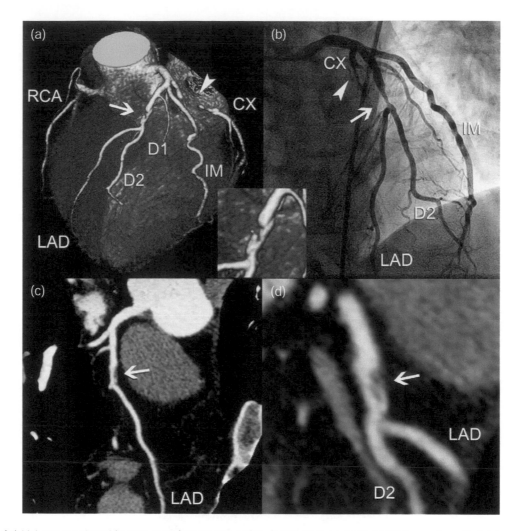

Figure 8 . 1 4(a) Volume-rendered image showing severe lesion (LAD) and occluded LCX (arrowhead). (b) Invasive coronary angiography confirming severe lesion in LAD (arrow) and occluded LCX (arrowhead). (c) Multiplanar intensity projection (MIP) demonstrating non-calcific obstructive plaque in LAD (arrow). (d) Higher magnification of severe plaque in LAD (arrow). RCA, right coronary artery; D1, first diagonal branch; D2, second diagonal branch; CX, circumflex artery; IM, intermediate branch.

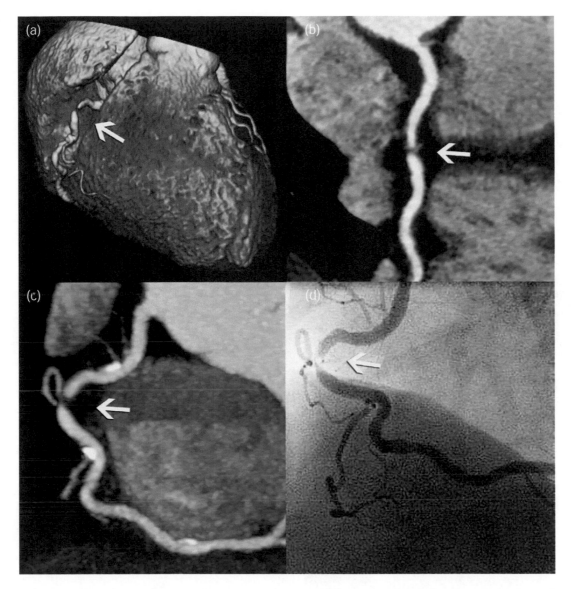

Figure 8 . 1 5a) Volume-rendered image showing severe lesion in right coronary artery (RCA) (arrow). (b) Curved multiplanar reconstruction showing severe lesion in RCA (arrow). (c) Maximum intensity projection demonstrating severe RCA lesion (arrow) with two non-obstructive calcified plaques (bright dots). (d) Corresponding invasive coronary angiography showing severe lesion in RCA (arrow).

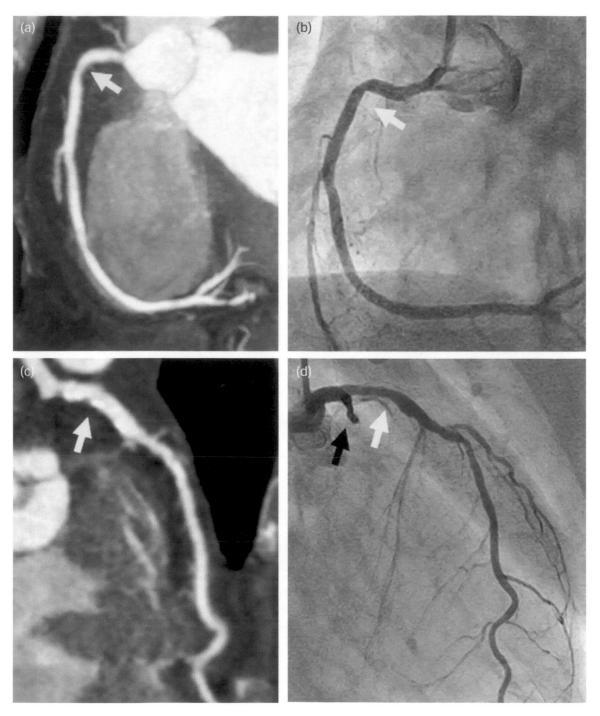

Figure 8 . 1 6 (a) Dual-source CT coronary angiography in a patient with a heart rate of 95 bpm. Mild disease is visualized in the right coronary artery (RCA) (arrow) on CT (a) and invasive coronary angiography (b). Mild disease is visualized in the left anterior descending coronary artery (LAD) on CT (c) and invasive coronary angiography (d)(arrows).

(Continued)

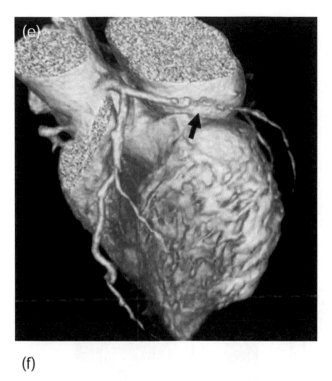

(f)

B_CorCTA 0.75 B30f 275ms - Phase Start: 275ms - IMA: 1 of 1
eartRate(bpm): Min: 92 Max: 101 Avg: 95 (RR: 630 ms)

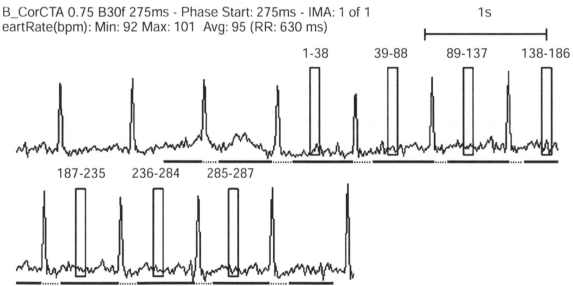

Figure 8 . 6 1Cont' d (e) Volume-rendered image showing total occlusion of the left circumflex artery. (f) Heart rate 95 bpm.

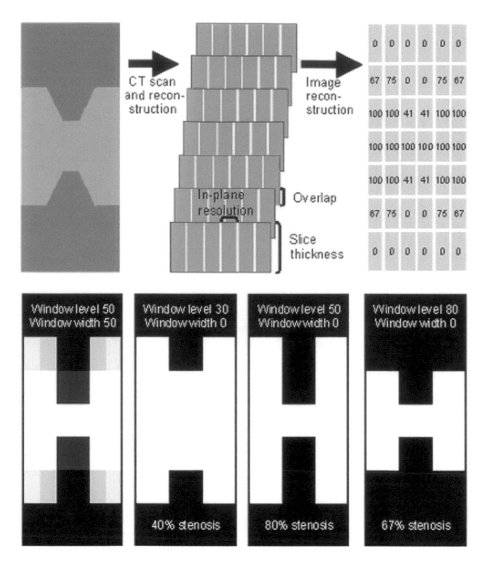

Figure 8.71 Stenosis severity depending on the window level/width settings. Imaging of small stenosed vessels with a limited spatial resolution is dependent on the window level and width settings. The vessel is scanned with a slice width of approximately one-half of the vessel width, for instance a 2.5-mm vessel with a 4× 1-mm detector collimation (1.25-mm effective slice thickness). Reconstruction of overlapping slices results in density measurement that depends on the amount of contrast-enhanced lumen (100) and non-enhanced vessel wall (0). The stenosis severity varies with the varying window level and width settings.

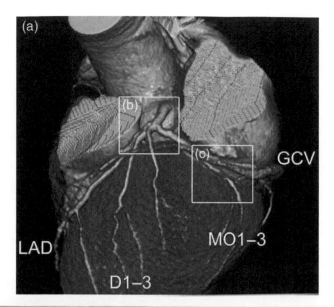

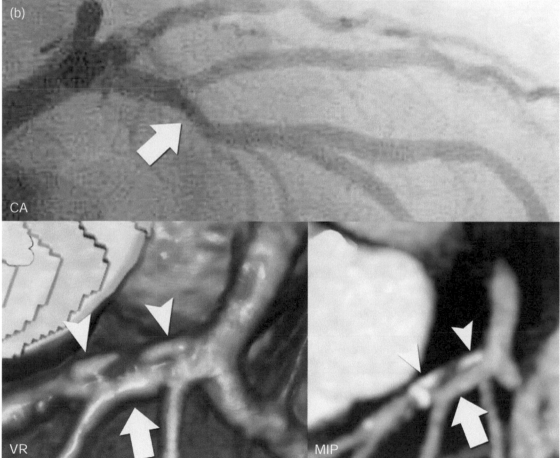

Figure 8 . 18 (a) Volume-rendered image (left lateral view) providing an anatomical overview of the left coronary artery. The boxes indicate the location of more-detailed images shown in Figure 8.18b and 8.18c. (b) Detailed image of the proximal left anterior descending coronary artery (LAD). Severe calcifications (arrowheads) cause blooming artifacts on CT and result in overestimation of the degree of stenosis.

(Continued)

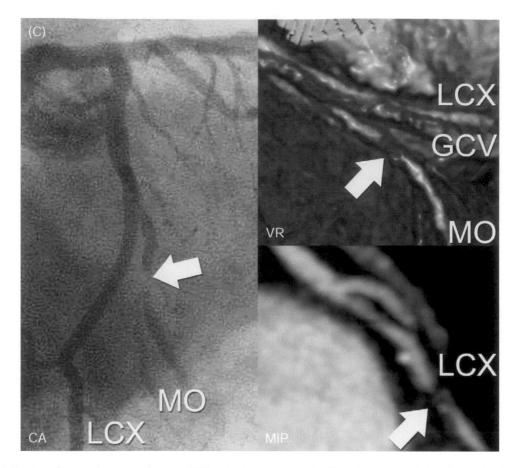

Figure 8 . 1Cont' d The invasive angiography image (CA) only shows a non-significant coronary lesion (arrow), whereas the volume-rendered (VR) and maximum intensity projection (MIP) CT images suggest a (false positive) significant lesion (arrows). (c) Detailed image of the marginal obtuse (MO) branch. This lesion predominantly consists of non-calcified plaque tissue, and the CT images do not suffer from blooming artifacts. The CA shows a significant lesion, which is also represented on the VR and MIP CT images. Note: the great cardiac vein (GCV) obscures the visualization of the proximal part of the MO on the VR image. D1– 3 first, second, and thir d diagonal branch; MO1– 3 first, second, and thir d marginal branch; LCX, left circumflex coronary artery.

T ble 8 . 8 Diagnostic performance of dual-source CT coronary angiography: patient and segment analysis

Author	Year	Patients (n)	Segments excluded (n)	Sensitivity (%)	Specificity (%)	PPV (%)	NPV (%)
Patient-based analysis							
Weustink et al[52]	2007	100	0	99 (76/77)	87 (20/23)	96 (76/79)	95 (20/21)
Leber et al[53]	2007	88	2	95 (20/21)	90 (60/67)	74 (20/27)	99 (60/61)
Segment-based analysis							
Weustink et al[52]	2007	1489	0	95 (208/220)	95 (1200/1269)	75 (208/277)	99 (1200/1212)
Leber et al[53]	2007	1232	0	90 (38/42)	98 (1165/1174)	81 (38/47)	99 (1165/1169)

PPV, positive predictive value; NPV, negative predictive value.

T ble 8 . 9 Factors influencing the image interpretability

Fixed scanner criteria

Temporal resolution
Spatial resolution
Contrast-to-noise

Fixed patient criteria

Arrhythmia
Patient size
Coronary size
Coronary calcification
Ability to hold breath
Metal objects: stents, pacemaker wires, etc.

Modifiable criteria

Contrast-enhancement protocol
Heart rate
Scan protocol: collimation, tube output
ECG gating
Patient population
Patient anxiety

Investigator related criteria

Experience
Confidence

T ble 8 . 1 0 Remaining CT problems/limitations

Fast heart rate (>70 bpm) (dual-source CT is much less problematic)

Persistent irregular heart rhythm (atrial fibrillation)

Small coronary arteries

Severely calcified coronary atherosclerosis

Coronary stents (small sized <2.5 mm)

Metal objects: prosthetic valves, pacemaker wires, etc. causing artifacts

High body mass index (>35 BMI)

Respiratory impairment and related motion artifacts

Renal dysfunction and contrast medium intolerance

such as beta-blockers, particularly in patients with higher heart rates, to reduce the occurrence of motion artifacts, and improve the diagnostic accuracy of MSCT coronary angiography.

CONCLUSION

CT coronary angiography is considered to be a significant breakthrough diagnostic modality to non-invasively assess the coronary lumen. It is expected that further technical improvements will soon be implemented to make this technique a reliable clinical diagnostic tool in a broad spectrum of patients. Remaining problems to be solved are further reduction of cardiac motion artifacts, despite the recent introduction of the 64-slice dual-source CT scan; the radiation exposure should be further reduced; ways should be found to handle obscuring calcium image artifacts; and, eventually, it should also be possible for patients with an irregular heart rhythm to be imaged. Many single and multicenter studies need to be performed in a wide spectrum of patients with different prevalences of coronary artery disease to convincingly demonstrate safety and reliability of non-invasive CT coronary angiography in clinical practice.

REFERENCES

1. Moshage WE, Achenbach S, Seese B, Bachmann K, Kirchgeorg M. Coronary artery stenoses: three-dimensional imaging with electrocardiographically triggered, contrast agent-enhanced, electron-beam CT. Radiology 1995; 196: 707–14.
2. Achenbach S, Moshage W, Ropers D et al. Value of electron-beam computed tomography for the noninvasive detection of high-grade coronary-artery stenoses and occlusions. N Engl J Med 1998; 339: 1964–71.
3. Rensing BJ, Bongaerts A, van Geuns RJ et al. Intravenous coronary angiography by electron beam computed tomography: a clinical evaluation. Circulation 1998; 98: 2509–12.
4. Reddy G, Chernoff DM, Adams JR et al. Coronary artery stenoses: assessment with contrast-enhanced electron-beam CT and axial reconstructions. Radiology 1998; 208: 167–72.
5. Schmermund A, Rensing BJ, Sheedy PF et al. Intravenous electron-beam computed tomographic coronary angiography for segmental analysis of coronary artery stenoses. J Am Coll Cardiol 1998; 31: 1547–54.
6. Nakanishi T, Ito K, Imazu M et al. Evaluation of coronary artery stenoses using electron-beam CT and multiplanar reformation. J Comput Assist Tomogr 1997; 21: 121–27.
7. Budoff MJ, Oudiz RJ, Zalace CP et al. Intravenous three-dimensional coronary angiography using contrast-enhanced electron beam computed tomography. Am J Cardiol 1999; 83: 840–45.

8. Moshage W, Ropers D, Daniel WG, Achenbach S. Noninvasive imaging of coronary arteries with electron beam tomography (EBCT). Z Kardiol 2000; 89 (Suppl 1): 15–20. [in German]

9. Achenbach S, Ropers D, Regenfus M et al. Contrast enhanced electron beam computed tomography to analyse the coronary arteries in patients after acute myocardial infarction. Heart 2000; 84: 489–93.

10. Lu B, Zhuang N, Mao SS et al. Image quality of three-dimensional electron beam coronary angiography. J Comput Assist Tomogr 2002; 26: 202–9.

11. Nieman K, Oudkerk M, Rensing BJ et al. Coronary angiography with multi-slice computed tomography. Lancet 2001; 357: 599–603.

12. Achenbach S, Giesler T, Ropers D et al. Detection of coronary artery stenoses by contrast-enhanced, retrospectively electrocardiographically-gated, multislice spiral computed tomography. Circulation 2001; 103: 2535–38.

13. Knez A, Becker CR, Leber A et al. Usefulness of multislice spiral computed tomography angiography for determination of coronary artery stenoses. Am J Cardiol 2001; 88: 1191–94.

14. Vogl TJ, Abolmaali ND, Diebold T et al. Techniques for the detection of coronary atherosclerosis: multi-detector row CT coronary angiography. Radiology 2002; 223: 212–20.

15. Nieman K, Rensing BJ, van Geuns RJM et al. Usefulness of multislice computed tomography for detecting obstructive coronary artery disease. Am J Cardiol 2002; 89: 913–18.

16. Kopp AF, Schröder S, Küttner A et al. Non-invasive coronary angiography with high resolution multidetector-row computed tomography: results in 102 patients. Eur Heart J 2002; 23: 1714–25.

17. Giesler T, Baum U, Ropers D et al. Noninvasive visualization of coronary arteries using contrast-enhanced multidetector CT: influence of heart rate on image quality and stenosis detection. AJR Am J Roentgenol 2002; 179: 911–16.

18. Nieman K, Rensing BJ, van Geuns RJ et al. Non-invasive coronary angiography with multislice spiral computed tomography: impact of heart rate. Heart 2002; 88: 470–74.

19. Kuettner A, Kopp AF, Schroeder S et al. Diagnostic accuracy of multidetector computed tomography coronary angiography in patients with angiographically proven coronary artery disease. J Am Coll Cardiol 2004; 43: 831–9.

20. Maruyama T, Yoshizumi T, Tamura R et al. Comparison of visibility and diagnostic capability of noninvasive coronary angiography by eight-slice multidetector-row computed tomography versus conventional coronary angiography. Am J Cardiol 2004; 93: 537–42.

21. de Feyter PJ, Weustink A, Alberghina F et al. Computed tomography of the coronary arteries. SA Heart 2007; 4: 12–18.

22. Nieman K, Cademartiri F, Lemos PA et al. Reliable noninvasive coronary angiography with fast submillimeter multislice spiral computed tomography. Circulation 2002; 106: 2051–54.

23. Mollet, NR, Cademartiri F, Nieman K et al. Multislice spiral CT coronary angiography in patients with stable angina pectoris. J Am Coll Cardiol 2004; 43: 2265–70.

24. Martuscelli E, Romagnoli A, D'Eliseo A et al. Accuracy of thin-slice computed tomography in the detection of coronary stenoses. Euro Heart J 2004; 25: 1043–48.

25. Kuettner A, Trabold T, Schroeder S et al. Non-invasive detection of coronary lesions using 16-slice MDCT technology: initial clinical results. J Am Coll Cardiol 2004; 44: 1230–7.

26. Leta R, Carreras F, Alomar X et al. Non-invasive coronary angiography with 16 multidetector-row spiral computed tomography: a comparative study with invasive coronary angiography. Rev Esp Cardiol 2004; 57: 217–24. [in Spanish]

27. Hoffmann U, Moselewski F, Cury R et al. Predictive value of 16-slice multidetector spiral computed tomography to detect signifi-cant obstructive coronary artery disease in patients at high risk for coronary artery disease. Patient-versus segment-based analysis. Circulation 2004; 110: 2638–43.

28. Mollet NR, Cademartiri F, Krestin G et al. Improved diagnostic accuracy with 16-row multi-slice computed tomography coronary angiography. J Am Coll Cardiol 2005; 45: 128–32.

29. Kuettner A, Beck T, Drosch T et al. Diagnostic accuracy of noninvasive coronary imaging using 16-detector slice spiral computed tomography with 188 ms temporal resolution. J Am Coll Cardiol 2005; 45: 123–7.

30. Cademartiri F, Runza G, Marano R et al. Diagnostic accuracy of 16-row multislice CT angiography in the evaluation of coronary segments. Radiol Med (Torino) 2005; 109: 91–7.

31. Schuijf JD, Bax JJ, Salm LP et al. Noninvasive coronary imaging and assessment of left ventricular function using 16-slice computed tomography. Am J Cardiol 2005; 95: 571–4.

32. Kefer J, Coche E, Legros G et al. Head-to-head comparison of three-dimensional navigator-gated magnetic resonance imaging and 16-slice computed tomography to detect coronary artery stenosis in patients. J Am Coll Cardiol 2005; 46: 92–100.

33. Hoffmann MH, Shi H, Schmitz BL et al. Noninvasive coronary angiography with multislice computed tomography. JAMA 2005; 293: 2471–8.

34. Kuettner A, Beck T, Drosch T et al. Image quality and diagnostic accuracy of non-invasive coronary imaging with 16 detector slice spiral computed tomography with 188 ms temporal resolution. Heart 2005; 91: 938–41.

35. Achenbach S, Ropers D, Pohle FK et al. Detection of coronary artery stenoses using multi-detector CT with 16 x 0.75 collimation and 375 ms rotation. Eur Heart J 2005; 26: 1978–86.

36. Leschka S, Alkadhi H, Plass A et al. Accuracy of MSCT coronary angiography with 64-slice technology: first experience. Eur Heart J 2005; 26: 1482–7.

37. Leber AW, Knez A, von Ziegler F et al. Quantification of obstructive and nonobstructive coronary lesions by 64-slice computed tomography: a comparative study with quantitative coronary angiography and intravascular ultrasound. J Am Coll Cardiol 2005; 46: 147–54.

38. Raff GL, Gallagher MJ, O'Neill WW et al. Diagnostic accuracy of noninvasive coronary angiography using 64-slice spiral computed tomography. J Am Coll Cardiol 2005; 46: 552–7.

39. Mollet NR, Cademartiri F, van Mieghem CA et al. High-resolution spiral computed tomography coronary angiography in patients referred for diagnostic conventional coronary angiography. Circulation 2005; 112: 2318–23.

40. Ropers D, Rixe J, Anders K et al. Usefulness of multidetector row spiral computed tomography with 64- x 0.6-mm collimation and 330-ms rotation for the noninvasive detection of significant coronary artery stenoses. Am J Cardiol 2006; 97: 343–8.

41. Schuijf JD, Mollet NR, Cademartiri F, et al. Do risk factors influence the diagnostic accuracy of noninvasive coronary angiography with multislice computed tomography? J Nucl Cardiol 2006; 13: 635–41.

42. Ong TK, Chin SP, Liew CK et al. Accuracy of 64-row multidetector computed tomography in detecting coronary artery disease in 134 symptomatic patients: influence of calcification. Am Heart J 2006; 151: 1323.e1–6.

43. Ehara M, Surmely JF, Kawai M et al. Diagnostic accuracy of 64-slice computed tomography for detecting angiographically significant coronary artery stenosis in an unselected consecutive patient population. Circulation J 2006; 70: 564–71.

44. Nikolaou K, Flohr T, Knez A et al. Advances in cardiac CT imaging: 64-slice scanner. Int J Cardiovasc Imaging 2004; 20: 535–40.

45. Herzog C, Zwerner P, Doll J et al. Significant coronary artery stenosis: comparison on per-patient and per-vessel or per-segment basis at 64-section CT angiography. Radiology 2007; 244: 112–20.

46. Mühlenbruch G, Seyfarth T, Pregalathan N, Mahnken A. Diagnostic value of 64-slice multi-detector row cardiac CTA in symptomatic patients. Eur Radiol 2007; 17: 603–9.

47. Oncel D, Oncel G, Tastan A, Tamci B. Detection of significant coronary artery stenosis with 64-section MDCT angiography. Eur Heart J 2007; 62: 394–405.

48. Flohr T, McCollough C, Bruder et al. First performance evaluation of a dual-source CT (DSCT) system. Eur Radiol 2006; 16: 256–68.

49. Scheffel H, Alkadhi H, Plass A et al. Accuracy of dual-source CT coronary angiography: first experience in a high pre-test probability population without heart rate control. Eur Radiol 2006; 16: 2739–47.

50. Achenbach S, Ropers D, Kuettner A et al. Contrast-enhanced coronary artery visualization by dual-source computed tomography – initial experience. Eur J Radiol 2006; 57: 331–35.

51. Johnson T, Nikolaou K, Wintersperger B et al. Dual-source CT cardiac imaging: initial experience. Eur Radiol 2006; 16: 1409–15.

52. Weustink A, Meijboom W, Mollet N et al. Reliable high-speed coronary computed tomography in symptomatic patients. J Am Coll Cardiol 2007; 50: 786–94.

53. Leber A, Johnson T, Becker A et al. Diagnostic accuracy of dual-source multi-slice CT-coronary angiography in patients with an intermediate pretest likelihood for coronary artery disease. Eur Heart J 2007; 28: 2354–60.

CHAPTER 9

Coronary plaque imaging

Direct non-invasive imaging of coronary calcific and non-calcific atherosclerotic plaques may significantly improve risk stratification of adverse coronary events and may prove useful in the better understanding of the development and progression of coronary atherosclerosis.

COMPOSITION OF CORONARY PLAQUES ASSESSED BY MSCT

Spiral CT coronary angiography is able to identify advanced coronary plaques. These plaques can be either non-obstructive due to arterial wall compensatory remodeling or may impact on the coronary lumen (Figure 9.1). The CT scanner permits assessment of the extent, severity, and localization of coronary plaques[1–10]. Furthermore, the CT scanner can distinguish between the various components of advanced plaques which have different X-ray density values. Lipid and fibrous tissue are low-density structures and calcium is a high-density structure, whereas a very low-density obstruction in the setting of an acute coronary syndrome may represent a thrombotic occlusion (Figures 9.2–9.5). In a comparative study of the histology and in vivo MSCT imaging of large carotid plaques in patients who underwent carotid endarterectomy, CT scanning was able to distinguish between lipid tissue that had a mean attenuation value of 39 ± 12 HU and fibrous tissue with a mean value of 90 ± 24 HU[10]. Schroeder et al were the first to demonstrate that the distinction between lipid and fibrous plaques was also possible in smaller coronary plaques[2]. These results were confirmed by the study of

Leber et al who, in an elegant study, demonstrated that the density measurements between lipid and fibrous plaques were different[11] (Table 9.1). Both studies correlated the coronary lesion echogenicity of intravascular ultrasound (IVUS) and CT density measurement, thereby taking IVUS as the reference standard to distinguish between lipid and fibrous tissue. It is of note that IVUS does not equate with histology; however, it is the best possible assumption in the setting of in vivo coronary plaque imaging. Furthermore, it should be appreciated that the density values of lipid and fibrous plaques overlap significantly, which makes the identification of an individual plaque unreliable.

DETECTION OF CORONARY PLAQUES BY MSCT

The diagnostic value of MSCT in detecting coronary plaques has been reported for non-calcific and calcific plaques[7,11]. The sensitivity was dependent on the plaque composition with lower sensitivity

Table 9.1 Plaque composition with contrast-enhanced CT coronary plaque imaging

IVUS	MSCT study	
	Schroeder et al (n = 17) (HU ± SD)	Leber et al (n = 37) (HU ± SD)
Hypoechoic	14 ± 26	49 ± 22
Hyperechoic	91 ± 21	91 ± 22
Calcified	419 ± 194	391 ± 156

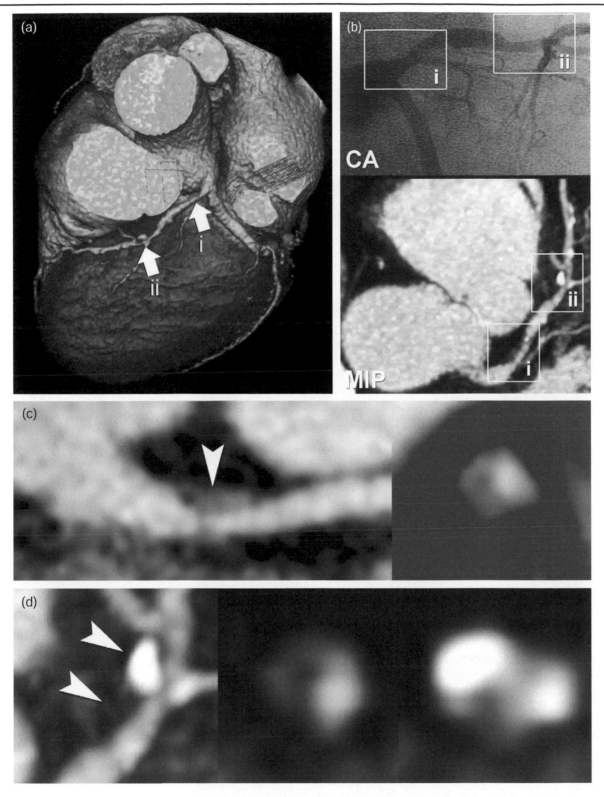

Figure 9 . 1(a) Volume-rendered image showing significant obstructive lesions in the proximal and mid-part of the left anterior descending coronary artery (arrows i and ii). (b) Invasive diagnostic angiogram (CA) and corresponding maximum intensity projection MSCT image (MIP). The lesions are highlighted in boxes (i) and (ii). MSCT coronary angiography provides not only information regarding the coronary lumen but also about coronary plaques: non-calcific plaque (i) and mixed (calcific/non-calcific) plaque (ii). (c) Multiplanar reconstructed image (left panel) of the proximal coronary lesion showing a non-calcified plaque. The arrowhead indicates the location of the cross-sectional image of the plaque (right panel), again showing the contrast-enhanced lumen and adjacent non-calcified plaque tissue. (d) Multiplanar reconstructed image (left panel) of the distal coronary lesion showing a mixed plaque. The arrowheads indicate cross-sectional images of the plaque at the level of the non-calcified plaque tissue (middle panel) and the calcified plaque tissue (right panel).

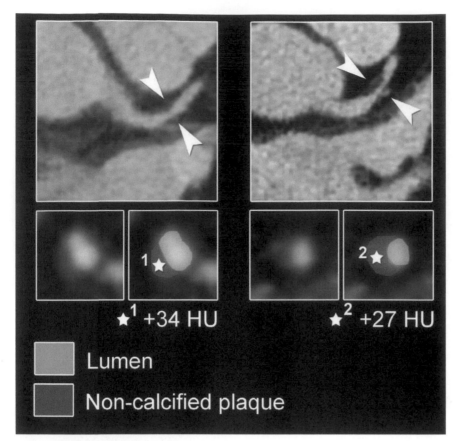

★¹ +34 HU   ★² +27 HU

Lumen

Non-calcified plaque

Figure 9 2 Non-significant (left panels) and significant obstructive (right panels) non-calcified plaques. The arrowheads indicate the location of cross-sectional images of the plaques (lower panels). The HU values measured within the plaques are in the range of lipid plaque tissue.

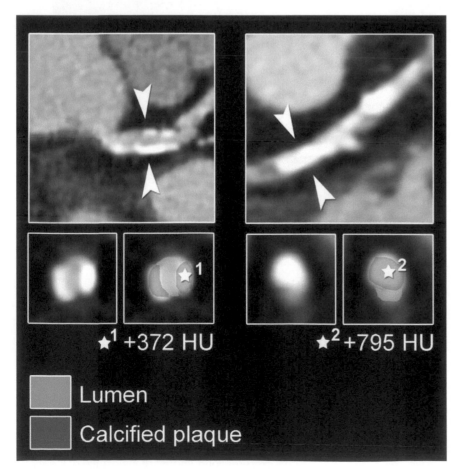

★¹ +372 HU   ★² +795 HU

Lumen

Calcified plaque

Figure 9 3 Non-significant (left panels) and significant obstructive (right panels) calcified plaques. The arrowheads indicate the location of cross-sectional images of the plaques (lower panels). The HU values measured within the plaques are in the range of calcified plaque tissue.

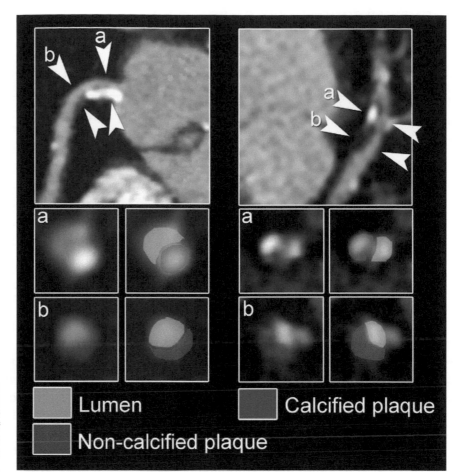

Figure 9 . 4 Non-significant (left panels) and significant obstructive (right panels) mixed plaques. The arrowheads indicate the location of cross-sectional images of the plaques (lower panels), showing the presence of both non-calcified (a) and calcified (b) plaque tissue components.

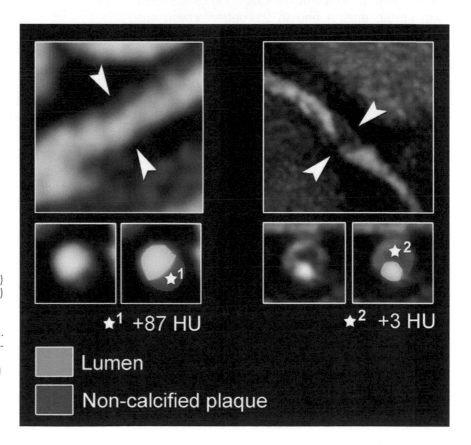

Figure 9 . 5 Non-significant (left panels) and significant obstructive (right panels) non-calcified plaques. The arrowheads indicate the location of cross-sectional images of the plaques (lower panels). The HU values measured within the non-significant lesion are in the range of fibrous plaque tissue. However , the HU values measured within the significant lesion in this patient with unstable angina suggest the presence of a thrombotic plaque.

T ble 9 . 2 Diagnostic value of MSCT to detect coronary plaques

IVUS plaque	Achenbach et al[7] (n = 22) sensitivity	IVU S	Leber et al[11] (n = 37) sensitivity
Mixed	78% (35/45)	Hypoechoic	78% (62/80)
Non-calcific	53% (8/15)	Hyperechoic	78% (87/112)
Calcified	92% (33/36)	Calcified	95% (150/158)
Any plaque	82% (41/50)	Any plaque	86% (299/350)
Exclusion plaque (specificity)	88% (29/33)		92% (484/525)

for non-calcified plaques and very high sensitivity for calcified plaques (Table 9.2). The specificity ranged from 88 to 92%. Plaques that were not detected were smaller and located in smaller vessels (Table 9.3).

Nikolaou et al reported the prevalence of coronary calcific and non-calcific plaques in 179 patients. Coronary calcific lesions were detected in 73% of the patients and non-calcific plaques were seen in 30%.[3]

Leber et al reported the distribution of calcific, mixed, and non-calcific plaques in 19 patients with stable angina and in 21 patients who survived an acute myocardial infarction (Table 9.4)[4]. The acute myocardial infarction patients had fewer calcific and more non-calcific lesions than the stable angina patients.

Mollet et al investigated 78 patients with MSCT to assess the MSCT–determined coronary plaque burden, which was defined as plaque extent, distribution, severity, and type of plaque. The results and an example of a patient with a high MSCT coronary plaque burden are shown in Figures 9.6–9.10[9].

REMODELING OF CORONARY PLAQUES

Coronary artery wall expansive remodeling occurs in the earlier phases of the development of coronary atherosclerosis, and enlargement of the whole vessel tends to preserve the normal size of the coronary lumen. Achenbach et al demonstrated that MSCT can identify coronary plaques with positive (expansive) vessel wall remodeling and negative (shrinkage) remodeling (Figure 9.11)[8].

MSCT IDENTIFICATION OF VULNERABLE PLAQUES

It has been shown that plaque composition, morphology, and expansive coronary wall remodeling may be more important predictors of plaque vulnerability and clinical behavior than the degree of coronary stenosis[12–18].

It has been suggested that non-calcified plaques are associated with plaque rupture. Hausleiter et al investigated 161 patients with an intermediate

Table 9.3 MSCT: characteristics of detected and non-detected plaques

	Non-detected plaques	Detected plaques
Plaque thickness (mm)	0.9 ± 0.3	1.5 ± 0.3
External diameter (mm)	3.6 ± 1.1	4.5 ± 1.2
Plaque volume (mm³)	47 ± 11	76 ± 10
Plaque area (mm²)	8 ± 3	11 ± 4

T ble 9 . 4 Prevalence of MSCT coronary plaque types[4]

	Stable angina (n = 19)	Acute myocardial infarction (n = 21)
Plaques/patient (n)	12 ± 6	10 ± 5
Calcific plaque (%)	79	56
Mixed plaque (%)	13	18
Non-calcific plaque (%)	7	24

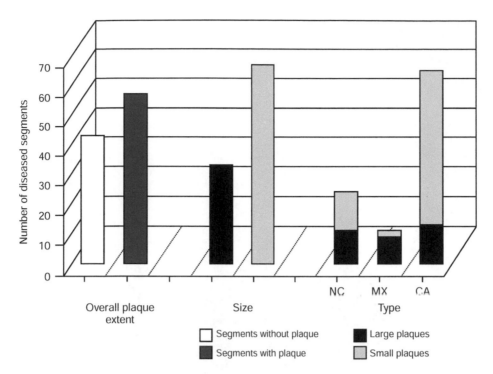

Figure 9 . 6 Results of plaque extent (number of diseased segments), size (large or small), type (non-calcified (NC), mixed (MX), and calcified (CA)), and number of plaques per patient assessed with MSCT coronary angiography in 78 patients with stable angina pectoris yielding a total of 855 segments. Overall, there were 6.2 ± 2.9 plaques per patient.

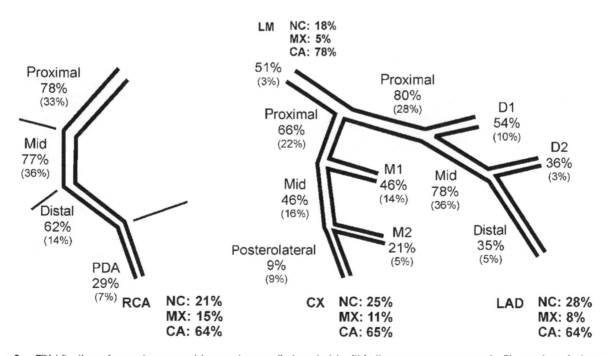

Figure 9 . 7 Distribution of any plaque and large plaques (in brackets) within the coronary segments. Plaque type is shown per vessel. Plaques are predominantly located in the proximal and mid-segments of the main coronary vessels. NC, non-calcified plaque; MX, mixed plaque; CA, calcified plaque; D1, first diagonal branch; D2, second diagonal branch; M1, first marginal branch; M2, second marginal branch; LM, left main coronary artery; LAD, left anterior descending coronary artery; CX, circumflex coronary artery; PDA, posterior descending artery.

129

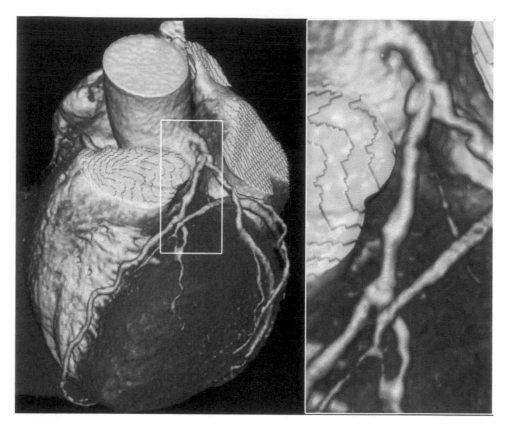

Figure 9 . 8 Volume-rendered image of a patient with a high plaque burden in the left anterior descending artery assessed with MSCT, coronary angiography. This image processing technique only provides information regarding the coronary lumen and coronary calcifications, whereas non-calcified plaque tissue components are not visualized.

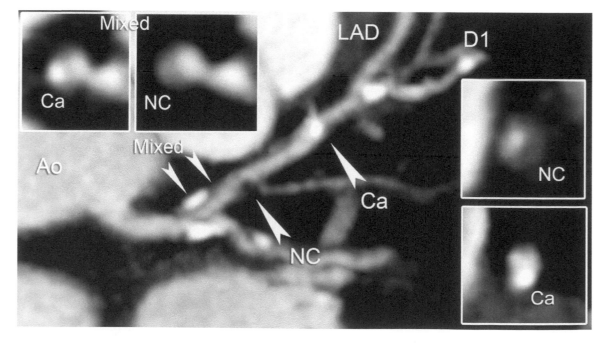

Figure 9 . 9 Maximum intensity projection and cross-sectional multiplanar reconstructed (inserts) MSCT images of the left main and proximal part of the left anterior descending coronary artery (LAD) of the same patient. The LAD is severely diseased and different types of plaques are visualized including mixed calcified (Ca), and non-calcified (NC) plaques. Ao, aorta; D1, first diagonal branch. Arrowheads denote site of cross-sectional images.

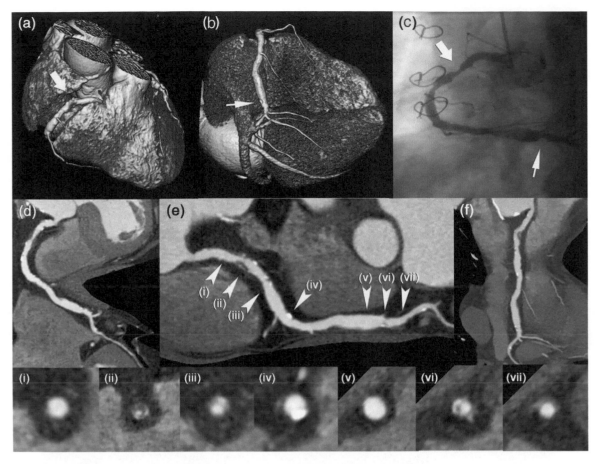

Figure 9.10 (a) and (b) Volume-rendered images showing right coronary artery (RCA) stenosis (arrows). (c) Stenosis confirmed by invasive coronary angiography. (d) and (e) Maximum intensity projections showing multiple plaques (i–vii) and corresponding cross-sections. (f) Curved multiplanar reconstruction showing proximal non-calcified plaque.

risk for coronary artery disease and non-calcified plaques were detected in 30% (48/161) of patients, but in only 6.2% (10/161) of the patients was a non-calcified plaque present as the only manifestation of coronary artery disease[19]. Hoffmann et al compared the CT characteristics of culprit lesions in patients with an acute coronary syndrome with culprit lesions in patients with stable angina[20]. They showed that unstable plaques were larger (17.5 ± 6 versus 13.5 ± 10 mm^2) and had a higher remodeling index (1.4 versus 1.2) than stable plaques. Motoyama et al compared unstable and stable lesions in 38 patients with acute coronary syndrome and 33 patients with stable angina pectoris[21]. They found a higher frequency of positive remodeling (87% versus 12%; $p<0.002$), low

density plaques (79% versus 9%; $p<0.001$) and spotty calcification (63% versus 21%; $p<0.001$) in unstable plaques compared with stable plaques.

Non-invasive MSCT plaque imaging can play a role in the identification of non-obstructive high-risk coronary plaques. This can be illustrated in the case history of a patient who was admitted with transient acute chest pain and ECG changes (Figure 9.12). The MSCT coronary angiogram showed a non-significant mid-left anterior descending coronary artery lesion as did the diagnostic invasive coronary angiogram. Non-invasive MSCT clearly showed a non-calcific plaque with vessel remodeling, which was confirmed with intracoronary ultrasound. This patient was treated with aspirin and aggressive statin therapy.

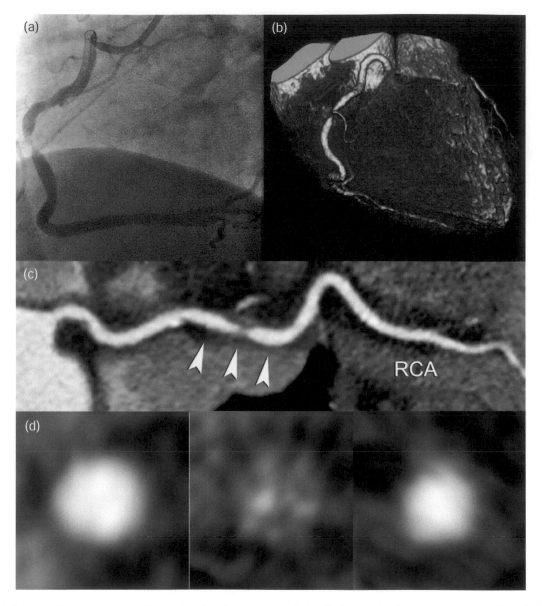

Figure 9 . 1 1a) Invasive coronary angiography showing a severe lesion in the mid-right coronary artery (RCA). (b) Volume-rendered image showing a severe RCA lesion. (c) Curved multiplanar reconstruction showing severe RCA lesion which shows positive remodeling (arrows). (d) Corresponding cross-sections.

LIMITATIONS OF MSCT PLAQUE IMAGING

The resolution of the current MSCT scanners fails to detect the very early stages of coronary atherosclerosis development. More advanced coronary plaques can be detected, but MSCT substantially underestimates the plaque volume as compared with intracoronary ultrasound[7].

The volume of calcific plaques can be overestimated due to partial voluming, and there often appears to be a dark circumferential artifact around the calcium which obscures identification of the adjacent tissue and, thus, may underestimate the presence of mixed plaques, and does not allow plaques with deep or superficial layers of calcium to be distinguished as can be seen by intracoronary ultrasound.

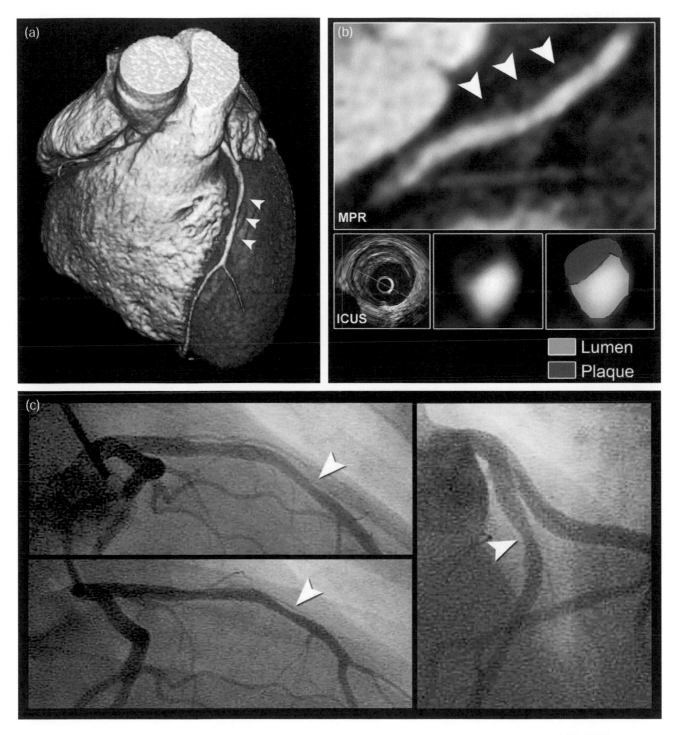

Figure 9 . 1 2a) Volume-rendered image showing only mild narrowing of the left anterior descending coronary artery (arrowheads), whereas the other coronary arteries were completely nor mal (not shown). (b) Multiplanar reconstructed image (MPR) of the proximal left anterior descending coronary artery. The arrowheads indicate the presence of a non-calcified plaque with positive vessel remodeling, which was confir med with intracoronary ultrasound (ICUS). Cross-sectional MSCT images also show the presence of a non-calcified plaque without encroachment of the lumen (lower panels). (c) Invasive coronary angiogram confirming the presence of a non-significant lesion in the proximal part of the left anterior descending coronary artery in different projections.

CONCLUSION

Non-invasive CT assessment of the coronary plaque burden appears to be a useful addition to the diagnostic armamentarium in cardiological practice (Table 9.5). It will increase our understanding of the development and progression of coronary atherosclerosis, and it may carry additional prognostic information. In patients with moderate - to high - quality MSCT images (poor-quality images were excluded) comparative studies with IVUS demonstrated that calcified plaques can be detected with a high sensitivity (>90%), but non-calcified plaque detection is less reliable with sensitivities ranging from 53 to 78% (Figure 9.13). The specificity ranged between 88 and 92%. Smaller non-calcific plaques were not reliably detected and the volume and area of plaques were significantly underestimated.

Non-invasive CT assessment of coronary plaques of the clinically relevant parts of the entire coronary tree (as opposed to intracoronary diagnostic tools) may be useful in the identification of a vulnerable plaque (Table 9.6). Non-invasive detection may further guide invasive diagnostic tools. Early non-invasive detection of coronary plaques may eventually improve management of both individuals with subclinically coronary artery disease and asymptomatic patients with known coronary artery disease.

Table 9 . 5 CT coronary plaque imaging

Non-contrast enhanced imaging (EBCT-MSCT): coronary calcium quantification
Predict presence of significant coronary obstruction
Risk stratification
Contrast enhanced imaging (MSCT): coronary lumen and plaque imaging
Number of plaques (extent)
Plaque distribution (RCA, left main, LAD, LCX)
Plaque type:
calcific
non-calcific
mixed
thrombotic in ACS
Lumen obstruction
non-obstructive
$\geq$ 50%
total occlusion
Vessel wall remodeling
May have improved risk stratification?

EBCT, electron beam CT; MSCT, multislice CT; RCA, right coronary artery; LAD, left anterior descending artery; LCX, left circumflex artery; ACS, acute coronary syndrome.

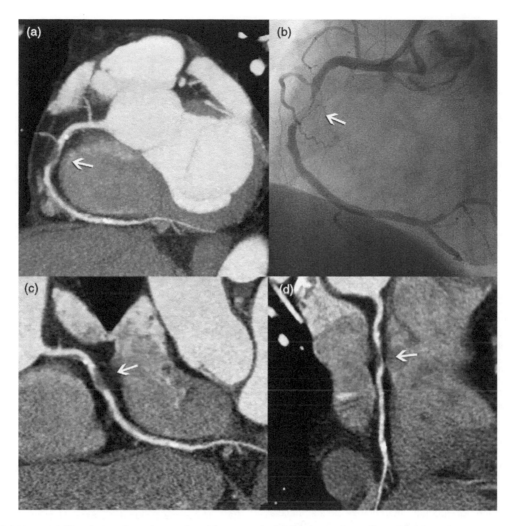

Figure 9 . 1 ₃a) Non-calcific obstructive plaque in mid-segment of RCA (arrow) confirmed by invasive coronary angiography (b) and also shown in curved multiplanar reconstructions (c) and (d).

T ble 9 . 6 Vulnerable plaque features: non-invasive and invasive diagnosis

	MSCT	Invasive tools
Plaque components		
lipid	Low density	Angioscopy/IVUS
fibrous	Moderate density	IVUS
calcific	High density	IVUS
Severe narrowing	+	Coronary angiography
Remodeling	±	IVUS
Fibrous cap	−	OCT
Inflammation	−	Thermography
Deformability	−	Palpography

IVUS, intravascular ultrasound; OCT, optical coherence tomography.

REFERENCES

1. Becker CR, Knez A, Ohnesorge B, Schoepf UJ, Reiser MF. Imaging of noncalcified coronary plaques using helical CT with retrospective ECG gating. AJR Am J Roentgenol 2000; 175: 423–4.

2. Schroeder S, Kopp AF, Baumbach A et al. Noninvasive detection and evaluation of atherosclerotic coronary plaques with multislice computed tomography. J Am Coll Cardiol 2001; 37: 1430–5.

3. Nikolaou K, Sagmeister S, Knez A et al. Multidetector-row computed tomography of the coronary arteries: predictive value and quantitative assessment of non-calcified vessel-wall changes. Eur Radiol 2003; 13: 2505–12.

4. Leber AW, Knez A, White CW et al. Composition of coronary atherosclerotic plaques in patients with acute myocardial infarction and stable angina pectoris determined by ontrast-enhanced multislice computed tomography. Am J Cardiol 2003; 91: 714–18.

5. Caussin C, Ohanessian A, Lancelin B et al. Coronary plaque burden detected by multislice computed tomography after acute myocardial infarction with near-normal coronary arteries by angiography. Am J Cardiol 2003; 92: 849–52.

6. Becker CR, Nikolaou K, Muders M, et al. Ex vivo coronary atherosclerotic plaque characterization with multi-detector-row CT. Eur Radiol 2003; 13: 2094–8.

7. Achenbach S, Moselewski F, Ropers D et al. Detection of calcified and noncalcified coronary atherosclerotic plaque by contrast-enhanced, submillimeter multidetector spiral computed tomography: a segment-based comparison with intravascular ultrasound. Circulation 2004; 109: 14–17.

8. Achenbach S, Ropers D, Hoffmann U et al. Assessment of coronary remodeling in stenotic and nonstenotic coronary atherosclerotic lesions by multidetector spiral computed tomography. J Am Coll Cardiol 2004; 43: 842–7.

9. Mollet NRA, Cademarkiri F, Nieman K et al. Non-invasive assessment of coronary plaque burden using multislice computed tomography. Am J Cardiol 2005; 95: 1165–9.

10. Estes JM, Quist WC, Lo Gerfo FW, Costello P. Noninvasive characterization of plaque morphology using helical computed tomography. J Cardiovasc Surg (Torino) 1998; 39: 527–34.

11. Leber AW, Knez A, Becker A et al. Accuracy of multidetector spiral computed tomography in identifying and differentiating the composition of coronary atherosclerotic plaques; A comparative study with intracoronary ultrasound. J Am Coll Cardiol 2004; 43: 1241–7.

12. Varnava AM, Mills PG, Davies MJ. Relationship between coronary artery remodeling and plaque vulnerability. Circulation 2002; 105: 939–43.

13. Pasterkamp G, Schoneveld AH, van der Wal AC et al. Relation of arterial geometry to luminal narrowing and histologic markers for plaque vulnerability: the remodeling paradox. J Am Coll Cardiol 1998; 32: 655–62.

14. Takano M, Mizuno K, Okamatsu K et al. Mechanical and structural characteristics of vulnerable plaques: analysis by coronary angioscopy and intravascular ultrasound. J Am Coll Cardiol 2001; 38: 99–104.

15. Nakamura M, Nishikawa H, Mukai S et al. Impact of coronary artery remodeling on clinical presentation of coronary artery disease: an intravascular ultrasound study. J Am Coll Cardiol 2001; 37: 63–9.

16. Schoenhagen P, Ziada KM, Kapadia SR et al. Extent and direction of arterial remodeling in stable versus unstable coronary syndromes: an intravascular ultrasound study. Circulation 2000; 101: 598–603.

17. Schoenhagen P, Tuzcu EM, Stillman AE et al. Non-invasive assessment of plaque morphology and remodeling in mildly stenotic coronary segments: comparison of 16-slice computed tomography and intravascular ultrasound. Coron Artery Dis 2003; 14: 459–62.

18. Gyongyosi M, Yang P, Hassan A et al. Intravascular ultrasound predictors of major adverse cardiac events in patients with unstable angina. Clin Cardiol 2000; 23: 507–15.

19. Hausleiter J, Meyer T, Hadamitzky M et al. Prevalence of non-calcified coronary plaques by 64-slice computed tomography in patients with an intermediate risk for significant coronary artery disease. J Am Coll Cardiol 2006; 48: 312–18.

20. Hoffmann U, Moselewski F, Nieman K et al. Noninvasive assessment of plaque morphology and composition in culprit and stable lesions in acute coronary syndrome and stable lesions in stable angina by multidetector computed tomography. J Am Coll Cardiol 2006; 47: 1655–62.

21. Motoyama S, Kondo T, Sarai M et al. Multislice computed tomographic characteristics of coronary lesions in acute coronary syndromes. J Am Coll Cardiol 2007; 50: 319–26.

CHAPTER 10

Coronary calcification

Imaging of coronary arteries has been a major focus of clinicians interested in cardiovascular disease for a long time. The search for, in particular, non-invasive methods has led to the development of electron beam computed tomography (EBCT), a non-invasive imaging modality, which is able to detect and quantify coronary calcification. The recently introduced multislice CT (MSCT) scanners, which have an improved resolution, are able to detect both calcific and non-calcific plaques. The predictive value of coronary calcification has been almost exclusively established using EBCT technology and, to date, no long-term risk stratification studies are available using MSCT; however, it is expected that direct, non-invasive imaging of coronary calcific and non-calcific atherosclerotic plaques may potentially improve risk stratification for asymptomatic individuals or in patients with known coronary artery disease.

CORONARY CALCIFICATION

Coronary calcification is an active process and the development of coronary artery calcification is intimately associated with the development of coronary atherosclerotic plaques[1]. Calcification does not occur in normal coronary artery walls and the presence of coronary calcification is pathognomonic for the presence of coronary atherosclerosis[2–10] (Figure 10.1). The presence of coronary calcification is associated with coronary plaque size; however, not all plaques are calcified, and in a histological study the total calcium area was approximately 20% of the total atherosclerotic plaque area[4,5]. The degree of lumen encroachment by a calcific plaque is determined by variations of vessel wall remodeling (vessel enlargement), and there is only a weak relation between presence and size of a site-specific calcific plaque and the site of luminal narrowing. It remains to be determined whether a calcific plaque is indeed a vulnerable plaque, even though calcium is often found in ruptured plaques, and therefore CT calcium scanning cannot distinguish between stable and unstable plaques[4,5,9,10]. For many years, EBCT has been used for the detection and quantification of coronary calcium. Coronary calcium deposits have a high X-ray density which is approximately 2–10-fold higher than the low-density adjacent non-calcific tissue and surrounding fat tissue. For the purpose of CT scanning a calcific plaque is defined as a hyperattenuating coronary lesion above a threshold of 130 HU with an area of at least 3 adjacent pixels ($>1\,mm^3$). Agatston et al developed a calcium scoring algorithm for EBCT images that is now widely used in research and clinical practice (Figure 10.2)[11]. The calcium score is derived from the product of the area of calcification (mm^3) and a factor determined by the maximal X-ray density within that area. The Agatston score is derived using a data acquisition protocol with a slice thickness of 3 mm. The calcium score can be calculated per coronary segment, per coronary vessel (right coronary artery, left anterior descending, and left circumflex artery), or for the entire coronary tree.

The Agatston score is susceptible to partial voluming effects and has limited reproducibility. Alternative quantification methods include

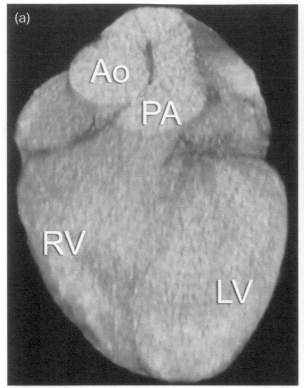

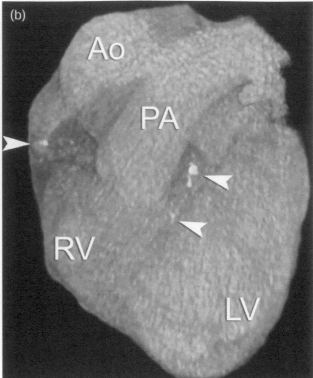

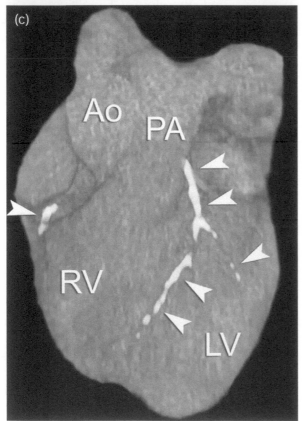

Figure 1 0 . Volume-rendered images of (a) no calcium, (b) moderate amount of calcium, and (c) high amount of calcium. Ao, aorta; PA, pulmonary artery; RV, right ventricle; and LV, left ventricle.

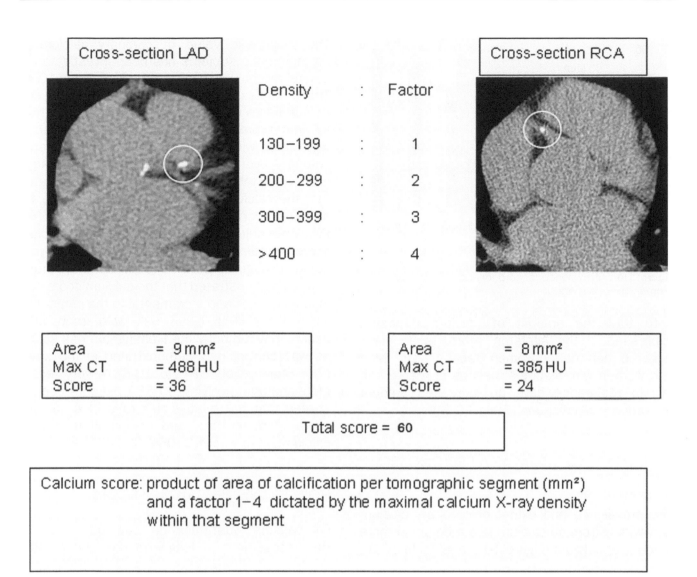

Figure 1 0 2 Coronary calcium scoring – Agatston score. LAD, left anterior descending artery; RCA, right coronary artery.

assessment of the calcified volume and the mass of calcium[12,13]. The calcium volume score is calculated as the sum of the calcified area multiplied with the image increment or Σ area (n) increment[12]. The volume measurement is less susceptible to partial volume effects and allows quantification independent of section thickness or image overlap. The calcium mass is proportional to the volume of the lesion multiplied by the average CT density of the lesion and a calibration factor C or mass C × average CT density × volume lesion. In this case the CT scanner should be calibrated to an external calibration phantom which must be included in the scan field. Calcium mass is a physical measurement

(mg calcium) which can be used across different CT systems and scanning techniques.

In spite of the potential advantages of these newer quantification methods, regarding problems of measurement variability or scanner type dependency, almost no prospective studies on the predictive value of calcium quantification using these two methods are available and nearly all reported studies are based on the 'Agatston' score.

The prevalence of coronary calcium is strongly related to age, with sharply increasing prevalences after age 50 in men and age 60 in women; however, at the ages of 65–70 the prevalences are almost equal (Figure 10.3)[14]. It is of

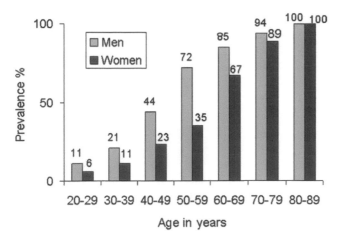

Figure 1 0 . Prevalence of coronary calcium in men or women at various ages.

note that the amount of calcium deposits, expressed in the Agatston score, is generally larger in men than in women (Table 10.1)[15]. Men and women with diabetes mellitus or markers of insulin resistance have an increased amount of coronary calcification (Table 10.2)[16].

CORONARY CALCIUM AS A PROGNOSTIC INDICATOR

The prevalence and extent of coronary calcium vary widely from no calcium to a medium or large amount of calcium (Figure 10.1 and Table 10.3).

The prognostic value of coronary calcium in asymptomatic subjects has been investigated in several recent large-scale studies[17–23] (Table 10.4). These studies indicated that calcium scoring can be used as a risk factor and, in particular, a high calcium score, adjusted for age and gender, is associated with a relatively high risk of adverse coronary events. Two recently published large-scale long-term studies clearly demonstrated that the calcium score was highly predictive for all-cause mortality (Tables 10.5 and 10.6)[17,23]. Even after adjustment of risk and age, the calcium score remained highly predictive of 10-year survival (Figure 10.4)[23]. Furthermore, these studies demonstrated that the calcium score was independent of and incremental to the prognostic value of the Framingham risk factor score and, hence, may remodify the Framingham risk score, as was convincingly demonstrated in the study from Shaw et al[17] (Figure 10.5). A very recent meta-analysis involving 30 854 patients demonstrated that the relative risk ratio of a calcium score of more than zero compared to a zero calcium score was 4.3 (95% CI 3–55.2)[24].

HOW TO USE THE CALCIUM SCORE

CT calcium quantification can be used for the assessment of long-term risk and primary

T ble 1 0 . EBCT calcium score centiles for 25 251 men and 9995 women within age strata. From reference 15, with per mission

	Age (years)								
Calcium scores	<40	40–44	45–49	50–54	55–59	60–64	65–69	70–74	>74
Men (n)	3504	4238	4940	4825	3472	2288	1209	540	235
25th centile	0	0	0	1	4	13	32	64	166
50th centile	1	1	3	15	48	113	180	310	473
75th centile	3	9	36	103	215	410	566	892	1071
90th centile	14	59	154	332	554	994	1299	1774	1982
Women (n)	641	1024	1634	2184	1835	1334	731	438	174
25th centile	0	0	0	0	0	0	1	3	9
50th centile	0	0	0	0	1	3	24	52	75
75th centile	1	1	2	5	23	57	145	210	241
90th centile	3	4	22	55	121	193	410	631	709

T ble 1 0 . 2 Median coronary artery calcium (CAC) scores of men and women with and without diabetes [16]

Age group (years)	Diabetes		No diabetes		p value
	n	Median CAC score	n	Median CAC score	
Men					
<40	46	4	3005	1	<0.001
40– 44	63	13	3653	1	<0.001
45– 49	100	9.5	4322	3	0.001
50– 54	144	42	4142	14	<0.001
55– 59	160	111	2192	43	<0.001
60– 64	117	192	1860	105	<0.001
65-69	72	378	955	152	<0.001
³70	45	343	592	301	0.77
Total	747	63	21 441	6	<0.001
Women					
<40	21	1	514	0	<0.001
40– 44	32	0	846	0	0.14
45– 49	32	1	1398	0	0.01
50– 54	74	8.5	1826	0	<0.001
55– 59	52	7.5	1522	1	<0.001
60– 64	47	21	1105	2	0.003
65– 69	34	104	712	5	0.006
³70	36	114	465	52	0.54
Total	328	5	8388	1	<0.001

Mann-Whitney U test was used to compare CAC scores between diabetic and non-diabetic subjects within each 5-year age group. The analyses were performed separately for men and women.

T ble 1 0 . 3 Age-related calcium prevalence, mean total calcium score, and lesion number

Age (years)	Male			Female		
	Calcium prevalence (%)	Total calcium score (mean ±SD)	Number of lesions (mean ±SD)	Calcium prevalence (%)	Total calcium score (mean ±SD)	Number of lesions (mean ±SD)
0– 29	11	0.5±3.0	0.2±0.6	6	0.06± 0.20	0.06±0.24
30– 39	21	8±35*	0.7±2.1	11	2±10*	0.35±1.70
40– 49	44	28±112*	1.8±3.9*	23	11±46*	0.6±1.9*
50– 59	72	140±324	6.1±8.6*	35	63±487*	1.8±5.8*
60– 69	85	239±371	10.1±12.7	67	122±274*	5.0±6.9*
70– 79	94	425±422*	13.7±10.3*	89	243±332*	7.6±7.8*
80– 89	100	468±13.9		100	249±136	100±3.7

*p<0.05 for age-matched group of opposite sex. Adapted from Janowitz, Am J Cardiol 1993; 72: 247.

Table 10. EBCT predictive value in asymptomatic populations

Study	n	Mean age (years)	Follow-up years (%)	Calcium score value	Comp. group for RR calculation	Relative risk ratio	Endpoint
Shaw et al[17]	10 377	53±0.1	5 (100)	401– 1000	≤10	6.2	All-cause mortality
Park et al[18]	967	67±1.4	6.4 (100)	>142	<3.7		MI coronary death
Arad et al[19]	4613	59 ±6	4.3 (94)	³ 100	<100	9.2	Fatal MI/death
Taylor et al[20]	1627	43 ±3	3 (99)	>0	0	11.8	Death/MI/UA
Vliegenthart et al[21]	1795	71±6	3.3 (99)	>1000	0– 100	8.1	MI/mortality
LaMonte et al[22a]	Men 6835	54±10	3.5 (70)	Top tertile	0	8.7*	Death/MI
	Women 3911			Top tertile	0	6.3	Death/MI
Budoff et al[23]	25 253	56±11	6.8 (100)	0	>10	1.7	All-cause mortality

*per 1000 person years; only men; ªLamonte et al partly self-reported.
MI, myocardial infarction; UA, unstable angina.

prevention of future adverse coronary events. However, calcium scoring should not be performed as a 'stand-alone' test but should be integrated into risk assessment with the well-recognized traditional risk factors. Asymptomatic individuals can be categorized into three levels of risk[25–31]. Individuals considered to be at high risk are defined as having a risk of 20% or more of a coronary event within 10 years. This risk is similar to the level of risk in patients with known coronary artery disease, and according to the guidelines from the National Cholesterol Education Program (NCEP) this risk level is a target for intensive cholesterol reduction[25]. It is estimated that approximately 25% of adults fall into this category[28,29]. Intermediate risk is defined as a risk of a coronary

event of 10–20% within 10 years, and about 40% of adults over 20 years of age fall into this category. Low risk is defined as a risk of a coronary event within 10 years of less than 10%. About 35% of adults over 20 years of age have low risk[28,29].

The assessment of coronary calcium scoring in asymptomatic individuals, in order to be useful, must be able to improve the prediction of the risk of coronary events, as established with known risk factors. It may be assumed that, because the calcium scoring test is not 100% sensitive and specific for the prediction of future adverse coronary events, a positive test will not be able to increase the risk of the prescan low-risk individuals to a high-risk category requiring

Table 105. Prognostic value of coronary calcium score for all-cause mortality in study of Shaw et al[17] (10 377 asymptomatic individuals). Total deaths 2.4% (n = 249)

Calcium score	Number of individuals (%)	All-cause deaths (%)	RRR	Adjusted RRR
≤10	5946 (57)	1.0 (62)	Ñ	Ñ
11– 100	2044 (20)	2.6 (53)	2.5	1.7
101– 400	1432 (14)	3.8 (54)	3.6	1.8
401– 1000	623 (6.0)	6.3 (39)	6.2	2.6
>1000	332 (3.2)	12.3 (41)	12.3	4.0

Table 10. Coronary calcification predictive of all-cause mortality in study of Budoff et al[23] (25 253 asymptomatic individuals). All-cause deaths 2% (n = 510)

Calcium score	Number of individuals (%)	RRR	Adjusted RRR
0	11 046 (44)	Ñ	Ñ
1– 10	3567 (14)	2.6	1.5
11– 100	5033 (20)	6.7	3.6
101– 400	3177 (13)	13	3.9
401– 1000	1469 (6)	23	6.2
>1000	965 (4)	38	9.4

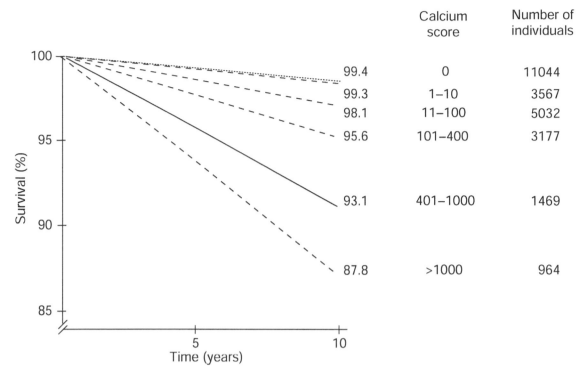

	Calcium score	Number of individuals
99.4	0	11044
99.3	1–10	3567
98.1	11–100	5032
95.6	101–400	3177
93.1	401–1000	1469
87.8	>1000	964

Figure 1 0 4 Risk-adjusted (including age) 10-year survival[23].

preventive measures[25,30]. Furthermore, a negative calcium scan in a prescan high-risk population will not reduce this risk to a level at which preventive interventions can be withheld[25,30]. However, a calcium scan may be useful in an intermediate-risk group of individuals. Here, a

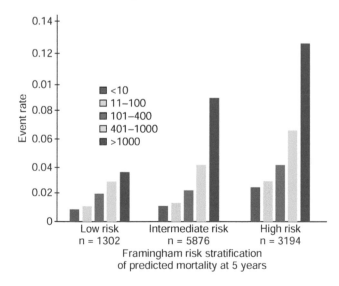

Figure 1 0 . 5 Calcium score remodification of Framingham risk score in a high-risk asymptomatic population (n = 10 377) with a mean age of 53 years (60% male) n[17].

positive or negative calcium scan may reclassify individuals to a higher- or lower-risk group, respectively, and thus provide further support for either instituting or withholding long-term preventive measures (Figure 10.6)[32]. Greenland and Gaziano in a landmark article presented a practical approach taking into account a pretest risk assessment and how the outcome of a calcium scan can influence clinical decision making[33]. A pretest risk assessment can be derived from the risk assessment of the Framingham Heart Study or the European guidelines on cardiovascular disease prevention in clinical practice[25,34]. Greenland and Gaziano provided a straightforward simple way to assess risk by counting risk factors. Individuals with zero or one risk factor are considered to be at low risk <10% within 10 years, and individuals with three or more risk factors or diabetics are considered at high risk >20% within 10 years[33]. It has been shown that a calcium score of more than 80 has a sensitivity of 85% and a specificity of 75% to predict the occurrence of clinical coronary events including death, non-fatal myocardial infarction, and clinically indicated revascularization[35]. According to the calculations of Greenland

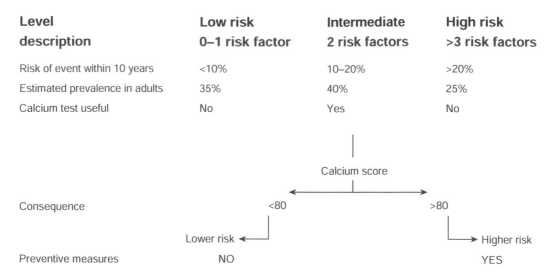

Level description	Low risk 0–1 risk factor	Intermediate 2 risk factors	High risk >3 risk factors
Risk of event within 10 years	<10%	10–20%	>20%
Estimated prevalence in adults	35%	40%	25%
Calcium test useful	No	Yes	No

Figure 1 0 6 Approach to calcium CT scan testing. Adapted from reference 32, with per mission.

and Gaziano a calcium score of less than 80 significantly reduced the risk of a coronary event within 10 years in the intermediate-risk group to less than 5% and, thus, to no need for preventive risk measures, whereas a calcium scan of more than 80 significantly increased the risk in the intermediate-risk group to >20% and, thus, to a category of individuals where preventive measures are warranted (Table 10.7). Recent studies demonstrated that a high calcium score was associated with independent additional risk in the intermediate-risk group as determined by the Framingham risk score[17,20–23,36]. This lends further support to the theory that a high calcium score can modify predicted risk, which is useful in an intermediate-risk group.

This approach is in accord with the statement of the Writing Group which suggested that in individuals at intermediate risk a calcium score may be useful to adjust classification of an individual to a lower-risk category if there is no calcium, or to a higher-risk category if calcium is present[32].

In conclusion, the presence of coronary calcium is a predictor of adverse coronary events. Calcification is neither a marker for plaque vulnerability nor for plaque stability. However, the greater is the overall calcium burden, which correlates with a greater overall coronary plaque burden, the greater is the likelihood of an adverse coronary event. The absence of calcium does not exclude the presence of coronary atherosclerosis but is associated with a low likelihood of advanced coronary atherosclerosis and

T ble 1 0 . Probability of a coronary event within 10 years calculated on the basis of results of EBCT[33]

Pretest probability of a coronary event within 10 years (%)	Probability of a coronary event within 10 years according to results of EBCT (%)	
	Calcium score ≥80	Calcium score <80
1.0	3.0	0.2
2.0	6.5	0.4
3.0	9.5	0.6
4.0	12.5	0.9
5.0	15.0	1.0
6.0	18.0	1.2
7.0	20.0	1.4
10.0	27.0	2.2
15.0	38.0	3.4
20.0	46.0	4.8

a very low likelihood of an adverse coronary event. The American College of Cardiology (ACC)/ American Heart Association (AHA) consensus conference and the European Guidelines do not recommend calcium screening with CT of the general population[8,34].

CORONARY CALCIUM TO PREDICT SIGNIFICANT CORONARY OBSTRUCTIONS

The greater is the amount of calcium, the greater is the likelihood of a significant coronary obstruction, which however, is not site specific. Calcium prediction for the presence of a significant coronary obstruction was established in 4394 patients (67% males), mean age 55.3 years, who all underwent coronary angiography with a prevalence of significant coronary artery disease of 52%[9]. The ability of the presence of calcium to predict a significant obstruction was high with a sensitivity of 93%, but with a low specificity of 45% and a predictive accuracy of 70% (Table 10.8). Haberl et al[37] performed a comparative study between the calcium score in men and women and the outcome of invasive coronary angiography. They calculated the likelihood of the presence or absence of a significant coronary stenosis in relation to gender and age. The outcome is depicted in Figures 10.7 and 10.8. These data may be helpful to estimate the likelihood of the presence of a significant coronary

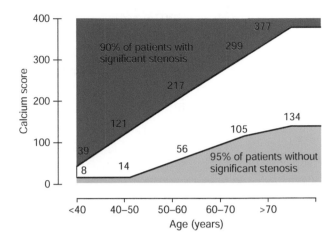

Figure 1 0 . *C*alcium score to predict presence or absence of significant stenosis in men. From reference 37, with permission.

stenosis; they may also be helpful to adjust the sometimes difficult interpretation of a contrast-enhanced MSCT coronary angiogram of a patient with severe calcifications, which precludes accurate assessment of the coronary lumen. However, one should keep in mind that there is not a direct one-to-one correlation between the site of detected coronary calcium and luminal disease.

CORONARY CALCIUM TO PREDICT ADVERSE EVENTS IN PATIENTS WHO HAVE UNDERGONE INVASIVE CORONARY ANGIOGRAPHY

Symptomatic patients who have undergone invasive coronary angiography have been shown to be at high risk. However, the risk of these patients is further significantly increased by 3–6 times if coronary calcium is present compared with the risk in patients with no coronary calcium (Table 10.9)[38,39].

CONCLUSION

A high coronary calcium score, adjusted for age and sex, is an independent risk factor for adverse coronary events and may be helpful to remodify

T ble 1 08. Coronary calcium to predict significant (>50% diameter stenosis) coronary obstruction[8,37]

Subjects (n)	4.394
Male %	67
Mean age (years)	55.3
Prevalence CAD %	52
Coronary calcium diagnostic performance	
Sensitivity (%)	93
Specificity (%)	45
Predictive accuracy (%)	70

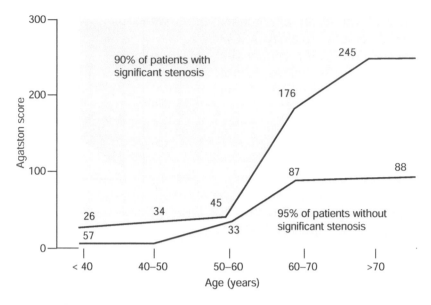

Figure 1 0 . Calcium score to predict likelihood of presence or absence of significant stenosis in women. From reference 37, with permission.

T ble 1 0 . Predictive value of calcium after diagnostic coronary angiography

	Detrano et al[38] (n=422)	Keelan et al[39] (n=288)
Age (years)	55±12	56±11
Follow-up (months)	30±13	71
Death/myocardial infarction (n)	13/8	22
Coronary calcium score (Agatston)	³75	³10
Risk	6 : 1*	3.2*

*Compared to patients with lower calcium threshold or no presence of calcium.

risk in individuals at intermediate risk in whom there is uncertainty about the institution of preventive measures[24,25,40].

REFERENCES

1. Fuster V, Moreno PR, Fayad ZA, Corti R, Badimon JJ. Atherothrombosis and high-risk plaque: part I: evolving concepts. J Am Coll Cardiol 2005;46: 937–54.
2. Rifkin RD, Parisi AF, Folland E. Coronary calcification in the diagnosis of coronary artery disease. Am J Cardiol 1979; 44: 141–7.
3. McCarthy JH, Palmer FJ. Incidence and significance of coronary artery calcification. Br Heart J 1974; 36: 499–506.
4. Rumberger JA, Simons DB, Fitzpatrick LA et al. Coronary artery calcium area by electron-beam computed tomography and coronary atherosclerotic plaque area. A histopathologic correlative study. Circulation 1995; 92: 2157–62.
5. Sangiorgi G, Rumberger JA, Severson A et al. Arterial calcification and not lumen stenosis is highly correlated with atherosclerotic plaque burden in humans: a histologic study of 723 coronary artery segments using nondecalcifying methodology. J Am Coll Cardiol 1998; 89: 36–44.
6. Mautner SL, Mautner GC, Froehlich J et al. Coronary artery disease: prediction with in vitro electron beam CT. Radiology 1994; 192: 625–30.
7. Simons DB, Schwartz RS, Edwards WD et al. Noninvasive definition of anatomic coronary artery disease by ultrafast computed tomographic scanning: a quantitative pathologic comparison study. J Am Coll Cardiol 1992; 20: 1118–26.
8. O'Rourke RA, Brundage BH, Froelicher VF et al. American College of Cardiology/American Heart Association Expert Consensus document on electron-beam computed tomography for the diagnosis and prognosis of coronary artery disease. Circulation 2000; 102: 126 40.
9. Schmermund A, Baumgart D, Gorge G et al. Coronary artery calcium in acute coronary syndromes: a comparative study of electron-beam computed tomography, coronary angiography, and intracoronary ultrasound in survivors of acute myocardial infarction and unstable angina. Circulation 1997; 96: 1461–69.
10. Schmermund A, Schwartz RS, Adamzik M et al. Coronary atherosclerosis in unheralded sudden coronary death under age 50: histo-pathologic comparison with 'healthy' subjects dying out of hospital. Atherosclerosis 2001; 155: 499–508.
11. Agatston AS, Janowitz WR, Hildner FJ et al. Quantification of coronary artery calcium using ultrafast computed tomography. J Am Coll Cardiol 1990; 15: 827–32.
12. Callister TQ, Cooil B, Raya SP et al. Coronary artery disease: improved reproducibility of calcium scoring with an electron-beam CT volumetric method. Radiology 1998; 208: 807–14.
13. Hong C, Becker CR, Schoepf UJ et al. Coronary artery calcium: absolute quantification in nonenhanced and

contrast-enhanced multi-detector row CT studies. Radiology 2002; 223: 474–80.

14. Janowitz WR, Agatston AS, Kaplan G, Viamonte M Jr. Differences in prevalence and extent of coronary artery calcium detected by ultrafast computed tomography in asymptomatic men and women. Am J Cardiol 1993; 72: 247–54.

15. Hoff JA, Chomka EV, Krainik AJ et al. Age and gender distributions of coronary artery calcium detected by electron beam tomography in 35,246 adults. Am J Cardiol 2001; 87: 1335–9.

16. Hoff JA, Quinn L, Sevrukov A et al. The prevalence of coronary artery calcium among diabetic individuals without known coronary artery disease. J Am Coll Cardiol 2003; 41: 1008–12.

17. Shaw LJ, Raggi P, Schisterman E, Berman DS, Callister TQ. Prognostic value of cardiac risk factors and coronary artery calcium screening for all-cause mortality. Radiology 2003; 228: 826–33.

18. Park R, Detrano R, Xiang M et al. Combined use of computed tomography coronary calcium scores and C-reactive protein levels in predicting cardiovascular events in nondiabetic individuals. Circulation 2002; 106: 2073–7.

19. Arad Y, Goodman KJ, Roth M, Newstein D, Guerci AD. Coronary calcification, coronary disease risk factors, C-reactive protein, and atherosclerotic cardiovascular disease events: the St. Francis Heart Study. J Am Coll Cardiol 2005; 46: 158–65.

20. Taylor AJ, Bindeman J, Feuerstein I et al. Coronary calcium independently predicts incident premature coronary heart disease over measured cardiovascular risk factors: mean three-year outcomes in the Prospective Army Coronary Calcium (PACC) project. J Am Coll Cardiol 2005; 46: 807–14.

21. Vliegenthart R, Oudkerk M, Hofman A et al. Coronary calcification improves cardiovascular risk prediction in the elderly. Circulation 2005; 112: 572–7.

22. LaMonte MJ, FitzGerald SJ, Church TS et al. Coronary artery calcium score and coronary heart disease events in a large cohort of asymptomatic men and women. Am J Epidemiol 2005; 162: 421–9.

23. Budoff MJ, Shaw LJ, Liu ST et al. Long-term prognosis associated with coronary calcification: observations from a registry of 25 253 patients. J Am Coll Cardiol 2007; 49: 1871–3.

24. Greenland P, Bonow RO, Brundage BH et al. American College of Cardiology Foundation Clinical Expert Consensus Task Force (ACCF/AHA Writing Committee to Update the 2000 Expert Consensus Document on Electron Beam Computed Tomography); Society of Atherosclerosis Imaging and Prevention; Society of Cardiovascular Computed Tomography. ACCF/AHA 2007 clinical expert consensus document on coronary artery calcium scoring by computed tomography in global cardiovascular risk assessment and in evaluation of patients with chest pain: a report of the American College of Cardiology Foundation Clinical Expert Consensus Task Force (ACCF/AHA Writing Committee to Update the 2000 Expert Consensus Document on Electron Beam Computed Tomography) developed in collaboration with the Society of Atherosclerosis Imaging and Prevention and the Society of Cardiovascular Computed Tomography. J Am Coll Cardiol 2007; 49: 378–402.

25. Expert Panel on Detection, Evaluation and Treatment of High Blood Cholesterol in Adults. Executive summary of the Third Report of the National Cholesterol Education Program (NCEP) JAMA 2001; 285: 2486–97.

26. Pearson TA, Blair SN, Daniels SR et al. AHA guidelines for primary prevention of cardiovascular disease and stroke: 2002 update; consensus panel guide to comprehensive risk reduction for adult patients without coronary or other atherosclerotic vascular diseases. Circulation 2002; 106: 388–91.

27. Smith SC, Blair SN, Bonow RO et al. AHA/ACC scientific statement: AHA/ACC guidelines for preventing heart attack and death in patients with atherosclerotic cardiovascular disease: 2001 update: a statement for healthcare professionals from the American Heart Association and the American College of Cardiology. Circulation 2001; 104: 1577–9.

28. Jacobson TA, Griffiths GG, Varas C et al. Impact of evidence-based "clinical judgment" on the number of American adults requiring lipid-lowering therapy based on updated NHANES III data. National Health and Nutrition Examination Survey. Arch Intern Med 2000; 160: 1361–9.

29. Greenland P, Smith SC Jr, Grundy SM. Improving coronary heart disease risk assessment in asymptomatic people: role of traditional risk factors and noninvasive cardiovascular tests. Circulation 2001; 104: 1863–7.

30. Grundy SM. Primary prevention of coronary heart disease: integrating risk assessment with intervention. Circulation 1999; 100: 988–98.

31. Smith SC Jr, Greenland P, Grundy SM, AHA Conference Proceedings. Prevention conference V: Beyond secondary prevention: Identifying the high-risk patient for primary prevention: executive summary. American Heart Association. Circulation 2000; 101: 111–16.

32. Greenland P, Abrams J, Aurigemma GP et al. Prevention Conference V: Beyond secondary prevention: identifying the high-risk patient for primary prevention: noninvasive tests of atherosclerotic burden: Writing Group III. Circulation 2000; 101: e16–e22.

33. Greenland P, Gaziano JM. Clinical practice. Selecting asymptomatic patients for coronary computed tomography or electrocardiographic exercise testing. N Engl J Med 2003; 349: 465–73.

34. De Backer G, Amrosioni E, Borch-Johnson K et al. European Guidelines on cardiovascular disease prevention in clinical practice. Eur J Cardiovasc Prevent Rehabil 2003; 10: 1–10.

35. Greenland P, LaBree L, Azen SP, Doherty TM, Detrano RC. Coronary artery calcium score combined with Framingham score for risk prediction in asymptomatic individuals. JAMA 2004; 291: 210–15.

36. Arad Y, Spadaro LA, Goodman K, Newstein D, Guerci AD. Prediction of coronary events with electron beam computed tomography. J Am Coll Caroliol 2000; 36: 1253–60.

37. Haberl R, Becker A, Leber A et al. Correlation of coronary calcification and angiographically documented stenoses in patients with suspected coronary artery disease: results of 1764 patients. J Am Coll Cardiol 2001; 37: 451–7.

38. Detrano R, Hsiai T, Wang, S et al. Prognostic value of coronary calcification and angiographic stenoses in patients undergoing coronary angiography. J Am Coll Cardiol 1996; 27: 285–90.

39. Keelan PC, Bielak LF, Ashai K et al. Long-term prognostic value of coronary calcification detected by electron-beam computed tomography in patients undergoing coronary angiography. Circulation 2001; 104: 412–17.

40. Budoff MJ. Atherosclerosis imaging and calcified plaque: coronary artery disease risk assessment. Prog Cardiovasc Dis 2003; 46: 135–48.

CHAPTER 11

Assessment of coronary stents

Since the publication in 1993 of two landmark randomized clinical trials showing the superior outcome of coronary stent implantation as compared with balloon angioplasty[1,2], percutaneous coronary interventions (PCIs) using stents have become the preferred revascularization strategy for patients with obstructive coronary artery disease. Currently, coronary stents are used in 85–90% of PCIs[3]. The almost systematic use of coronary stents abolished the occurrence of acute vessel recoil and constrictive remodeling associated with balloon angioplasty[4], but introduced the issue of stent thrombosis and the more prevalent problem of restenosis, due to the excessive growth of neointimal hyperplasia inside the stent or within the borders of the stent. The introduction of drug-eluting stents (DES), in 2003, resulted in an important reduction of restenosis rates after PCI. Nevertheless, clinically significant restenosis occurs in on average 10% of patients treated with DES. This figure increases to 20–30% in patients treated with bare metal stents, i.e. stents without drug coating[5]. The recurrence of anginal symptoms after PCI is usually related to the progression of coronary artery disease in non-revascularized vessel segments or owing to the appearance of in-stent restenosis. Traditionally, patients who present with recurrent symptoms after PCI are investigated using a number of non-invasive functional tests. However, the diagnostic performance of these functional tests for the evaluation of symptomatic patients after PCI is suboptimal[6], and as a result a substantial proportion of patients end up having an invasive coronary angiogram. Multislice computed tomography (MSCT) has developed into a reliable non-invasive alternative to assess the patency of the coronary arteries. However, coronary stents have been notoriously difficult to assess by CT owing to the occurrence of stent-related high-density artifacts.

The metallic composition of stents causes high-density artifacts, causing the stent struts to appear much larger than they actually are, thereby impairing the assessability of the lumen inside the stent (Figure 11.1)[7]. This artifact is known as 'blooming effect'. The amount of 'blooming effect' and, thus, artificial lumen narrowing is correlated to the amount and density of the metal. Stents that are composed of metal with high density such as tantalum or gold cause more blooming effect than stainless steel stents (Figure 11.2)[8]. The 'blooming effect' is a fairly constant phenomenon and, therefore, less evident in large diameter stents. In general, stents with a diameter of less than 3 mm and/or strut thickness of 140 µm or more are often uninterpretable[9,10]. Other factors affecting the visibility of the in-stent lumen are the scanner technology and the type of stent. An in vitro evaluation of 68 different metallic stent types that were implanted in a 3-mm coronary artery phantom showed that even when using a 64-slice scanner, which provides the highest spatial resolution to date, factors such as stent material and strut thickness have an important impact on stent assessability[8]. In an ideal in vitro situation using (z-)ultra high 0.3 mm spatial resolution the in-stent lumen is well appreciated (Figure 11.3).

Coronary stents are easily recognized in vivo on both non-enhanced and contrast-enhanced CT images because the density of the stents is

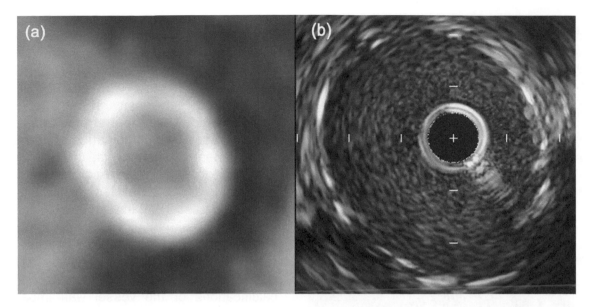

Figure 11.1a) CT cross-sectional image of a 3.5-mm Express® (Boston Scientific, Natick MA, USA) stent in the left main coronary artery. (b) Corresponding intravascular ultrasound (IVUS) cross-sectional image. The actual size of the metallic stent struts is magnified on CT due to the blooming effect.

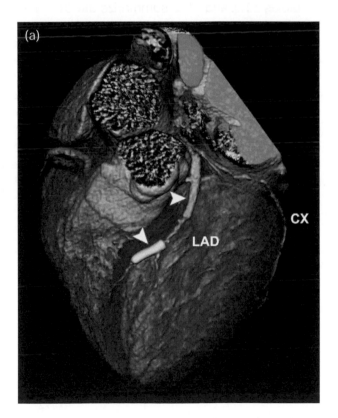

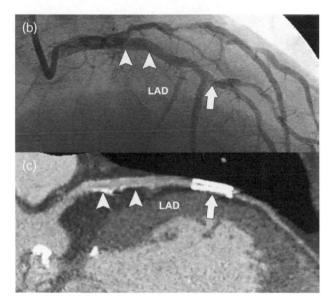

Figure 11.2a) Volume-rendered CT image of a patient, who in the course of a few years, underwent stenting of the left anterior descending coronary artery (LAD) on two occasions. Two different stent types (arrowheads) were implanted: the more distal stent is a gold-coated NIR® stent, and the more proximal stent is an Express stent. (b) Invasive coronary angiogram focusing on the LAD in which both stents show good patency. (c) Curved multiplanar CT reconstruction showing both the Express stent (arrowheads) and the gold-coated NIR ¨ (Medinol, Maple Grove MN,USA). stent (arrow). Due to its high metal density, the gold-coated stent is showing an important blooming effect, thereby almost completely obscuring the underlying lumen. CX, circumflex artery.

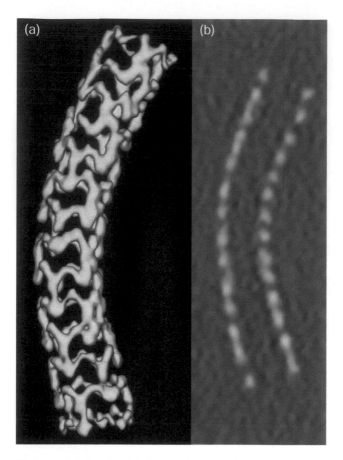

Figure 1 1 3 Ex vivo 64-slice CT image of a 3-mm Express stent implanted in the coronary artery of a pig's heart. The stent strut morphology can be recognized as shown in the three-dimensonal reconstruction (a). Also, the lumen within the stent is easily assessable as shown in the longitudinal through-plane reconstruction (b).

higher than any other tissue in or around the heart, including the contrast-enhanced lumen[11,12]. In vivo MSCT stent imaging suffers from the same stent-related imaging degrading artifacts as those seen in the in vitro situation. Again, the stent-related high-density artifacts enlarge the apparent size of the stent struts. This 'blooming effect' caused by a combination of partial voluming and beam hardening is, in particular, quite disturbing in smaller-sized coronary stents with thick struts and relatively less disturbing in larger stents (at least 3 mm in diameter) (Figure 11.4). In the in vivo situation, additional factors further affect stent assessability: (1) the tissues surrounding the heart cause X-ray scattering and a reduction in the contrast to noise; (2) severe calcifications of the vessel wall impair lumen assessability; and (3) cardiac motion artifacts, particular with high heart rates, further reduce reliable assessment of coronary stents.

Tables 11.1 and 11.2 summarize the CT studies that have evaluated patients with previous stent implantation. In the early studies, using four-slice MSCT technology, it was not possible to visualize the lumen within the stent[13,14]. A rough distinction between stent occlusion and patency of the stented segment was based on the absence and presence, respectively, of contrast enhancement distal to the stent. Direct assessment of the coronary stent lumen became possible with 16-slice and 64-slice CT technology (Figure 11.5)[9,10,15–26].

T ble 1 1 . Diagnostic performance of four- and 16-slice MSCT to detect coronary in-stent restenosis, with conventional angiography as the standard of reference

Study	Scanner type	Patients (n)	Stents (n)	Stent types (n)*	Not assessable (%)	Lumen assessable	Sensitivity/ specificity (%)†
Kruger et al[13]	4-slice	20	32	4	0	–	Ñ
Maintz et al[14]	4-slice	29	47	13	19	–	Ñ
Hong et al[15]	16-slice	19	26	3	23	+	Ñ
Schuijf et al[9]	16-slice	22	65	14	23	+	78/100
Cademartiri et al[16]	16-slice	51	76	Ñ	2	+	83/98
Gilard et al[17]	16-slice	29	29ᵃ	Ñ	7	+	100/92
Gaspar et al[18]	40-slice	65	111	Ñ	4	+	74/83
Kitagawa et al[19]	16-slice	42	61	14	31	+	Ñ
Gilard et al[10]	16-slice	143	232	10	45	+	Ñ

*Total number of different stent types; stent-based analysis; ᵃstudy that only included patients with stents in the left main coronary artery.

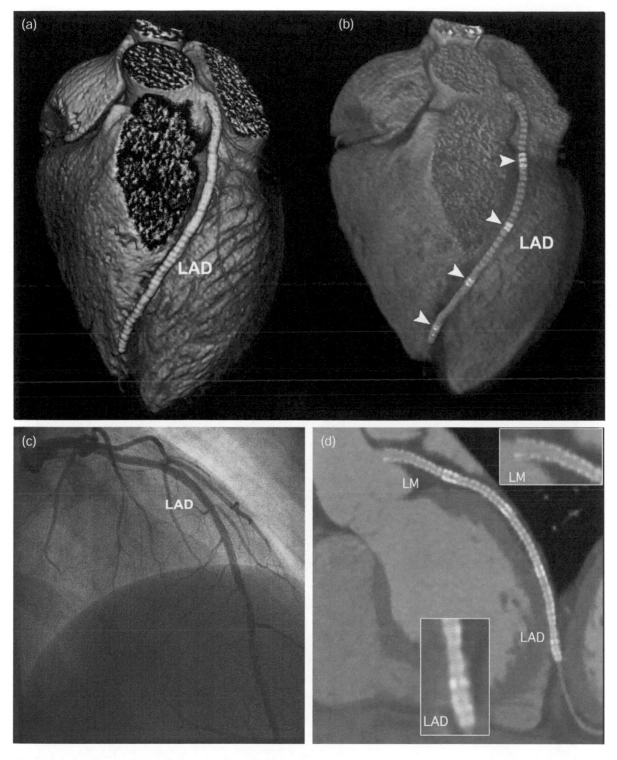

Figure 1 1 . 4 a) Volume-rendered CT image of a patient in whom 5 Bx velocity Cypher ® stents had been implanted to treat a catheter-induced dissection of the left main (LM) and left anterior descending (LAD) coronary artery. (b) Identical volume-rendered CT image as in (a) but using different window level settings (1000 HU), thereby highlighting the overlapping portions of the stents (arrowheads). (c) Invasive coronary angiogram of the LAD after 1-year follow-up. The stents are widely patent. (d) Curved multiplanar CT image of the LAD. Only the lumen of the very proximal stent (3.5 mm in diameter) in the LM can be reliably assessed. The most distal stent (2.25 mm in diameter) in the LAD does not allow interpretation of the in-stent lumen.

Table 11. Diagnostic performance of 64-slice MSCT to detect coronary in-stent restenosis, with conventional angiography as the standard of reference

Study	Scanner type	Patients (n)	Stents (n)	Stent types (n)*	Not assessable (%)	Lumen assessable	Sensitivity/ specificity (%)†
Van Mieghem et al[20]	64-slice[a]	70	162	2	0	+	100/91*
Oncel et al[21]	64-slice	30	39	9	0	+	89/95
Rixe et al[22]	64-slice	64	102	5	42	+	86/98
Ehara et al[23]	64-slice	81	163	16	20	+	91/93
Cademartiri et al[24]	64-slice	182	192	10	7	+	95/93
Carbone et al[25]	64-slice	41	88	–	28	+	79/84
Pugliese et al[26]	64-slice	100	247	8	5	+	94/92

*Total number of different stent types; stent-based analysis; [a]study also only included patients scanned with 16-slice CT technology; **patient-based analysis; study performed using dual-source CT technology.

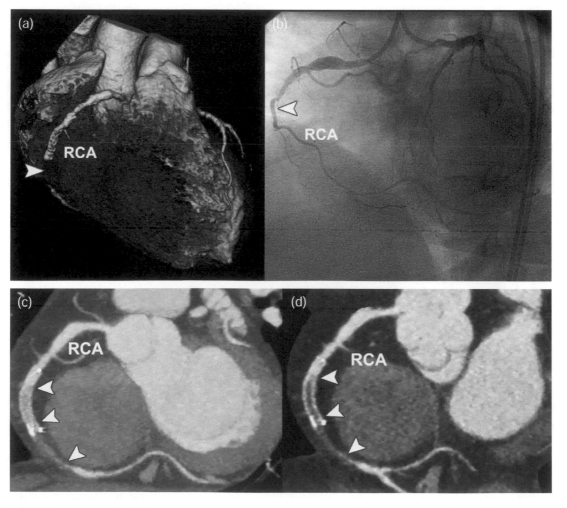

Figure 11. (a) Volume-rendered CT image showing an occlusion (arrowhead) in the mid-part of the right coronary artery (RCA). (b) The corresponding invasive angiogram shows the entry point of the occlusion (arrowhead) at the origin of the margo acutis. (c) Maximal intensity projection and (d) multiplanar reconstruction of the RCA showing that the occlusion starts within a previously implanted stent (upper two arrowheads) extending distally into the non-stented part of the vessel (lower arrowhead).

However, published results have been very heterogeneous owing to the fact that different stent types and stents with various diameters, as low as 2.25 mm, have been included. Promising results have been reported in patients who underwent previous left main stenting, in whom MSCT may offer special value as a reliable technique for angiographic follow-up[17,20]. Post-stent implantation assessment with MSCT may be useful to assess the correct position and patency of the stent (Figure 11.6), but unfortunately fails to identify the more subtle post-stent implantation problems (Table 11.3).

Table 11.3. MSCT coronary stent assessment

Possible
Patency/occlusion
Neointimal hyperplasia in large stents
In-stent restenosis in large stents
Stent position in ostial lesions
Stent overlap
Not possible
Neointimal hyperplasia in small stents
Stent malapposition
Stent underexpansion

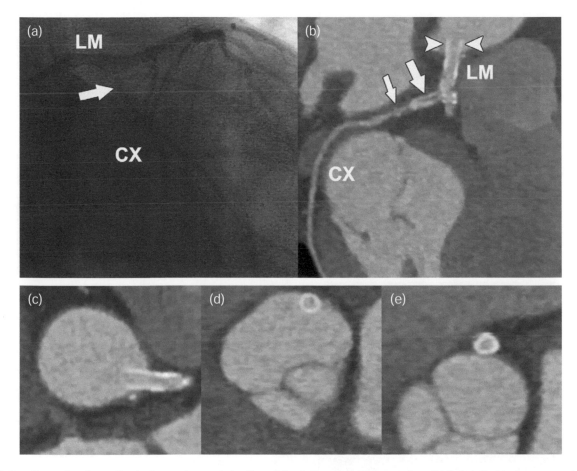

Figure 11. Example of a patient who underwent stenting of the left main coronary artery (LM). (a) Owing to recurrent angina, a control invasive angiogram was performed. It was not possible to engage the diagnostic catheter well into the origin of the left coronary artery. This resulted in a poor opacification of the entire left coronary system. Restenosis of the stent in the proximal part of the circumflex artery (CX) was suspected. (b) Curved multiplanar reconstruction of the LM and CX. This image clearly shows protrusion of the stent in to the ascending aorta (arrowheads) and explains the difficulties when cannulating the left coronary artery. The stent in the CX shows restenosis (large arrow). Furthermore, there is a significant stenosis of the CX at the distal stent edge (smaller arrow). (c) Axial view of the stent protruding in the ascending aorta. (d) Cross-sectional view of the stent in the aorta. (e) Cross-sectional view of the stent within the LM.

Requirements for reliable coronary stent imaging are MSCT scanners with thinner detectors to reduce partial volume effects, higher temporal resolution to reduce motion artifacts, and dedicated filtering of the acquired data to correct for high-density artifacts. The recent trend towards using thin-strut metal stents and the introduction of low-density metal stents such as nitinol- or cobalt-chromium stents within the field of interventional cardiology, is another effective means to improve stent imaging.[27–29] Very recent studies are evaluating the effectiveness of non-metallic biodegradable stents, the use of which would overcome completely the problem of metal-related artifacts[30] (Figure 11.7).

CONCLUSION

Current 16- and 64-slice CT technology allows reliable assessment of large-diameter (≥3 mm) coronary artery stents. Metal-related artifacts preclude the correct evaluation of stents with smaller diameters. In parallel with new technical developments in MSCT technology, the preferable use of thin-strut or low-density metal stents will further improve overall stent imaging.

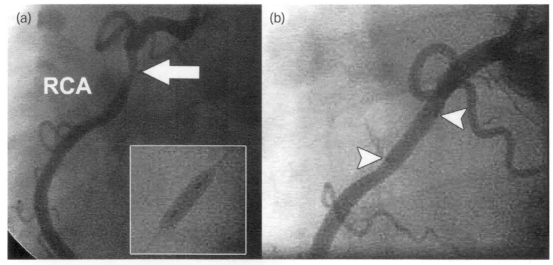

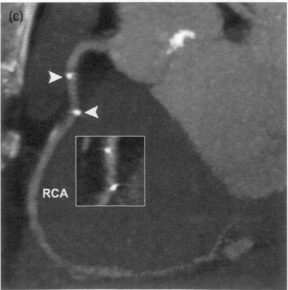

Figure 11.7 a) Invasive angiogram showing a significant stenosis in the proximal part of the right coronary artery (RCA). A biodegradable stent, composed of a polylactic acid polymer with nitinol markers at both ends, was implanted (inset). (b) Angiographic image post-stent implantation. The markers of the stent are visible (arrowheads). (c) Maximal intensity projection showing the position of the stent in the RCA. Note that only the markers of the stent are visible. The markers, which consist of metal (nitinol), appear oversized due to the blooming effect.

REFERENCES

1. Serruys PW, de Jaegere P, Kiemeneij F et al. A comparison of balloon-expandable-stent implantation with balloon angioplasty in patients with coronary artery disease. Benestent Study Group. N Engl J Med 1994; 331: 489–95.
2. Fischman DL, Leon MB, Baim DS et al. A randomized comparison of coronary-stent placement and balloon angioplasty in the treatment of coronary artery disease. Stent Restenosis Study Investigators. N Engl J Med 1994; 331: 496–501.
3. Rosamond W, Flegal K, Friday G et al. Heart disease and stroke statistics–2007 update: a report from the American Heart Association Statistics Committee and Stroke Statistics Subcommittee. Circulation 2007; 115: e69–171.
4. Togni M, Balmer F, Pfiffner D et al. Percutaneous coronary interventions in Europe 1992–2001. Eur Heart J 2004; 25: 1208–13.
5. Babapulle MN, Joseph L, Belisle P et al. A hierarchical Bayesian meta-analysis of randomised clinical trials of drug-eluting stents. Lancet 2004; 364: 583–91
6. Dori G, Denekamp Y, Fishman S et al. Exercise stress testing, myocardial perfusion imaging and stress echocardiography for detecting restenosis after successful percutaneous transluminal coronary angioplasty: a review of performance. J Intern Med 2003; 253: 253–62.
7. Mahnken AH, Buecker A, Wildberger JE et al. Coronary artery stents in multislice computed tomography: in vitro artifact evaluation. Invest Radiol 2004; 39: 27–33.
8. Maintz D, Seifarth H, Raupach R et al. 64-slice multidetector coronary CT angiography: in vitro evaluation of 68 different stents. Eur Radiol 2006; 16: 818–26.
9. Schuijf JD, Bax JJ, Jukema JW et al. Feasibility of assessment of coronary stent patency using 16-slice computed tomography. Am J Cardiol 2004; 94: 427–30.
10. Gilard M, Cornily JC, Pennec PY et al. Assessment of coronary artery stents by 16 slice computed tomography. Heart 2006; 92: 58–61.
11. Nieman K, Cademartiri F, Raaijmakers R et al. Noninvasive angiographic evaluation of coronary stents with multi-slice spiral computed tomography. Herz 2003; 28: 136–42.
12. Mohlenkamp S, Pump H, Baumgart D et al. Minimally invasive evaluation of coronary stents with electron beam computed tomography: In vivo and in vitro experience. Catheter Cardiovasc Interv 1999; 48: 39–47.
13. Kruger S, Mahnken AH, Sinha AM et al. Multislice spiral computed tomography for the detection of coronary stent restenosis and patency. Int J Cardiol 2003; 89: 67–72.
14. Maintz D, Grude M, Fallenberg EM et al. Assessment of coronary arterial stents by multislice-CT angiography. Acta Radiol 2003; 44: 597–603.
15. Hong C, Chrysant GS, Woodard PK et al. Coronary artery stent patency assessed with in-stent contrast enhancement measured at multi-detector row CT angiography: initial experience. Radiology 2004; 233: 286–91.
16. Cademartiri F, Mollet N, Lemos PA et al. Usefulness of multislice computed tomographic coronary angiography to assess in-stent restenosis. Am J Cardiol 2005; 96: 799–802.
17. Gilard M, Cornily JC, Rioufol G et al. Noninvasive assessment of left main coronary stent patency with 16-slice computed tomography. Am J Cardiol 2005; 95: 110–12.
18. Gaspar T, Halon DA, Lewis BS et al. Diagnosis of coronary in-stent restenosis with multidetector row spiral computed tomography. J Am Coll Cardiol 2005; 46: 1573–9.
19. Kitagawa T, Fujii T, Tomohiro Y et al. Noninvasive assessment of coronary stents in patients by 16-slice computed tomography. Int J Cardiol 2006; 109: 188–94.
20. Van Mieghem CA, Cademartiri F, Mollet NR et al. Multislice spiral computed tomography for the evaluation of stent patency after left main coronary artery stenting: a comparison with conventional coronary angiography and intravascular ultrasound. Circulation 2006; 114: 645–53.
21. Oncel D, Oncel G, Karaca M. Coronary stent patency and in-stent restenosis: determination with 64-section multidetector CT coronary angiography–initial experience. Radiology 2007; 242: 403–9.
22. Rixe J, Achenbach S, Ropers D et al. Assessment of coronary artery stent restenosis by 64-slice multi-detector computed tomography. Eur Heart J 2006; 27: 2567–72.
23. Ehara M, Kawai M, Surmely JF, et al. Diagnostic accuracy of coronary in-stent restenosis using 64-slice computed tomography: comparison with invasive coronary angiography. J Am Coll Cardiol 2007; 49: 951–9.
24. Cademartiri F, Schuijf JD, Pugliese F et al. Usefulness of 64-slice multislice computed tomography coronary angiography to assess in-stent restenosis. J Am Coll Cardiol 2007; 49: 2204–10.
25. Carbone I, Francone M, Algeri E et al. Non-invasive evaluation of coronary artery stent patency with retrospectively ECG-gated 64-slice CT angiography. Eur Radiol 2007; 18: 234–43.
26. Pugliese F, Weustink AC, Van Mieghem C et al. Dual-source coronary computed tomography angiography for detecting in-stent restenosis. Heart 2008; in press.
27. Pache J, Dibra A, Mehilli J et al. Drug-eluting stents compared with thin-strut bare stents for the reduction of restenosis: a prospective, randomized trial. Eur Heart J 2005; 26: 1262–8.
28. Kastrati A, Mehilli J, Dirschinger J et al. Intracoronary stenting and angiographic results: strut thickness effect on restenosis outcome (ISAR-STEREO) trial. Circulation 2001; 103: 2816–21.
29. Ortolani P, Marzocchi A, Marrozzini C et al. Randomized comparative trial of a thin-strut bare metal cobalt-chromium stent versus a sirolimus-eluting stent for coronary revascularization. Catheter Cardiovasc Interv 2007; 69: 790–8.
30. Erbel R, Di Mario C, Bartunek J et al. Temporary scaffolding of coronary arteries with bioabsorbable magnesium stents: a prospective, non-randomised multicentre trial. Lancet 2007; 369: 1869–75.

CHAPTER 12

Coronary bypass graft imaging

CORONARY BYPASS GRAFT SURGERY

One of the therapeutic options in patients with symptomatic coronary artery disease is coronary artery bypass graft (CABG) surgery. Depleted myocardium is reperfused by a surgically inserted vessel distal to the obstruction. Various materials can be used, but most are either saphenous vein or internal mammary artery grafts (Figures 12.1 and 12.2). Saphenous veins are free grafts that require surgical anastomosis to the (ascending) aorta. The internal mammary arteries can also be used for grafting, and have a much higher long-term patency rate. Mobilization of the internal mammary artery is a delicate procedure and involves clipping of the intercostal side branches. Single attached grafts are only inserted into a single coronary artery, while sequential grafts are inserted into two or more coronary artery branches. Up to 10% of grafts become occluded during the perioperative period[1]. After 10 years occlusion rates of 59% and 17% have been reported for venous and arterial grafts, respectively[2]. Of patients who undergo bypass surgery, 40% will experience recurrence of symptoms within 6 years, and 25% of bypass grafts are found to be occluded at follow-up 5 years after surgery[3–6]. Patients who have undergone CABG in the past will be older, often present with co-morbidity, and have a higher prevalence of valvular heart disease and ventricular dysfunction. Compared with non-CABG patients they will have a higher incidence of complications during invasive procedures, including cardiac catheterizations, and may therefore benefit more from non-invasive coronary angiography.

GRAFT IMAGING

Compared with the coronary arteries grafts have a larger diameter, are less calcified, and are more stationary, which makes them easier to image by CT. To include the proximal grafts the range of the scan needs to be extended in a caudal direction. To avoid artifacts due to high-concentration contrast medium at the site of the left internal mammary artery (LIMA) take-off, injection of contrast from the right side is recommended. Additionally, there are other factors associated with post-CABG patients that complicate interpretation of the CT images (Table 12.1). Surgical material such as sutures, clips and markers may cause artifacts and interfere with the interpretation of the grafts (Figure 12.3). While radiopaque material at the aortic anastomosis site of a venous graft is useful to guide future catheterization procedures, it may cause significant artifacts on CT and hinder evaluation of the proximal graft. Additionally, sternal suture wires and vascular clips can complicate assessment of the graft by CT. Using four-slice CT the proximal part of the mammary artery was often not included (Figure 12.4). With a 4×1.0-mm detector collimation complete acquisition would require a breathing pause of up to 50 s. To image the entire mammary artery, either a wider detector collimation was selected, or a protocol with a caudocranial scan direction that permits continuation of breathing near the end of the acquisition. Using 16- and 64-slice technology neither of these concessions is needed, and the entire graft can be acquired at high resolution during a manageable breath-hold time (Figure 12.5).

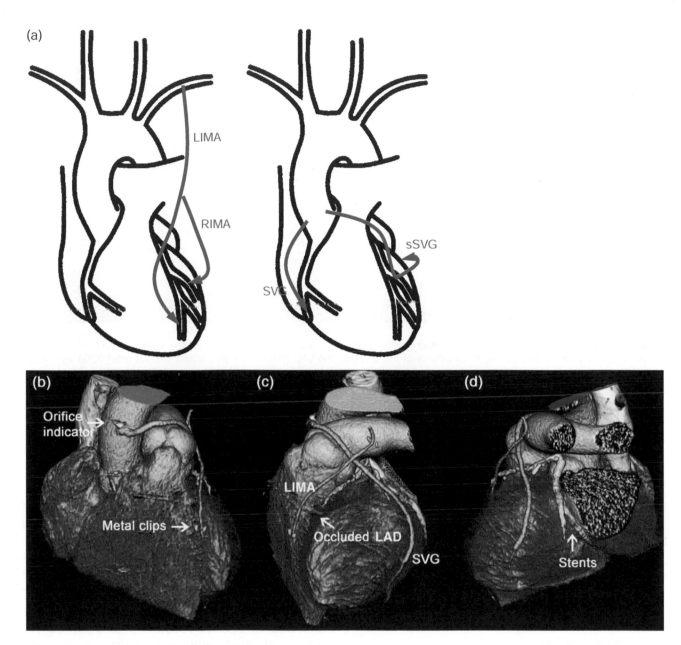

Figure 1 2 . 1a) Coronary bypass graft surgery. Both arterial and venous material can be used to bypass coronary lesions. The left internal mammary artery (LIMA) is often anastomosed to the left anterior descending coronary artery (LAD). The right internal mammary artery (RIMA) can be used similarly, or as a free graft with a proximal anastomosis to the aorta or the LIMA as a Y-graft. Venous grafts usually have a proximal anastomosis at the ascending aorta and one (saphenous vein graft, SVG) or several distal anastomoses (sSVG). Postsurgical revascularization: (b) volume-rendered anterior view; (c) anterolateral view; (d) lateral view LIMA on graft LAD, LIMA graft on right coronaryartery (RCA) (c), occluded LAD (Occl. LAD) (d) occluded venous graft (with stents) on circumflex and patent venous graft on posterolateral branch (arrow). SVG, saphenous vein graft.

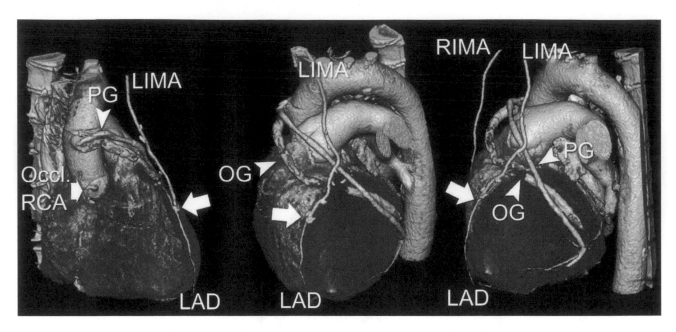

Figure 1 2 . Volume-rendered images showing a patent left internal mammary artery (LIMA) inserted into the left anterior descending coronary artery (LAD). Anastomosis of the LIMA on the LAD (arrow). An occluded venous graft (OG) with several stents, a redo patent venous graft inserted into a marginal branch, and an occluded right coronary artery (Occl. RCA) are also visualized. The right internal mammary artery (RIMA) is in situ. PG, patent graft.

T ble 1 2 . CT challenges in postsurgical patients

Population

Age and co-morbidity

Diffuse atherosclerotic disease

More frequent arrhythmia

Intracorporal metal

Vascular clips

Graft anastomosis indicator

Sternal sutures

Stents

Pacemaker and intracorporal defibrillator wires

Interpretation

Diffusely calcified coronary artery disease

Significance of (chronic) graft occlusion

Hemodynamic significance of findings

DIAGNOSTIC ACCURACY AFTER BYPASS GRAFT SURGERY

CT has been used to assess graft patency for more than two decades. Previously, electron beam CT as well as single-slice CT yielded reasonable sensitivity for the detection of complete graft occlusion (Figure 12.6)[7–14]. This fast CT technology, nevertheless, lacked sufficient coverage and/or spatial resolution to visualize non-occlusive graft disease. Although coverage remained a challenge, four-slice MSCT demonstrated robust three-dimensional angiographic imaging of bypass grafts, and was able to detect graft stenosis (Table 12.2)[15–18]. Sixteen-slice CT allowed complete coverage of the entire graft, and almost 100% accuracy to assess occlusive and stenotic disease in the proximal graft and graft body, although assessment of the anastomosis site remained suboptimal (Figure 12.7)[19–24]. Assessment of the distal anastomosis site seems to have improved according to recent studies using 64-slice CT, which show sensitivity of 96–100% and specificity of 89–97% to detect

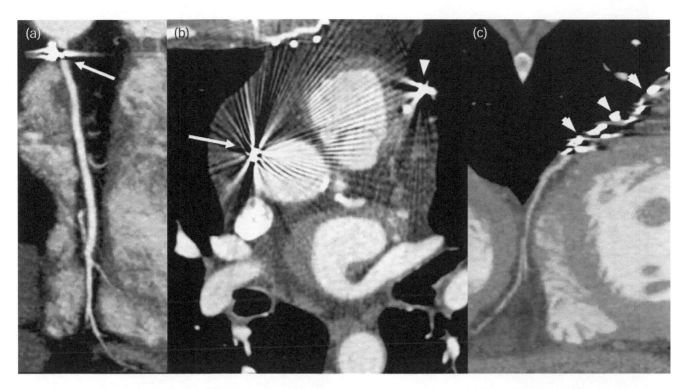

Figure 1 2 . 3 Artifacts caused by a metal indicator (arrow) (a) and (b) near the ostium of a venous graft to the right coronary artery, and surgical clips (arrowheads) (b) and (c) around a left internal mammary graft to the left anterior descending coronary artery.

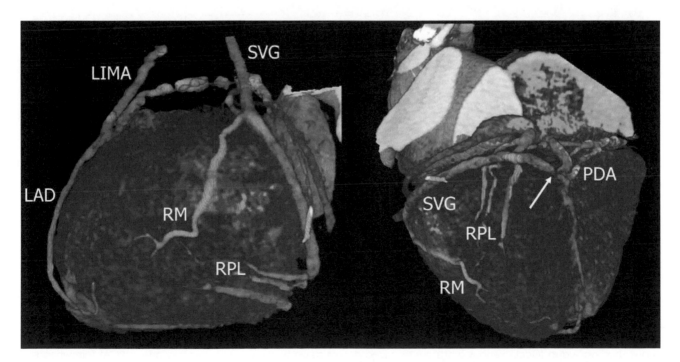

Figure 1 2 . 4 Four-slice CT angiography after bypass graft surgery. The left internal mammary artery graft (LIMA) is anastomosed to the left anterior descending coronary artery (LAD). A venous graft (SVG) is anastomosed to a marginal branch (RM), a posterolateral branch (RPL), and the posterior descending coronary branch (PDA). The last graft segment is significantly stenosed (arrow).

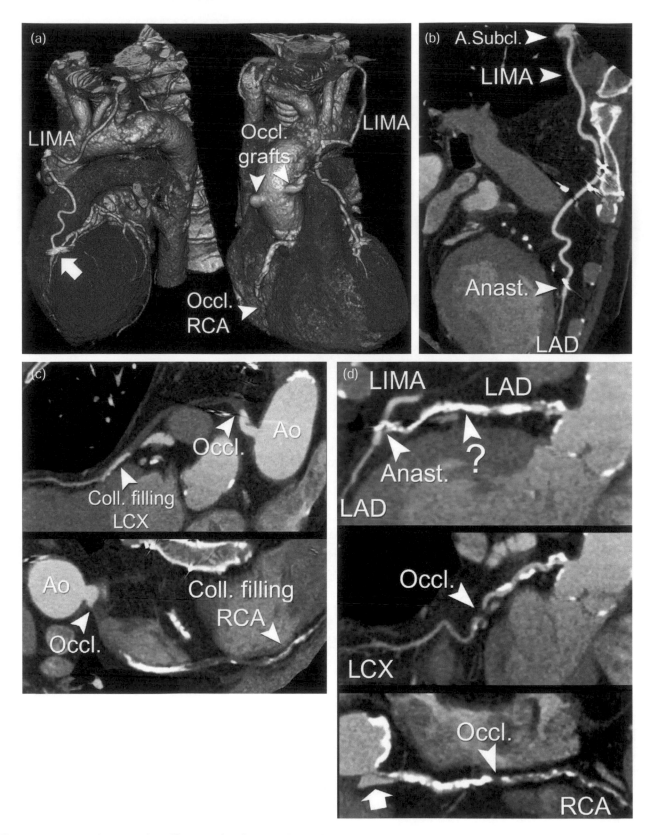

Figure 1 25. (a) Volume-rendered images showing a patent left internal mammary artery (LIMA) inserted into the left anterior descending coronary artery (LAD). However, the presence of a surgical clip precludes reliable visualization of the anastomosis (arrow). Two occluded (Occl.) venous grafts are visualized as well as an occluded right coronary artery (RCA) (arrowheads). (b) Curved multiplanar reconstructed image showing the LIMA and distal filling of the LAD. (c) Curved multiplanar reconstructed images of the occluded venous grafts (arrowheads) and collateral (Coll.) filling of the circumflex coronary artery (LCX) (upper panel) and right coronary artery (lower panel). (d) Curved multiplanar reconstructed images of the LAD (upper panel), LCX (middle panel), and RCA (lower panel). The occlusions within the non-calcified areas of the LCX and RCA are clearly visualized, whereas extensive calcification of the LAD precludes reliable evaluation of the coronary lumen (question mark). The arrow indicates the presence of an aneurysm of the RCA. Ao, aorta; A. Subcl, arteria sublavia; Anast, anastomosis.

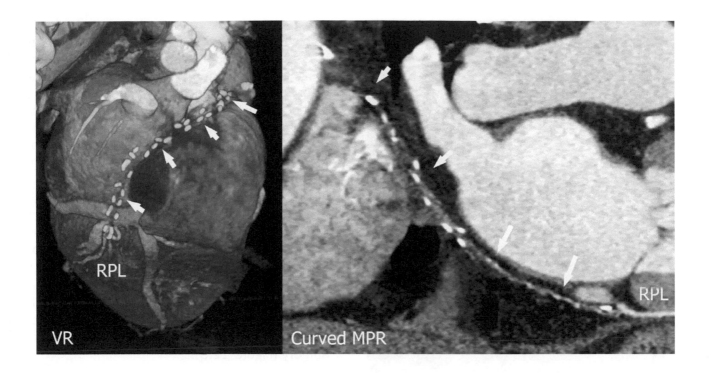

Figure 1 2 . Occluded free arterial graft (right internal mammary artery) from the aorta to the posterolateral branch (RPL) of the right coronary artery.

T ble 1 2 . Diagnostic accuracy of four-, 16-, and 64-slice CT

Study	CT slices/ detectors (n)	N	Graft type Arterial (n)	Venous (n)	Total occlusion Excluded (%)	Sensitivity (%)	Specificity (%)	Stenosis (50– 9%) Excluded (%)	Sensitivity (%)	Specificity (%)
Ropers et al[15]	4	65	43	162	0	97	98	38	75	92
Yoo et al*[16]	4	42	70	55	0	98	100			
Nieman et al[17†]	4	24	26	60	0	100	98	9	50	91
					5	94	98	5	86	93
Marano et al[18]	4	57	95	27	0	93	98	33	80	96
Schlosser et al[19]	16	51	40	91	6	100	100	26	67	95
Martuscelli et al[20]	16	96	85	166	13	100	100	0	90	100
Burgstahler et al[21‡]	16	13	11	32				5	100	93
Salm et al[22‡]	16	25	14	53				9	100	100
Anders et al[23†]	16	32	20	74	0	100	98	22	80	85
								16	82	88
Stauder et al[24‡]	16	20	16	34				12	98	95
Pache et al[25‡]	64	31	23	73				6	98	89
Malagutti et al[26]	64	52	45	64	0	96	100	0	100	94
Ropers et al[27]	64	50	37	101	0	100	100	0	100	94
Meyer et al[28‡]	64	138	147	259				2	97	97

*Only detection of total occlusion; readings by two observers; ᵠcombined results for graft occlusion and stenosis.

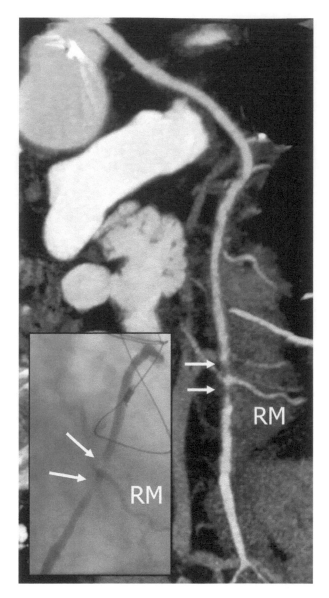

Figure 1 2 . Sequential venous graft with stenotic disease proximal and distal (arrows) to the anastomosis with a marginal branch (RM).

and accuracy to detect obstructive disease (Table 12.3)[17]. Assessment of the coronary arteries is complicated by diffuse, calcified atherosclerosis in older patients with advanced coronary artery disease. The coronary assessment can be divided in three: (1) coronary run-offs, the distal coronary branches that are supplied by the grafts; (2) non-grafted coronary branches, coronary arteries that were not revascularized during previous surgery; and (3) proximal branches of grafts that are significantly obstructed, which may be potential targets for percutaneous re-intervention. The coronary arteries were ignored in the largest 16-slice CT studies in post-CABG patients. New attempts with 64-slice CT show improved assessability of the coronary arteries[26,27]. Nevertheless, interpretability remains more challenging in these patients compared with patients without previous bypass graft surgery (Figure 12.9).

CLINICAL VALUE OF CT AFTER BYPASS GRAFT SURGERY

Ischemic symptoms in patients after bypass surgery can be caused by obstructive bypass graft disease or by progression of disease in the native coronary arteries. In fact, 5 years after bypass surgery, progression of coronary artery disease is more likely to be the cause of symptoms than is graft disease. Therefore, evaluation cannot be limited to the bypass grafts but should also include the coronary arteries. Malagutti et al found that there was limited accuracy for finding any relevant distal run-off disease (87%) or non-grafted coronary artery disease (83%); however, they were able to identify the obstructive lesion in any graft or coronary artery in the vast majority of cases (98% (CI 94–100%)), compared with invasive coronary angiography[26].

However, finding a significantly stenosed lesion, detected by either invasive or non-invasive angiography, does not automatically imply myocardial ischemia. Grafts may occlude without symptoms, for example in the presence of competitive flow via the native coronary artery (Figure 12.10). Alternatively, extensive collateral vascularization may have developed in these

any graft disease[25–28]. Because of their larger diameter, stented grafts are usually better assessable than stented coronary arteries (Figure 12.8).

ASSESSMENT OF THE CORONARY ARTERIES AFTER CORONARY ARTERY BYPASS GRAFT

Initial attempts to assess the coronary arteries by four-slice CT demonstrated poor interpretability

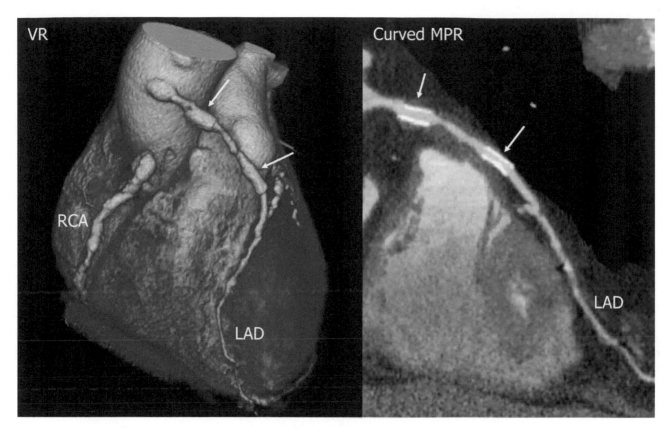

Figure 1 28. Venous graft anastomosed to the left anterior descending coronary artery (LAD), containing two stents (arrows). Despite the presence of diffuse graft disease, patency of both stents can be established.

T ble 1 2 . Detection of coronary artery stenosis (>50%) by CT after coronary artery bypass graft

Study	CT slices/detectors (n)	n	Excluded (%)	Sensitivity (%)	Specificity (%)	Accuracy (%)
Nieman et al[17]*	4	24	31	90	75	83
			34	79	72	76
Stauder et al[24]	16	20	31	92	77	87
Salm et al[22]	16	25	26	100	89	93
Malagutti, et al[26]	64	52	0	98	71	81
Ropers et al[27]	64	50	9	86	76	78

*Readings by two observers.

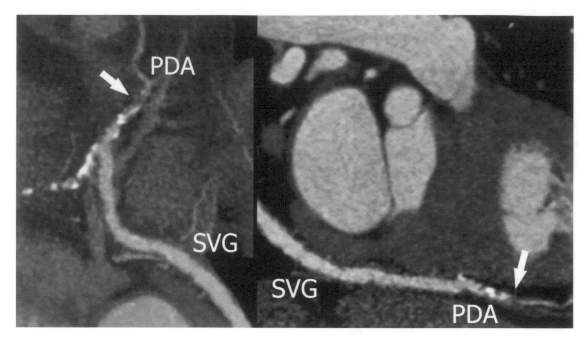

Figure 1 2 9 Coronary run-off disease. Distal to the venous graft anastomosis the posterior descending coronary artery PDA branch shows obstructive disease. SVG, saphenous vein graft.

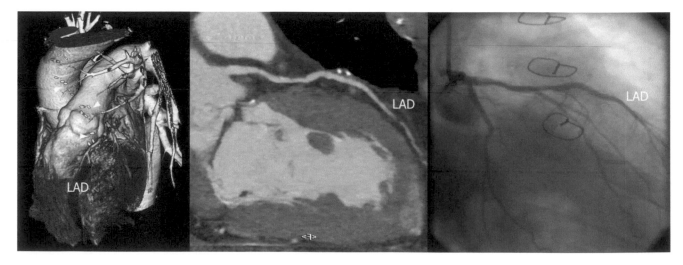

Figure 1 2 . 1 0 Occlusion of a left internal mammary graft (arrowheads indicating the surgical clips) to a left anterior descending coronary artery (LAD) without significant stenosis.

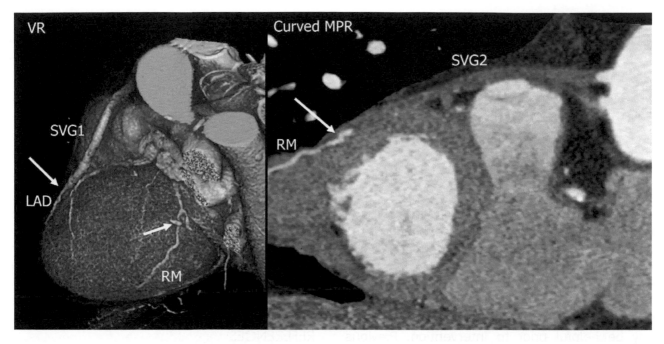

Figure 1 21.1 Separate venous grafts have been anastomosed (arrows) to the left anterior descending coronary artery (SVG1, LAD) and a marginal branch (SVG2, RM). Despite occlusion of the latter graft, the marginal branch is opacified, seemingly by collaterals.

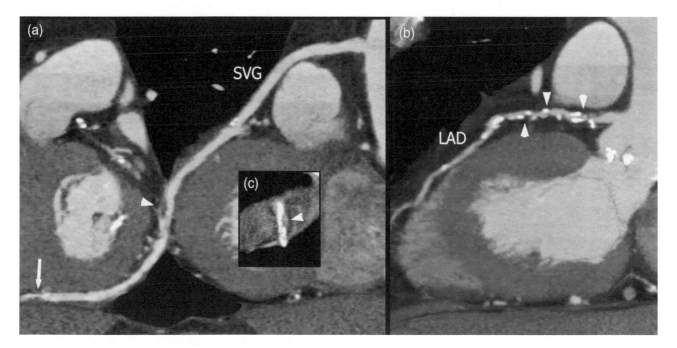

Figure 1 21.2 Diffuse disease after coronary artery bypass graft. The venous graft with several anastomoses along the postero-lateral wall of the left ventricle is moderately stenosed (arrowhead) (a) and (c). The posterior descending coronary artery shows a moderate lesion just distal of the anastomosis (arrow) (a). The non-grafted left anterior descending coronary artery (LAD) shows diffuse, calcified disease (arrowheads (b).

Table 12. Clinical applications of cardiac CT after bypass artery graft (CABG) surgery

Symptoms shortly after CABG

Contraindications to invasive angiography (aortic disease, aortic valve endocarditis)

Unknown graft anatomy, or failure to selectively inject the graft during surgery

Atypical symptoms or decreased left ventricular function after CABG

Graft localization prior to (redo) thoracic surgery

cases of chronic coronary artery disease (Figure 12.11), which makes assessment of the hemodynamic significance of a detected lesion even more difficult (Figure 12.12).

One advantage of CT is that it allows visualization of the heart beyond the coronary/graft lumen. Knowledge of the obstructive pathology may be helpful prior to intervention. Previous myocardial infarction may be identified, and left ventricular function can be accurately quantified[22]. Another advantage of CT is the ability to visualize complex graft anatomy. This is particularly useful when information about previous surgery is incomplete, or unusual techniques were used. If redo CABG is considered, CT will reveal the location and proximity of functioning graft to the sternum. If percutaneous reintervention is considered, CT may be helpful to assess native coronary artery disease, i.e. the nature and length of the occlusion, as an alternative target for stenting[26].

In some situations the assessment by CT can be limited to the bypass grafts, for example to evaluate surgical success early after the procedure[29]. Routine use of CT to image the bypass grafts, including left ventricular function, prior to scheduled catheter angiography has been suggested. This approach could reduce overall contrast dose and shorten catheterization procedure time (not radiation dose). A number of (developing) clinical indications of CT angiography after CABG are summarized in Table 12.4.

CONCLUSION

The accuracy of CT angiography to detect obstructive graft disease is almost 100%.

Comprehensive post-bypass surgery evaluation should also include the assessment of the native coronary arteries, which may prove challenging as a result of advanced, diffuse coronary artery disease.

REFERENCES

1. Bryan AJ, Angelini GD. The biology of saphenous vein occlusion: etiology and strategies for prevention. Curr Opin Cardiol 1994; 9: 641–9.
2. Barner HB, Standeven JW, Reese J. Twelve-year experience with internal mammary artery for coronary artery bypass. J Thoracic Cardiovasc Surg 1985; 90: 668–75.
3. Cameron A, Davis KB, Rogers WJ. Recurrence of angina after coronary artery bypass surgery: predictors and progression (CASS Registry). J Am Coll Cardiol 1995; 26: 895–9.
4. Fitzgibbon GM, Kafka HP, Leach AJ et al. Coronary bypass graft fate and patient outcome: angiographic follow-up of 5065 grafts related to survival and reoperation in 1388 patients during 25 years. J Am Coll Cardiol 1996; 28: 616–26.
5. Christenson JT, Simonet F, Schmuziger M. Sequential vein bypass grafting: tactics and long-term results. Cardiovasc Surg 1998; 6: 389–97.
6. Dion R, Glineur D, Derouck D et al. Complementary saphenous grafting: long-term follow-up. J Thorac Cardiovasc Surg 2001; 122: 296–304.
7. Bateman TM, Gray RJ, Whiting JS et al. Cine computed tomographic evaluation of aortocoronary bypass graft patency. J Am Coll Cardiol 1986; 8: 693–8.
8. Bateman TM, Gray RJ, Whiting JS et al. Prospective evaluation of ultrafast cardiac computed tomography for determination of coronary bypass graft patency. Circulation 1987; 75: 1018–24.
9. Stanford W, Brundage BH, MacMillan R et al. Sensitivity and specificity of assessing coronary bypass graft patency with ultrafast computed tomography: results of a multicenter study. J Am Coll Cardiol 1988; 12: 1–7.
10. Achenbach S, Moshage W, Ropers D. Non-invasive, three-dimensional visualization of coronary artery bypass grafts by electron beam tomography. Am J Cardiol 1997; 79: 856–61.
11. Ha JW, Cho SY, Shim WH et al. Non-invasive evaluation of coronary artery bypass graft patency using threedimensional angiography obtained with contrast-enhanced electron beam CT. Am J Roentgenol 1999; 172: 1055–9.
12. Lu B, Dai RP, Jing BL et al. Evaluation of coronary artery bypass graft patency using three-dimensional reconstruction and flow study on electron beam tomography. J Comput Assist Tomogr 2000; 24: 663–70.

13. Engelmann MG, von Smekal A, Knez A et al. Accuracy of spiral computed tomography for identifying arterial and venous coronary graft patency. Am J Cardiol 1997; 80: 569–74.
14. Tello R, Costello P, Ecker C, Hartnell G. Spiral CT evaluation of coronary artery bypass graft patency. J Comput Assist Tomogr 1993; 17: 253–9.
15. Ropers D, Ulzheimer S, Wenkel E et al. Investigation of aortocoronary artery bypass grafts by multislice computed tomography with electrocardiographic-gated image reconstruction. Am J Cardiol 2001; 88: 792–5.
16. Yoo KJ, Choi D, Choi BW et al. The comparison of the graft patency after coronary artery bypass grafting using coronary angiography and multislice computed tomography. Eur J Cardiothorac Surg 2003; 24: 86–91.
17. Nieman K, Pattynama PMT, Rensing BJ et al. CT angiographic evaluation of post-CABG patients: assessment of grafts and coronary arteries. Radiology 2003; 229: 749–56.
18. Marano R, Storto ML, Maddestra N, Bonomo L. Non-invasive assessment of coronary artery bypass graft with retrospectively ECG-gated four-row multi-detector spiral computed tomography. Eur Radiol 2004; 14: 1353–62.
19. Schlosser T, Konorza T, Hunold P et al. Noninvasive visualization of coronary artery bypass grafts using 16-detector row computed tomography. J Am Coll Cardiol 2004; 44: 1224–9.
20. Martuscelli E, Romagnoli A, D'Eliseo A et al. Evaluation of venous and arterial conduit patency by 16-slice spiral computed tomography. Circulation 2004; 110: 3234–8.
21. Burgstahler C, Beck T, Kuettner A et al. Non-invasive evaluation of coronary artery bypass grafts using 16-row multi-slice computed tomography with 188 ms temporal resolution. Int J Cardiol 2006; 106: 244–9.
22. Salm LP, Bax JJ, Jukema JW et al. Comprehensive assessment of patients after coronary artery bypass grafting by 16-detector-row computed tomography. Am Heart J 2005; 150: 775–81.
23. Anders K, Baum U, Schmid M et al. Coronary artery bypass graft (CABG) patency: assessment with high-resolution sub-millimeter 16-slice multidetector-row computed tomography (MDCT) versus coronary angiography. Eur J Radiol 2006; 57: 336–44.
24. Stauder NI, Kuttner A, Schroder S et al. Coronary artery bypass grafts: assessment of graft patency and native coronary artery lesions using 16-slice MDCT. Eur Radiol 2006; 16: 2512–20.
25. Pache G, Saueressig U, Frydrychowicz A et al. Initial experience with 64-slice cardiac CT: non-invasive visualization of coronary artery bypass grafts. Eur Heart J 2006; 27: 976–80.
26. Malagutti P, Nieman K, Meijboom WB et al. Use of 64-slice CT in symptomatic patients after coronary bypass surgery: evaluation of grafts and coronary arteries. Eur Heart J 2007; 28: 1879–85.
27. Ropers D, Pohle FK, Kuettner A et al. Diagnostic accuracy of noninvasive coronary angiography in patients after bypass surgery using 64-slice spiral computed tomography with 330-ms gantry rotation. Circulation 2006; 114: 2334–41.
28. Meyer TS, Martinoff S, Hadamitzky M et al. Improved noninvasive assessment of coronary artery bypass grafts with 64-slice computed tomographic angiography in an unselected patient population. J Am Coll Cardiol 2007; 49: 946–50.
29. Vernhet-Kavocsik H, Battistella P, Demaria R et al. Early post-operative assessment of coronary artery bypass graft patency and anatomy: value of contrast-enhanced 16-MDCT with retrospectively ECG-gated reconstructions. AJR Am J Roentgenol 2006; 186: 395–400.

CHAPTER 13

Pre-percutaneous coronary intervention assessment: chronic total occlusions and magnetic navigation

Percutaneous coronary intervention (PCI) of coronary stenoses has undergone dramatic evolution since its inception in 1977 and has become the dominant method of coronary revascularization in contemporary practice[1,2]. Coronary angioplasty was initially limited to patients with single-vessel disease with a single, discrete, non-calcified, proximal stenosis[3,4]. Remarkable improvements in techniques and technology have resulted in an enormous expansion in patient selection criteria. As a result, an increasing number of PCIs carried out today involve patients with increased risk of future cardiovascular complications and/or complex lesion morphology[5-7].

Complex lesion morphology can be defined as lesions anticipated to pose problems in terms of accessing, delivering a device to, or traversing the lesion. Chronic total occlusions (CTO), generally defined as complete obstructions of coronary arteries that are more than 3 months old, are regarded as one of the most complex lesion subtypes in contemporary PCI practice. A CTO is present in up to 52% of patients found to have significant coronary artery disease (defined as 70% or more diameter stenosis) on diagnostic catheterization[8]. Because of its procedural complexity, PCI still faces a not insignificant risk of failure in this lesion subtype and as a result many of the patients are managed with either medical therapy or referred directly for coronary bypass graft surgery. Despite the development of new devices and techniques, even in those patients selected to be suitable for PCI, published success rates have remained unchanged in recent years, averaging around 70%[9]. Before embarking on a potentially long procedure that can be costly and expose the operator and the patient to higher radiation doses, it would be beneficial to select carefully those CTO patients in whom PCI is likely to succeed. Several angiographic features, such as older age (i.e. 3 months or more) and length (i.e. more than 15 mm) of the occlusion, presence of bridging collaterals, and absence of a tapered segment at the entry point of the occlusion, have been identified as predictors for an unsuccessful percutaneous recanalization attempt[10] (Figures 13.1 and 13.2). However, in the presence of an occlusion it is difficult to ascertain the trajectory and length of the occluded segment. Furthermore, due to its purely luminographic properties the angiogram does not offer information on the tissue composition of the occluded vessel part (Figure 13.3). Conceptually, CT coronary angiography (CTCA) should be more informative than conventional coronary angiography (CCA) as it provides three-dimensional tomographic data and, thus, information regarding the plaque composition and course of the coronary arteries. To date, two studies have reported on the role of CTCA in predicting the outcome of attempted CTO recanalization and, therefore, identifying those patients most likely to benefit from attempted PCI. In both reports the presence of severe calcification identified on CTCA was an independent predictor of PCI failure[11,12]. The study by Mollet et al also found that the CTO lesion length could not be measured with CCA in a substantial number of cases (17%) and that the presence of a relatively long occlusion, i.e. more than 15 mm, on CTCA, was associated with higher PCI failure rate (Figure 13.4). Several reports have also suggested that CT images

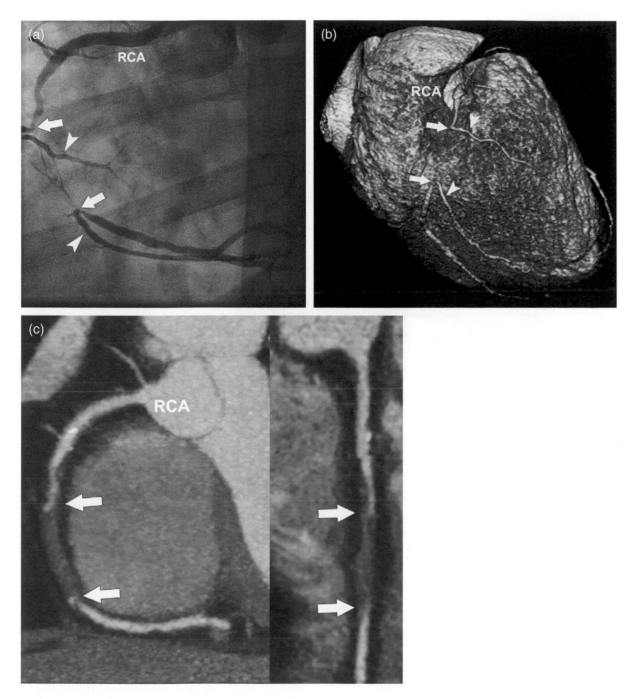

Figure 13.1 Invasive coronary angiography (a), volume-rendered image (b), and multiplanar reconstruction (c), showing chronic total occlusion of the right coronary artery(RCA). Note the non-calcified total occlusion. Arrows: proximal stump, distal stump. Arrowheads: proximal and distal side branch. Invasive coronary angiographic image corresponding with CT volume-rendered image.

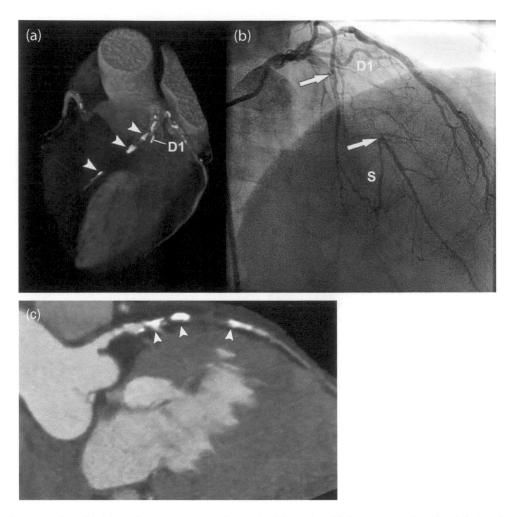

Figure 13.2 Volume-rendered (a), invasive coronary angiography (b), and multiplanar reconstruction (c), showing chronic total occlusion of the left anterior descending artery with severe calcification at the proximal and distal parts of the occluded segments. D1, first diagonal branch; septal branch; arrowheads, calcification; arrows, calcification.

could be helpful during the actual process of the PCI[13-15]. Since CTCA allows characterization of the length, course, and composition of the occluded coronary artery segment, it could serve as a guide for the interventional cardiologist. Thereby, the CT images may assist in the selection of a more targeted interventional strategy, for example the use of an ablative technique or very stiff penetrative wire in severely calcified occlusions, or may facilitate the operator steering the guidewire in the direction of the distal vessel beyond the occlusion.

Magnetic navigation represents a novel technology that has been introduced within the field of interventional cardiology with the aim of improving procedural success in coronary lesions with tortuous vessel anatomy and/or complex morphology. The magnet navigation system (MNS) consists of two permanent magnets that create a uniform magnetic field inside the chest of the patient and is integrated with a digital angiography system that provides the operator with a three-dimensional reconstructed image of the target vessel [16]. Using a computer interface

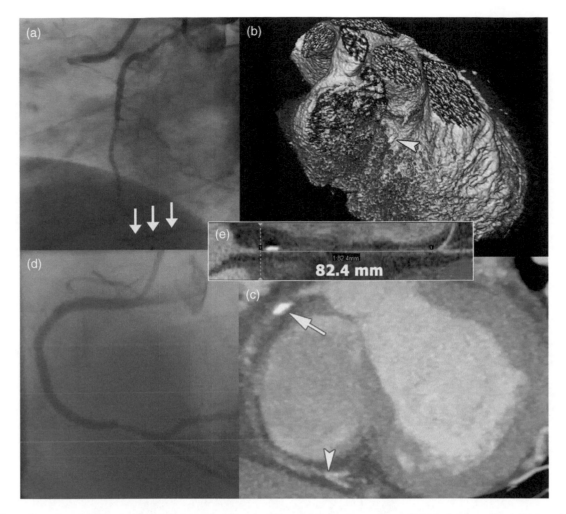

Figure 13.3 Chronic total occlusion of the proximal part of the right coronary artery (RCA). (a) Invasive bifemoral coronary angiography showing total occlusion of the proximal RCA and filling of the distal parts of the RCA by collaterals from the left anterior descending artery(arrows). (b) Volume-rendered image showing total occlusion of the RCA with a calcified RCA stump. (c) Multiplanar reconstruction showing total occlusion of the RCA. Arrow, calcification; arrowhead, filling of the distal part of the RCA. (d) Invasive coronary angiography post-stent implantation showing the total occluded vessel. (e) Total length of the occluded vessel segment is 82.4 mm.

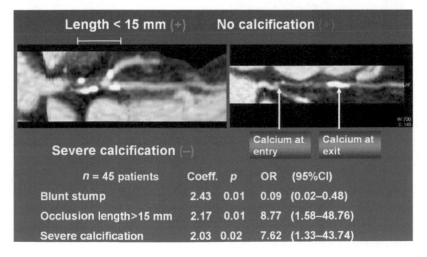

n = 45 patients	Coeff.	p	OR	(95%CI)
Blunt stump	2.43	0.01	0.09	(0.02–0.48)
Occlusion length>15 mm	2.17	0.01	8.77	(1.58–48.76)
Severe calcification	2.03	0.02	7.62	(1.33–43.74)

Figure 13.4 Chronic total occlusion predictors of success/failure in conventional and MSCT coronary angiogram.

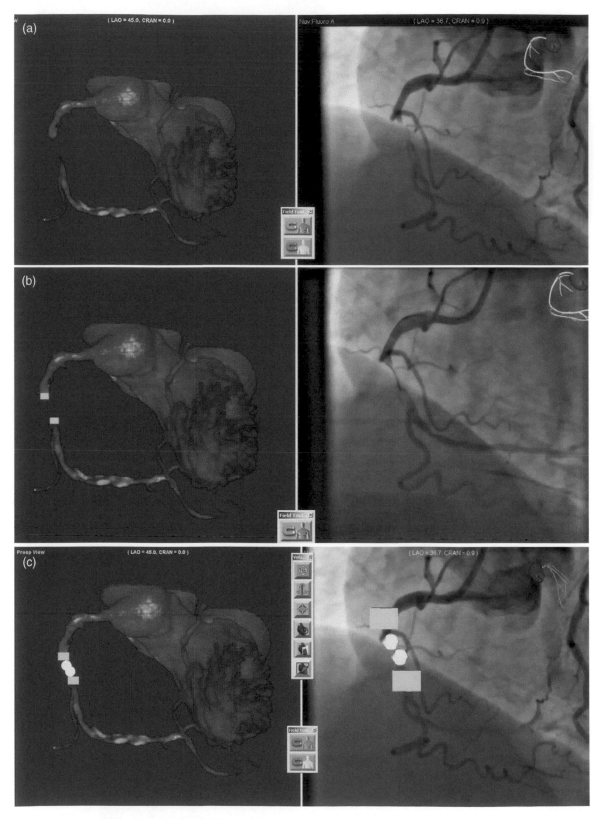

Figure 13.5 Fusion of CT images showing visualization of the ʋmissingʊsegment of the chronic total occlusion with fluoroscopy and creation of central line through missing segment. (A) Volume-rendered image of right coronary artery (left) with chronic total occlusion (missing segment). Corresponding invasive coronary angiography (right). (B) indication of proximal and distal stumps of occluded right coronary artery. (C)creation of center-line through missing segment.

system, the physician performing the PCI can manipulate the overall magnetic field vector, thus enabling the precise steering of the tip of a dedicated magnetically navigable guidewire through tortuous and angulated vessels into the distal vasculature. Interestingly, the MNS can integrate the DICOM (Digital Images and Communication in Medcine) images from a cardiac CT examination, which offers new opportunities when treating, for example, patients with CTOs[17]. Indeed, the ability to fuse the angiographic and CT data allows visualization of the 'missing angiographic segment' on the fluoroscopic screen (Figure 13.5). Furthermore, the magnetic-assisted wire manipulation allows precise steering and changing of the orientation of the guidewire tip according to the course of the vessel in the occlusion (Figure 13.6).

CONCLUSION

The field of interventional cardiology is moving towards the treatment of patients with complex coronary artery disease, often characterized by challenging lesion and vessel anatomical features. A preprocedural cardiac CT scan may provide useful information for selecting patients suitable for PCI of CTO or may be helpful for designing a dedicated therapeutic strategy. The integration of CT data in magnet navigation systems proves to be useful in patients with CTOs as it complements the angiographic information. Also, it may provide the operator with a three-dimensional vessel map, thereby offering the possibility of navigating the guidewire with a minimal amount of contrast and radiation.

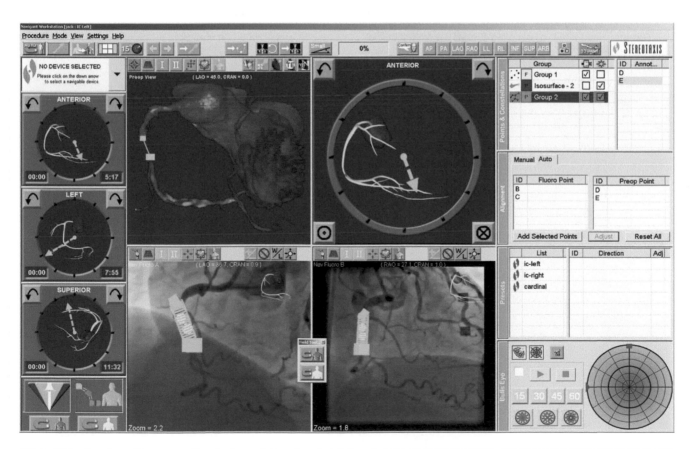

Figure 13.6 Steering of the magnetic wire through the chronic total occlusion based on the three-dimensional vector obtained by CT.

REFERENCES

1. Gruntzig A. Transluminal dilatation of coronary-artery stenosis. Lancet 1978; 1: 263.
2. Rosamond W, Flegal K, Friday G et al. Heart disease and stroke statistics–2007 update: a report from the American Heart Association Statistics Committee and Stroke Statistics Subcommittee. Circulation 2007; 115: e69–171.
3. Gruntzig AR, Senning A, Siegenthaler WE. Nonoperative dilatation of coronary-artery stenosis: percutaneous transluminal coronary angioplasty. N Engl J Med 1979; 301: 61–8.
4. Holmes DR Jr, Holubkov R, Vlietstra RE et al. Comparison of complications during percutaneous transluminal coronary angioplasty from 1977 to 1981 and from 1985 to 1986: the National Heart, Lung, and Blood Institute Percutaneous Transluminal Coronary Angioplasty Registry. J Am Coll Cardiol 1988; 12: 1149–55.
5. Srinivas VS, Brooks MM, Detre KM et al. Contemporary percutaneous coronary intervention versus balloon angioplasty for multivessel coronary artery disease: a comparison of the National Heart, Lung and Blood Institute Dynamic Registry and the Bypass Angioplasty Revascularization Investigation (BARI) study. Circulation 2002; 106: 1627–33.
6. Lemos PA, Serruys PW, van Domburg RT et al. Unrestricted utilization of sirolimus-eluting stents compared with conventional bare stent implan-tation in the "real world": the Rapamycin-Eluting Stent Evaluated At Rotterdam Cardiology Hospital (RESEARCH) registry. Circulation 2004; 109: 190–5.
7. Morrison DA, Sethi G, Sacks J et al. Percutaneous coronary intervention versus coronary artery bypass graft surgery for patients with medically refractory myocardial ischemia and risk factors for adverse outcomes with bypass: a multicenter, randomized trial. Investigators of the Department of Veterans Affairs Cooperative Study #385, the Angina With Extremely Serious Operative Mortality Evaluation (AWESOME). J Am Coll Cardiol 2001; 38: 143–9.
8. Christofferson RD, Lehmann KG, Martin GV et al. Effect of chronic total coronary occlusion on treatment strategy. Am J Cardiol 2005; 95: 1088–91.
9. Abbott JD, Kip KE, Vlachos HA et al. Recent trends in the percutaneous treatment of chronic total coronary occlusions. Am J Cardiol 2006; 97: 1691–6.
10. Puma JA, Sketch MH Jr, Tcheng JE et al. Percutaneous revascularization of chronic coronary occlusions: an overview. J Am Coll Cardiol 1995; 26: 1–11.
11. Mollet NR, Hoye A, Lemos PA et al. Value of preprocedure multislice computed tomographic coronary angiography to predict the outcome of percutaneous recanalization of chronic total occlusions. Am J Cardiol 2005; 95: 240–3.
12. Soon KH, Cox N, Wong A et al. CT coronary angiography predicts the outcome of percutaneous coronary intervention of chronic total occlusion. J Interv Cardiol 2007; 20: 359–66.
13. Soon KH, Selvanayagam JB, Cox N et al. Percutaneous revascularization of chronic total occlusions: review of the role of invasive and non-invasive imaging modalities. Int J Cardiol 2007; 116: 1–6.
14. Van Mieghem CA, van der Ent M, de Feyter PJ. Percutaneous coronary intervention for chronic total occlusions: value of preprocedural multislice CT guidance. Heart 2007; 93: 1492.
15. Yokoyama N, Yamamoto Y, Suzuki S et al. Impact of 16-slice computed tomography in percutaneous coronary intervention of chronic total occlusions. Catheter Cardiovasc Interv 2006; 68: 1–7.
16. Atmakuri SR, Lev EI, Alviar C et al. Initial experience with a magnetic navigation system for percutaneous coronary intervention in complex coronary artery lesions. J Am Coll Cardiol 2006; 47: 515–21.
17. Patterson MS, Schotten J, van Mieghem C et al. Magnetic navigation in percutaneous coronary intervention. J Interv Cardiol 2006; 19: 558–65.

CHAPTER 14

Coronary artery anomalies in the adult

Coronary artery anomalies are defined as abnormalities in the origin, course, or distribution of coronary arteries. They are a rare form of congenital heart disease that affects approximately 1% of the population [1-6]. They are often the cause of sudden sport-related death in the young.

ANATOMY

The majority of the coronary anomalies have an ectopic origin of the coronary artery and frequently have associated congenital heart defects including mitral valve prolapse, bicuspid aortic valve, tetralogy of Fallot, transposition of the great vessels, and aortic coarctation. Tetralogy of Fallot is associated with anomalous origin of the right coronary artery and transposition of the great arteries with a single coronary artery.

DIAGNOSIS OF CORONARY ANOMALIES

Traditionally the invasive technique of coronary angiography has been used to identify coronary anomalies. However, it is sometimes difficult to visualize the abnormal course and, in particular, the course of an anomalous artery running between the aorta and pulmonary trunk may be difficult and requires specific projections and skillful interpretation. Three-dimensional coronary image reconstruction, from data obtained with magnetic resonance imaging or CT, is extremely helpful and allows easy anatomical interpretation of the coronary anomalies [7-12]. Schmid et al investigated 35 patients with coronary anomalies [12]. The origin of all anomalous arteries and the exact course in all of the patients was correctly identified (Table 14.1). The anatomical identification of coronary anomalies with MSCT is shown to be relatively easy; however, it remains difficult to identify which individuals are actually at high risk of sudden death [13].

MALIGNANT CORONARY ANOMALY

Sudden death is often associated with two anomalies: (1) the left main artery and right coronary artery arising from the right aortic sinus, with the anomalous left main coronary artery coursing between the aorta and pulmonary trunk; and (2) the left main artery and right coronary artery originating from the left aortic sinus, with the anomalous right coronary artery coursing between the aorta and pulmonary trunk (Figures 14.1–14.4) [14].

Table 14.1 MSCT coronary anomalies. From reference 12

Origin of coronary anomaly	Number of patients
Right-sided origin left main	10
Right-sided origin left CX	10
Right-sided origin LAD	4
Left-sided origin RCA	6
Coronary fistula to pulmonary artery	4
Coronary fistula from CX to right atrium	1

CX, circumflex artery; LAD, left anterior descending artery; RCA, right coronary artery.

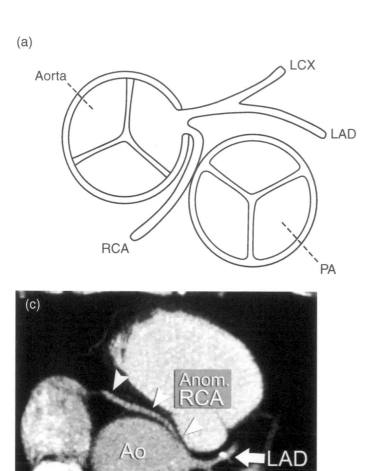

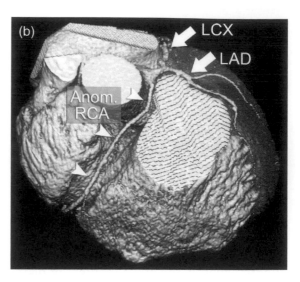

Figure 14.1 (a) Left main artery and right coronary artery (RCA)originating from the right aortic sinus. (b) Volume-rendered image showing anomalous RCA (Anom. RCA) originating from the left aortic sinus and coursing between the aorta (Ao) and pulmonary trunk. (c) Cross-sectional image showing abnormal origin of RCA from left aortic sinus and its course between aorta and pulmonary trunk. LCX, left circumflex artery; LAD, left anterior descending; PA, pulmonary artery.

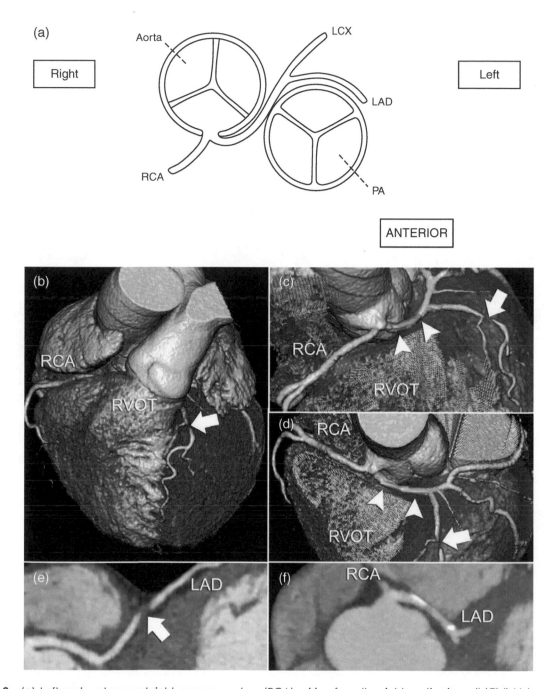

Figure 14.2 (a) Left main artery and right coronary artery (RCA) arising from the right aortic sinus. (b)Đ(d) Volume-rendered images showing left main artery and RCA arising from the right aortic sinus. The anomalous left main coronary artery courses between the aorta and pulmonary trunk (arrowheads). Note the severe lesion in left anterior descending (LAD) (arrow). (e) and (f) Multiplanar reconstructions showing left main coronary artery originating from right aortic sinus and coursing between the aorta and pulmonary trunk. Note the severe lesion in LAD (arrow). RVOT, right ventricle outflow track.

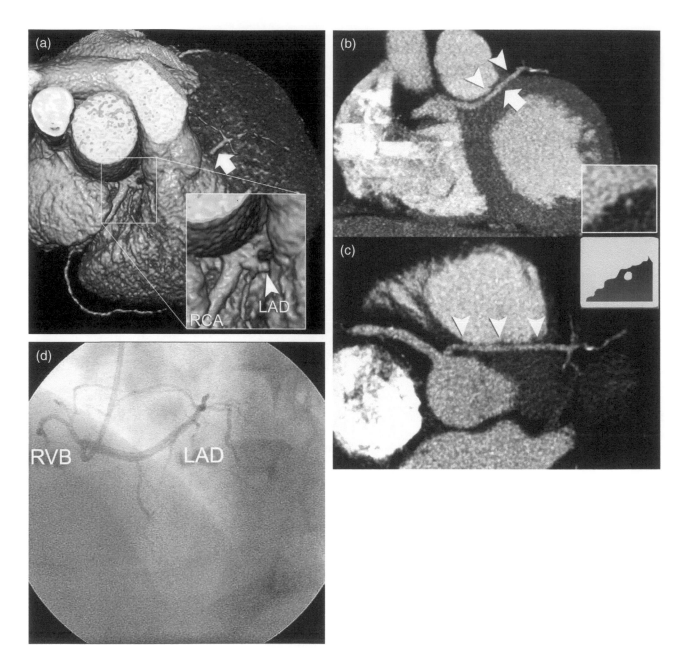

Figure 14.3 (a) Volume-rendered image showing the left main artery originating from the right aortic sinus and running between the aorta and pulmonary artery to the anterior left ventricle wall (arrow). (b) and (c) Multiplanar reconstructions showing the abnormal origin and course of the left main artery running between the aorta and pulmonary artery (arrowheads). (d) Corresponding invasive coronary angiogram. RCA, right coronary artery; LAD, left anterior descending; RVB, right ventricular branch.

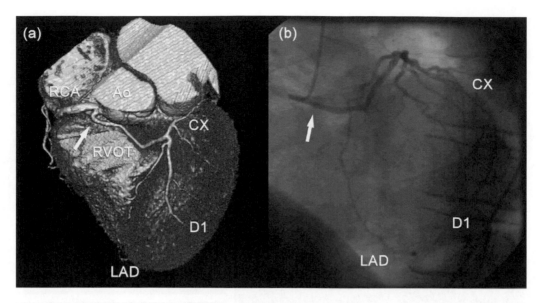

Figure 14.4 (a) Volume-rendered image showing the left main artery originating from the right aortic sinus and running between the aorta and pulmonary artery to the anterior left ventricle wall (arrow). (b) Corresponding invasive coronary angiogram. RCA, right coronary artery; Ao, Aorta; RVOT, right ventricular outflow tract; CX, circumflex coronary artery; L AD, left anterior descending coronary artery; D1, first diagonal.

BENIGN CORONARY ANOMALY

The majority of all coronary anomalies are benign and coincidental findings during coronar y angiography. One of the most frequently occurring anomalies is the left circumflex ar tery and right coronar y artery arising from the right aortic sinus. This anomaly is considered benign; however, awareness of this anomaly may be impor tant during cardiac surger y to institute appropriate m yocardial protection (Figures 14.5 and 14.6).

CORONARY ARTERY FISTULAE

Coronar y artery fistulae usually in volve the right coronary artery. The usual site of ter mination is in one or more low-pressure str uctures: right or left atrium, right ventricle, coronary sinus, pulmonary artery, or superior vena ca va. The fistulae appear as dilated (sometimes huge) tortuous communications betw een a coronar y artery and low-pressure cardiac str ucture (Figure 14.7–14.11).

CONCLUSION

Non-invasive CT scanning of the hear t allows correct identification of coronary anomalies and three-dimensional reconstr uction allows precise insight into the cour se of the coronar y anomalies to identify whether these anomalies are malignant or benign.

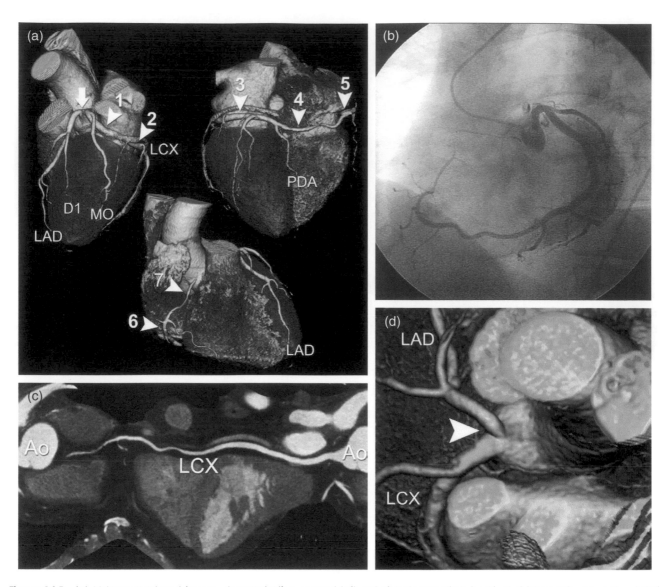

Figure 14.5 (a) Volume-rendered image demonstrating normal left anterior descending (LAD) and large left circumflex (LCX) (1) and (2) running over the diaphragm (3) to branch into a posterior descending artery (PDA) and running (4) and (5) further over the heart to end almost at the right aortic sinus (6) and (7). There is no right coronary artery. (b) Corresponding invasive coronary angiogram. (c) Curved multiplanar reconstruction demonstrating the course of the LCX from left aortic sinus to almost the right aortic sinus. (d) Volume-rendered image showing a separate ostium of the LAD and LCX. D1,first diagonal; MO, marginal obtuse.

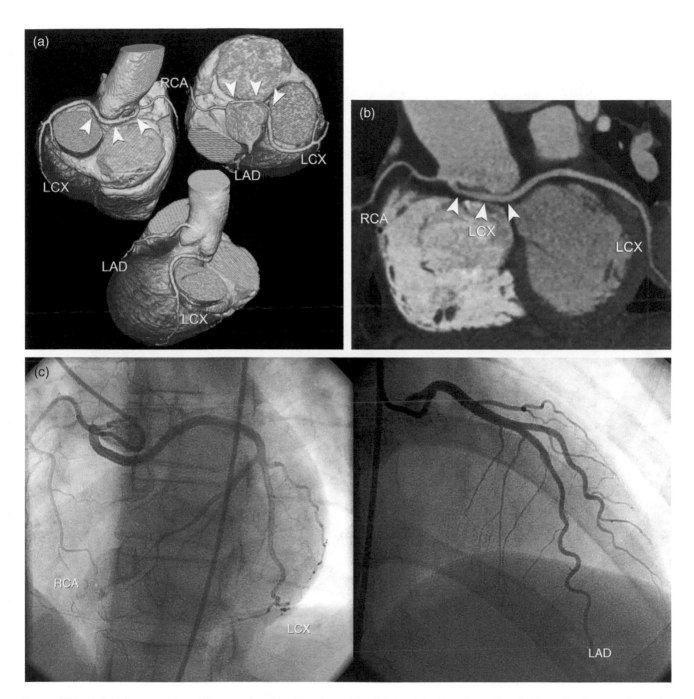

Figure 14.6 (a) Volume-rendered image showing left circumflex (LCX) originating from the right aortic sinus and running between the left atrium and aorta into the left atrioventricular groove. (b) Multiplanar reconstruction showing the L CX originating from the right aortic cusp and running to the left atrioventricular groove. (c) Corresponding invasive coronary angiograms. LAD, left anterior descending; RCA, right coronary artery.

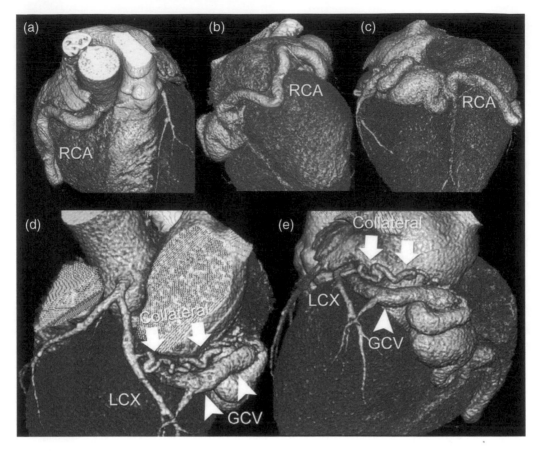

Figure 14.7 Volume-rendered images showing an enormous fistula from the right coronary artery (RCA) ending into the coronary sinus and a smaller fistula running from the left circumflex (LCX) to the coronary sinus. GCV, great cardiac vein.

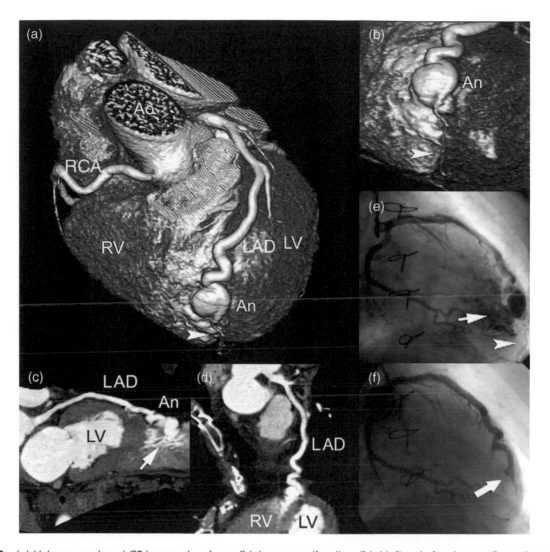

Figure 14.8 (a) Volume-rendered CT image showing a fistula connecting the distal left anterior descending artery (L AD) with the right ventricle (RV). (b) An aneurysmatic part of the LAD (An) and a hypoplastic distal segment can be seen (arrowhead). (c) and (d) CT images displaying the LAD throughout its course, ruling out significant lesions and ending in the RV where increased contrast enhancement can be seen (arrow). (e) Conventional coronary angiogram confirming the aneurysmatic part in the LAD with a hypoplastic distal segment (arrowhead) and its outflow in the right ventricle (RV) (arrow). (f) Conventional coronary angiogram showing the successful closure of the fistula revealing only a residual amount of contrast in the course of the former fistula (thick arrow).

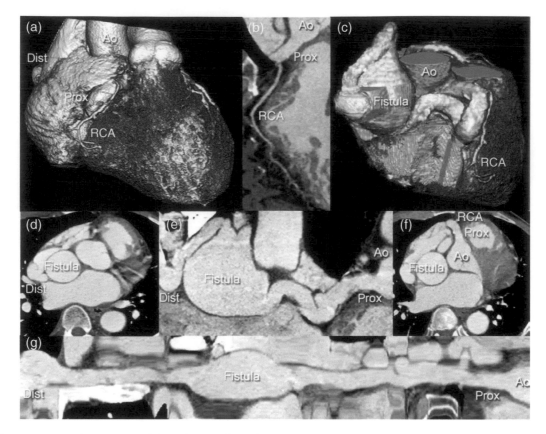

Figure 14.9 Volume-rendered image (a) and curved multiplanar reconstruction (b) showing the right coronary artery (RCA) originating from the proximal part of the fistula. (c) Removal of the right and left atria reveals the tortuous course of the fistula with the aneurysmatic dilatation beginning in the right sinus of Valsalva and ending in the right atria. (d) and (f) Axial slices showing the distal (d) and proximal (f) segments. Curved multiplanar reconstruction (e) and vessel-view (g) post-processing techniques showing the entire trajectory of the fistula. Ao, aorta; Prox, proximal part fistula; Dist, distal part fistula.

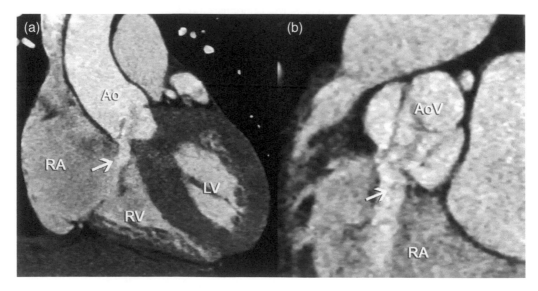

Figure 14.10 (a) Multiplanar CT image of a young woman with a bicuspid aortic valve showing a congenital fistula connecting from the aorta (Ao) to the right atrium (RA) (arrow). AoV, aortic valve; RV right ventricle; LV, left ventricle. (b) Blow-up of congenital fistula connecting aorta with right atrium.

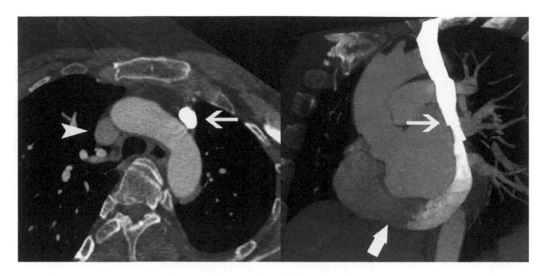

Figure 14.11 Multiplanar CT images of a patient with both a right (arrowhead) and left superior vena cava (arrow). The contrast was injected into the left arm. Note that the left superior vena cava drains into a dilated coronary sinus (thick arrow).

REFERENCES

1. Topaz O, DeMarchena EJ, Perin E et al. Anomalous coronary arteries: angiographic findings in 80 patients. Int J Cardiol 1992; 34: 129–38.
2. Yamanaka O, Hobbs RE. Coronary artery anomalies in 126,595 patients undergoing coronary arteriography. Cathet Cardiovasc Diagn 1990; 21: 28–40.
3. Taylor AJ, Rogan KM, Virmani R. Sudden cardiac death associated with isolated congenital coronary artery anomalies. J Am Coll Cardiol 1992; 20: 640–7.
4. Maron BJ, Shirani J, Poliac LC et al. Sudden death in young competitive athletes. Clinical, demographic, and pathological profiles. JAMA 1996; 276: 199–204.
5. Roberts WC. Major anomalies of coronary arterial origin seen in adulthood. Am Heart J 1986; 111: 941–63.
6. Taylor AJ, Virmani R. Coronary artery anomalies. Section 2, Chapter 2, page 201–11. In: Cardiology. eds Crawford MH, DiMarco JP. Paulus WJ. Edinburgh, London, Newyork, Oxford, Philadelphia, St Louis, Sydney, Toronto: Mosby, 2004.
7. Ropers D, Moshage W, Daniel WG, Jessl J, Gottwik M, Achenbach S. V isualization of coronary artery anomalies and their anatomic course by contrast-enhanced electron beam tomography and three-dimensional reconstruction. Am J Cardiol 2001; 87: 193–7.
8. Budoff MJ, Lu B, Shinbane JS et al. Methodology for improved detection of coronary stenoses with computed tomographic angiography. Am Heart J 2004; 148: 1085–90.
9. Shi H, Aschoff AJ, Brambs HJ, Hoffmann MH. Multislice CT imaging of anomalous coronary arteries. Eur Radiol 2004; 14: 2172–81.
10. Datta J, White CS, Gilkeson RC et al. Anomalous coronary arteries in adults: depiction at multi-detector row CT angiography. Radiology 2005; 235: 812–18.
11. Schmitt R, Froehner S, Brunn J et al. Congenital anomalies of the coronary arteries: imaging with contrast-enhanced, multidetector computed tomography. Eur Radiol 2005; 15: 1110–21.
12. Schmid M, Achenbach S, Ludwig J et al. V isualization of coronary artery anomalies by contrast-enhanced multi-detector row spiral computed tomography. Int J Cardiol 2006; 111: 430–5.
13. Maron BJ. Sudden death in young athletes. N Engl J Med 2003; 349:1064–75.
14. Angelini P. Coronary artery anomalies: an entity in search of an identity. Circulation 2007; 115: 1296–305.

Cardiac masses, intracardiac thrombi, and pericardial abnormalities

Cardiac masses, intracardiac thrombi, and pericardial abnormalities are infrequently occurring abnormalities, which can be identified b y CT cardiac imaging [1-4].

INTRACARDIAC TUMORS
(Figures 15.1–15.4)

Atrial myxomas account for 50% of intracardiac tumors. They are usually located in the left atrium attached to the atrial septum at the fossa o valis and are often pedunculated. Rhabdom yomas, fibromas, and lipomas are less frequently occurring benign cardiac tumor s. Metastatic tumor s most frequently arise from melanomas and lung and breast carcinomas. Intracavitary tumor masses appear as filling defects within the contrast-filled heart chambers, or are seen as filling deformities of the cardiac ca vities.

INTRACARDIAC THROMBI
(Figures 15.5–15.7)

Intracardiac thrombi are usually seen as filling defects within the contrast-filled cardiac chambers. In the left ventricle the y are usually located at the site of an infarcted m yocardium most frequently in the apex of the left ventricle following a large anterior wall myocardial infarction. Usually the thrombus is mural, but sometimes ma y be pedunculated. Long-standing thrombi can be calcified. The left atrial appendage is another frequently occurring site of intracardiac thrombus, in particular, in patients with mitral stenosis and atrial fibrillation.

PERICARDIAL ABNORMALITIES
(Figures 15.8 and 15.9)

The pericardium can usually be seen as a 1–2-mm thick, linear low-density structure lying between the mediastinal fat ventrally and the epicardial fat dor sally. Constrictive pericarditis causes a thick ening of the pericardium, which may be localized or diffuse and is often associated with tuberculosis, tumor infiltration, or infection. The thickened pericardium may cause constriction of the m yocardium which hamper s diastolic left ventricular filling. This should be differentiated from restrictive cardiomyopathy where the pericardium is nor mal.

Pericardial effusion, diffusely located, small in amounts or as massive fluid accumulation, is most readily seen on CT imaging.

Pericardial cysts are unusual but readily identifiable by CT because they are filled with low-density fluid that has an attenuation value (HU) similar to water.

Benign and malignant pericardial tumor s are rare.

CONCLUSION

MSCT is a useful, non-invasive technique for the evaluation of intracardiac masses, intracardiac thrombi, and pericardial disease.

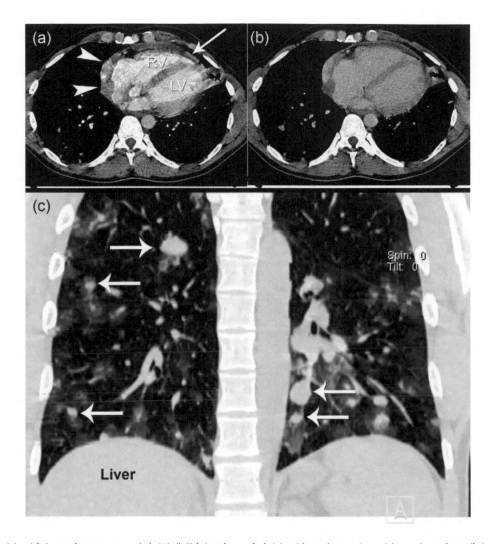

Figure 15.1 Right atrial angiosarcoma. (a) Wall thickening of right atrium (arrowheads) and pericardial effusion (arrow). (b) Delayed phase of enhancement. (c) Long metastases (arrows). RV, right ventricle, LV, left ventricle.

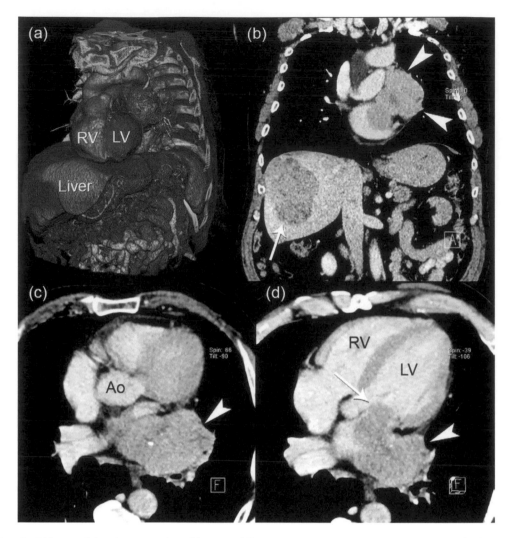

Figure 15.2 Carcinoid tumor. (a) Volume-rendered image of thorax and upper abdomen showing carcinoid tumor in right liver lobe and left atrium. (b) Volume-rendered image of carcinoid tumor in liver (arrow) and large tumor in left atrium (arrowheads). (c) and (d) Volume-rendered images of large carcinoid tumor in left atrium (arrowhead), almost totally occupying the left atrium, and bulging through the mitral valve (arrow). RV, right ventricle; LV, left ventricle.

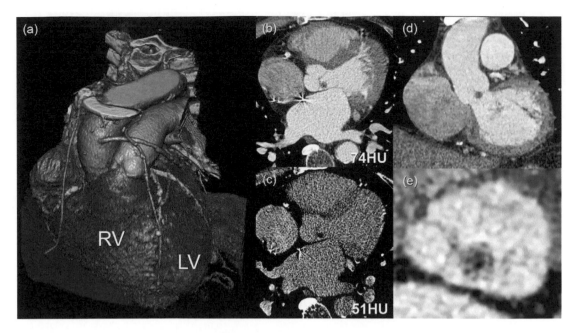

Figure 15.3 Aortic valve fibroelastoma. (a) Volume-rendered image of the heart showing venous bypass graft with anastomosis on left circumflex artery and left internal mammary artery with anastomosis on left anterior descending artery. (b), (c), and (d) Volume-rendered image of round filling defect in left aortic sinus attached to aortic valve. (e) Volume-rendered image enlargement showing filling defect. RV, right ventricle; LV, left ventricle.

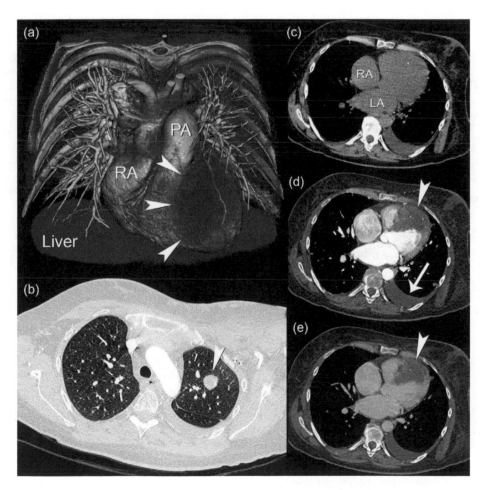

Figure 15.4 Breast carcinoma with metastasis in heart. (a) Volume-rendered image with metastasis of right and left ventricle (arrowheads). (b) Volume-rendered image of lung metastasis (arrowhead). (c), (d), and (e) Volume-rendered image of enormous filling defect in right and left ventricle (arrowheads) and pleural effusion (arrows). RA, right atrium; PA, pulmonary artery; LA, left atrium.

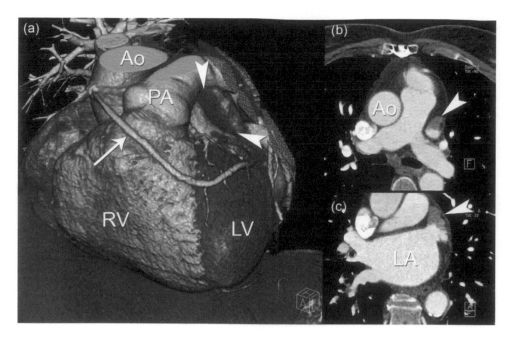

Figure 15.5 Left atrial thrombus. (a) Volume-rendered image showing venous bypass graft running from aorta (Ao) to left anterior descending, first diagonal and left circumflex (arrow). Left atrial appendage (arrowheads). (b) and (c) Volume-rendered image of filling defect of part of left atrial appendage (arrowheads). RV, right ventricle; LV, left ventricle; PA, pulmonary artery; LA, left atrium.

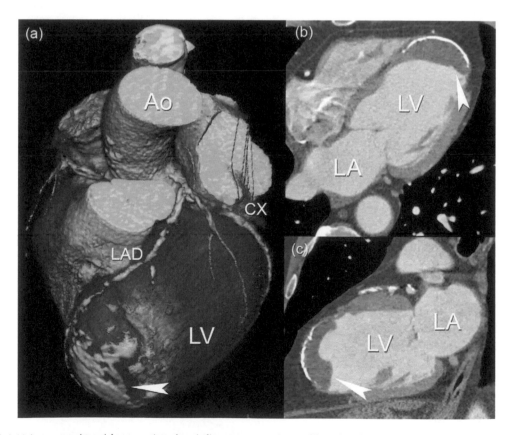

Figure 15.6 (a) Volume-rendered image showing left coronary artery with extensive coronary calcifications. Left ventricular apex is enlarged and calcified (arrowhead). (b) and (c) Volume-rendered image of extensive filling defect of apex of the left ventricle (LV) caused by organized thrombus (arrowheads). Note severe calcification of apex. LAD, left anterior descending; LCX, left circumflex; Ao, aorta; LA, left atrium.

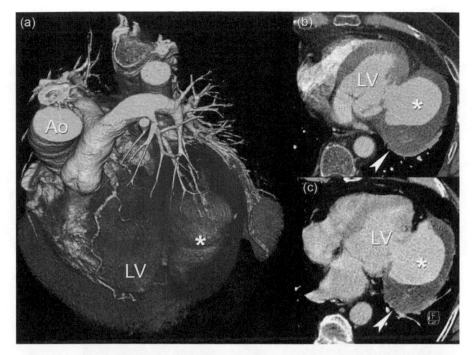

Figure 15.7 Left ventricular false aneurysm*. (a) Volume-rendered image. (b) and (c) Volume-rendered image of large false aneurysm with "short neck". The aneurysm is largely "filled" by organized thrombotic material (arrowhead). LV, left ventricle; Ao, aorta.

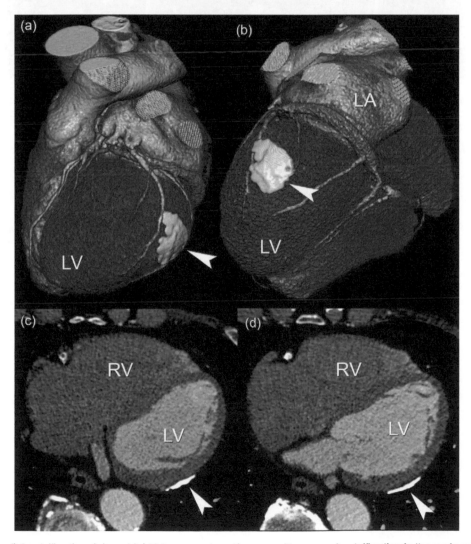

Figure 15.8 Pericardial calcification. (a) and (b) Volume-rendered images with areas of calcification in the pericardium (arrowheads). (c) and (d) Volume-rendered images of pericardial calcification (arrowheads). LV, left ventricle; LA, left atrium; RV, right ventricle.

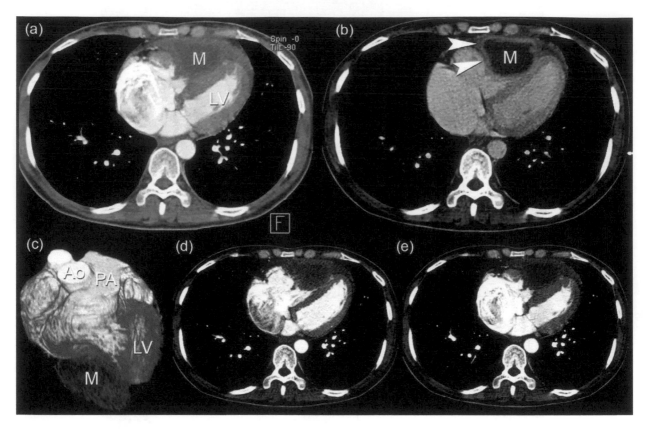

Figure 15.9   Pericardial abscess (M). (a)–(e) Volume-rendered images of pericardial non-contrast-filled abscess with surrounding rim of contrast enhancement (M) (arrowheads). The right ventricle is compressed. (c) Volume-rendered image showing abscess (M) involving pericardium and compression of right ventricle. LV, left ventricle; M, abscess (mass).

REFERENCES

1. Bleiweis MS, Georgiou D, Brundage BH. Detection of intracardiac masses by ultrafast computed tomography. Am J Card Imaging 1994; 8: 63–8.
2. Georgiou D, Bleiweis MS, Brundage BH. Ultra-fast computed tomography in the diagnosis of diseases of great vessels. Am J Card Imaging 1993; 7: 120–7.
3. Galvin JR, Gingrich RD, Hoffman E et al. Ultrafast computed tomography of the chest. Radiol Clin North Am 1994; 32: 775–93.
4. Lipton MJ, Higgins CB, Boyd DP. Computed tomography of the heart: evaluation of anatomy and function. J Am Coll Cardiol 1985; 5 (Suppl 1): 55S–69S.

CHAPTER 16

The great thoracic vessels

Aortic aneurysms and dissections are associated with significant morbidity and mor tality, and quick precise delineation of the underlying pathoanatomy is highly desirable and helpful for more favorable surgical management of these often critically ill patients.

For many years invasive contrast angiograph y has been the reference standard, but contrast angiography is limited because it shows only the lumen of the vessel and lacks the significant additional information of cross-sectional images and subsequent three-dimensional reconstr ucted images which are pro vided by CT angiograph y[1,2].

AORTIC ANEURYSM (Figures 16.1 and 16.2)

An aortic aneurysm is an abnor mal dilatation of the aorta, to at least 50% larger than normal.

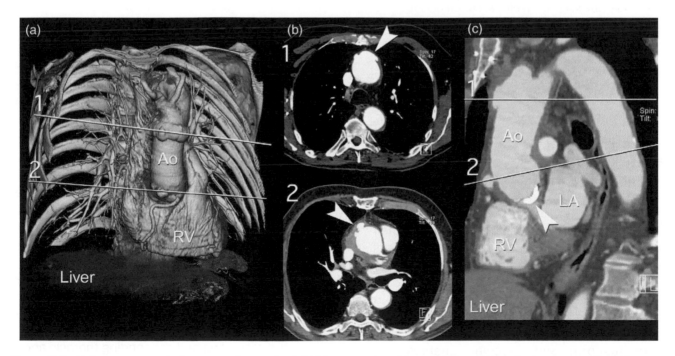

Figure 16.1 False aneurysms in the ascending aorta. (a) Volume-rendered image. (1) and (2) refer to cross-sectional images, (1) and (2) in (b), and show two false aneurysms (arrowhead). (c) Reformatted reconstruction, with calcified aortic valve (arrowhead). Ao, aorta; RV, right ventricle; LA, left atrium.

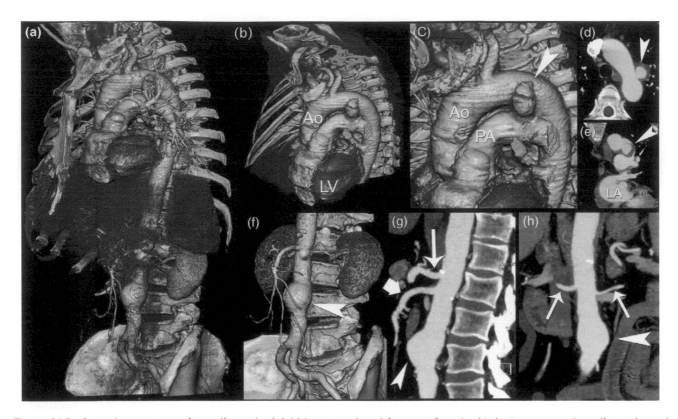

Figure 16.2 Saccular aneurysm in aortic arch. (a) Volume-rendered image of aorta (Ao). Aneurysm at aortic arch and abdominal aorta (f)–(h) fusiform aneurysm (arrowhead). (b)–(d) Enlargements of aortic arch saccular aneurysm (arrowhead) and fusiform abdominal aneurysm (arrowhead). (d) and (e) Contrast-enhanced multiplanar reconstructions of aortic arch with saccular aneurysm (arrowheads). (f), (g), and (h) Fusiform aneurysm (arrowhead) in abdominal aorta (arrowhead), below level of celiac trunk (thin arrow) and superior mesenteric artery (thick arrow). Fusiform aneurysm below renal arteries (arrows). PA, pulmonary artery; LV, left ventricle; LA, left artium.

The majority of aortic aneurysms are caused by atherosclerosis, while other causes include Marfan syndrome, cystic media necrosis, trauma, and post-stenotic dilatation of infectious mycotic disease.

Aneurysms are classified according to their shape, fusiform or saccular, and can be classified as true or false. A true aneurysm has an intact aortic wall, is usually fusiform, and is associated with atherosclerosis. A false aneurysm is caused by a disruption of the wall, is usually saccular, and is associated with infection or atherosclerosis. Both fusiform and saccular aneurysms may contain a thrombus. Aortic aneurysms have the tendency to expand.

AORTIC DISSECTION (Figures 16.3 and 16.4)

Aortic dissection is caused by a small tear in the intima, which propagates by dissecting the intima from the tunica media and the adventitia thus creating two channels: a false channel and a true channel[1,2]. The false channel is often large, may either become thrombosed or remain patent and may end blindly or re-enter the true lumen through a distal tear. Dissections can be classified according to the De Bakey classification or the Stanford classification. A dissection involving both the ascending and descending thoracic aorta is classified as De Bakey type I, if only the aorta ascendens is involved as De Bakey type II, and if

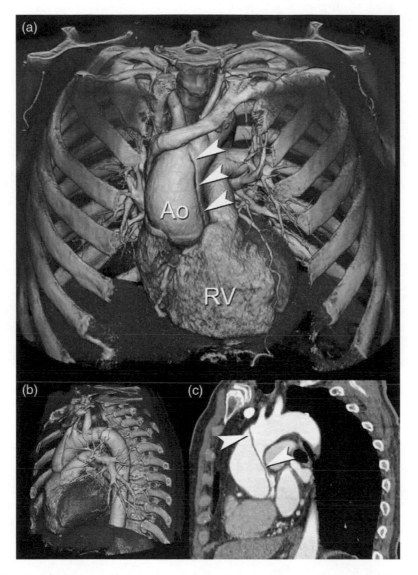

Figure 16.3 (a) and (b) Volume-rendered images of aorta showing dissection (arrowheads) in the ascending aorta during diastole. (c) Multiplanar reconstruction (during diastole) showing dissection in the ascending aorta (arrowheads). Ao, aorta; RV, right ventricle.

only the descending aorta is involved as De Bakey type III. The Stanford classification is based upon prognostic grounds. Type A involves dissection of the ascending aorta. These dissections have a worse prognose and require immediate surgery. Type B involves dissections of the descending aorta, which have a better prognosis. CT of an aortic dissection has typical features:

(1) Intimal flap separating the true and false lumen;
(2) Contrast enhancement occurs first in the true lumen and later in the false lumen;
(3) Inward displacement of intimal calcification by the false lumen;
(4) Often presence of thrombosis within the false lumen;
(5) Thickening of the aortic wall.

INTRAMURAL HEMORRHAGE OF THE AORTA

Intramural hemorrhage can be described as a dissection without initial tear which is now

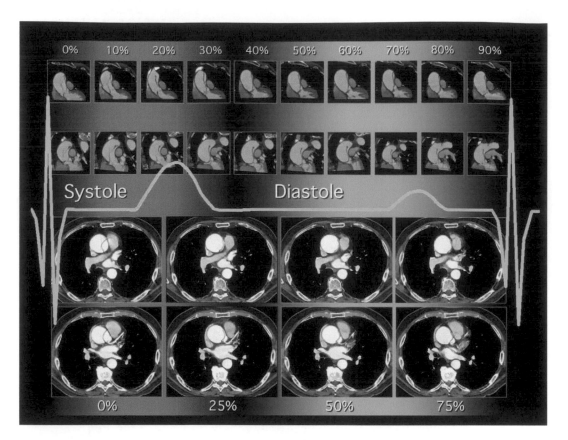

Figure 16.4 Dynamic representation of dissection in the ascending aorta. Large false lumen (left-side aorta) and small true lumen. The dissection is clearly visible during systole with small true lumen and large false lumen. During diastole the true lumen has almost disappeared because of increased blood flow and enlargement of the false lumen.

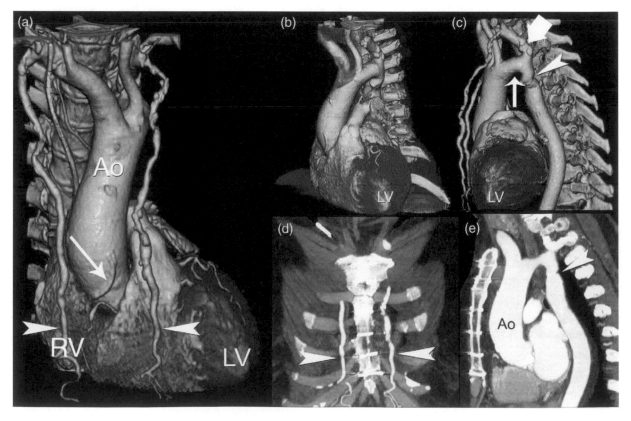

Figure 16.5 Coarctation aorta. (a) Volume-rendered image of an aorta (Ao) with a scar at the root of the aorta ascending (arrow) due to previous surgical incision (valve replacement and surgical repair of coarctation). The left internal mammary artery (LIMA) and right internal mammary artery (RIMA) (arrowheads). (b) and (c) Volume-rendered images of aorta showing coarctation of aorta with tubular aortic arch (arrow) and residual narrowing after surgical repair (arrowhead). Left subclavian artery with calcifications is shown (wide arrow). (d) Maximum intensity projection of LIMA and RIMA (arrowheads). (e) Maximum intensity projection of the aorta showing postsurgical situation at coarctation site (arrowhead). RV, right ventricle; LV, left ventricle.

considered an imminent precursor of aortic dissection. Aortic intramural hematoma is caused by rupture of the vaso vasorum in the medial wall layers[3]. CT allows identification of an intramural hemorrhage as a non-enhancing circular or crescent-shaped localized wall thickening, the high-density appearance of a fresh hematoma and absence of an intimal flap or tear. Thrombosis is identified by a multilayered appearance.

PENETRATING AORTIC ULCER

A penetrating aortic ulcer is an atheromatous plaque that ulcerates and disrupts the internal elastic lamina, and penetrates the aortic media and beyond[4]. On CT a penetrating aortic ulcer is diagnosed as a contrast-material filled outpouching in the aorta in the absence of a dissection flap or false lumen.

CONGENITAL AORTIC DISEASE
(Figures 16.5–16.8)

Patients with Marfan syndrome may show cardiovascular involvement with progressive aortic-root dilatation, with subsequent aortic insufficiency, dissection, or rupture. Coarctation of the aorta is associated with a localized narrowing of the aorta just distal to the ductus arteriosus. This anomaly is often associated with a bicuspid aortic valve. Both anomalies can be accurately identified by CT angiography.

PULMONARY EMBOLI (Figure 16.9)

Pulmonary emboli are seen as filling defects in the contrast-enhanced pulmonary arteries, and spiral CT has a high accuracy in identifying pulmonary emboli. CT scanning is excellent for the diagnosis of a central large pulmonary embolism but is less reliable for clinically important smaller pulmonary emboli in the peripheral pulmonary arteries [5,6].

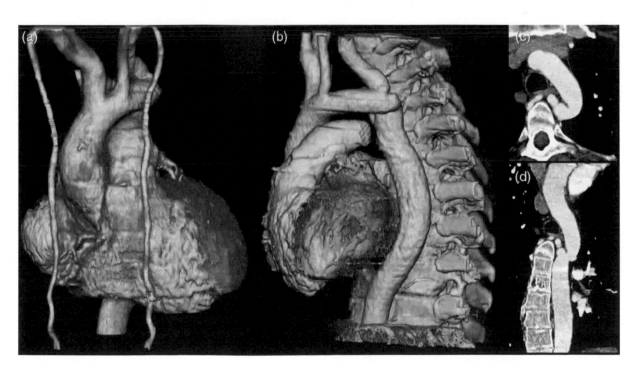

Figure 16.6 Coarctation of aorta. (a) and (b) Volume-rendered images of aorta from anterior and lateral views. (c) and (d) Multiplanar reconstructed images of aorta with coarctation of the aorta.

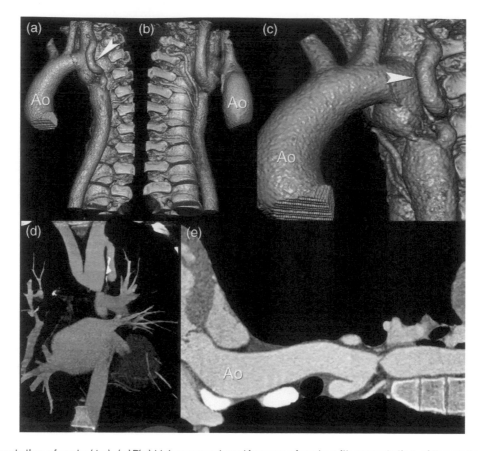

Figure 16.7 Coarctation of aorta (Ao). (a)Đ(c) Volume-rendered images of aorta with coarctation of the aorta. Bypass between left subclavian artery and thoracic aorta (arrowhead). (d) and (e) Maximum intensity projection and curved multiplanar reconstructed images of aorta showing clearly the coarctation with severe narrowing.

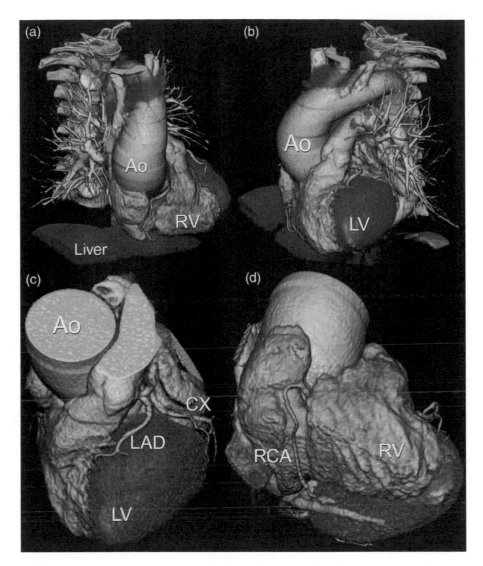

Figure 16.8 Dilatation of aortic root. (a)–(d) Volume-rendered images of heart and ascending aorta (Ao). The aortic root is dilated. LV, left ventricular; RV, right ventricular; Ao, aorta; LAD, left anterior descending; CX, left circumflex; RCA, right coronary artery.

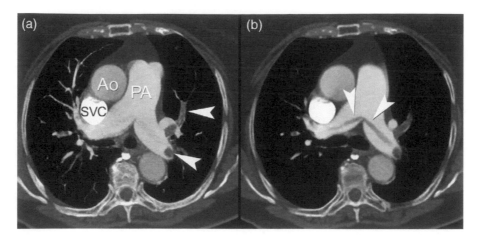

Figure 16.9 Pulmonary embolism. (a) Cross-sectional image of pulmonary artery (PA) and main branches. Filling defects in left pulmonary branch (lower arrowhead) and occluded smaller pulmonary branch (upper arrowhead). (b) Large filling defect at bifurcation of the main pulmonary artery (arrowheads). Ao, aorta; SVC, superior vena cava.

REFERENCES

1. Nienaber CA, Eagle KA. Aortic dissection: new frontiers in diagnosis and management: Part I: from etiology to diagnostic strategies. Circulation 2003; 108: 628–35.
2. Nienaber CA, Eagle KA. Aortic dissection: new frontiers in diagnosis and management: Part II: therapeutic management and follow-up. Circulation 2003; 108: 772–8.
3. Nienaber CA, von Kodolitsch Y, Petersen B et al. Intramural hemorrhage of the thoracic aorta. Diagnostic and therapeutic implications. Circulation 1995; 92: 1465–72.
4. Coady MA, Rizzo JA, Hammond GL et al. Penetrating ulcer of the thoracic aorta: what is it? How do we recognize it? How do we manage it? J Vasc Surg 1998; 27: 1006–15.
5. Drucker EA, Rivitz SM, Shepard JA et al. Acute pulmonary embolism: assessment of helical CT for diagnosis. Radiology 1998; 209: 235–41.
6. Rathbun SW, Raskob GE, Whitsett TL. Sensitivity and specificity of helical computed tomography in the diagnosis of pulmonary embolism: a systematic review. Ann Intern Med 2000; 132: 227–32.

CHAPTER 17

Computed tomography in the emergency department

Patients presenting with acute chest pain at an emergency department (ED) can pose a difficult diagnostic problem. Cur rent diagnostic algorithms in acute chest pain units aim to 'r ule out myocardial infarction', which requires ser ial negative electrocardiograms (ECG) and troponin tests (up to 6–12 h). This algorithm reduces the number of patients with a missed diagnosis of acute coronar y syndrome (A CS) and, consequently, incorrect dismissal from the emergency department to approximately 2% [1]. However, the majority of patients do not have an ACS, and the costs of triage of negative patients is estimated to be as high as 8 billion USD in the US annually [2]. Thus, a less time-consuming, non-invasive diagnostic method that is able to detect or r ule out an A CS in patients with acute chest pain of unknown origin would be highly desirable.

VALUE OF CT CORONARY CALCIUM SCORING IN PATIENTS WITH ACUTE CHEST PAIN

The presence of coronar y calcification as assessed by CT ma y increase the lik elihood that acute chest pain is caused by coronary artery disease. Younger patients with positive calcium scores (Agatston score more than zero) require further in-hospital diagnostic wor k-up, whereas in patients with absence of detectable coronar y calcification the likelihood of a flow-limiting coronar y stenosis is ver y low, and discharge of the patient may be safe (F igures 17.1–17.3) [3]. Calcium scoring performed in patients with acute chest pain

presenting at an emergency depar tment may also predict future adver se coronary events, including sudden cardiac death and non-fatal myocardial infarction. A positive calcium scoring scan is associated with a higher annualized event rate, while a negative scan is associated with a very low risk of future adverse coronary events (Table 17.1)[4,5] (Figure 17.4). T o date, only limited data are a vailable on the combined assessment of CT calcium scoring and CT coronary angiography in the setting of the e valuation of acute chest pain in an emergency depar tment. However, it seems reasonable to assume that the combined infor mation would be clinically relevant.

VALUE OF CT CORONARY ANGIOGRAPHY IN PATIENTS WITH ACUTE CHEST PAIN

CT coronary angiography to rule out myocardial infarction

CT coronary angiography can be of use to r ule out the presence of m yocardial infarction in patients suspected of ha ving an acute coronar y syndrome, combined with negative ECG and biomarker tests at time of admission to the emergency department (Figures 17.5 and 17.6). Hoffmann et al studied a group of 103 consecutive patients in whom m yocardial infarction could not initially be r uled out, requiring further ECG and troponin testing [6]. CT coronar y angiography was performed on a verage within 4 h after presentation at the emergency depar tment. The presence of non-obstr uctive coronary plaque could be

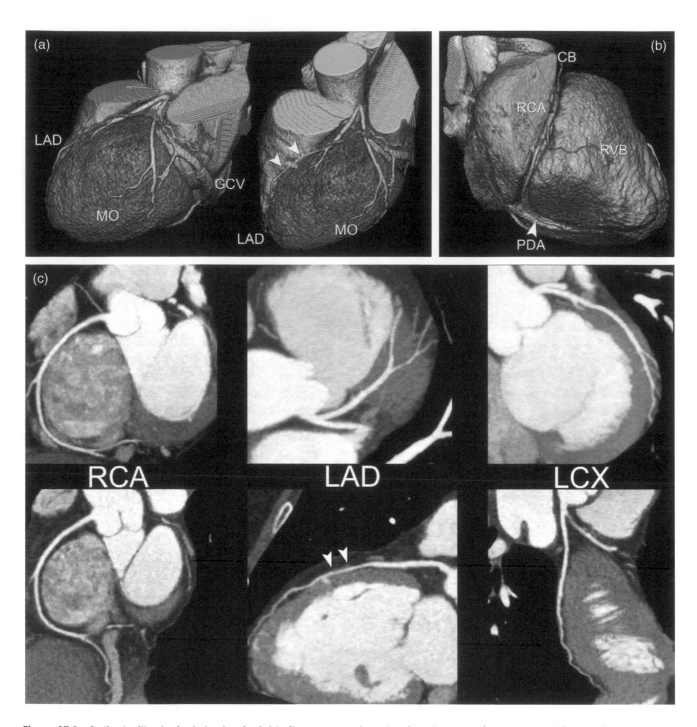

Figure 17.1 Patient with atypical chest pain. (a) Left coronary artery showing absence of coronary calcium and no coronary artery lumen abnormalities. Left anterior descending (LAD) runs in the myocardium (arrowheads). (b) Right coronary artery (RCA) with no abnormalities. (c) Multiplanar reconstruction showing intramyocardial course of LAD (arrowheads). MO, marginal obtuse; GCV, great cardiac vein; RVB, right ventricular branch; PDA, posterior descending artery (arrowhead); LCX, left circumflex.

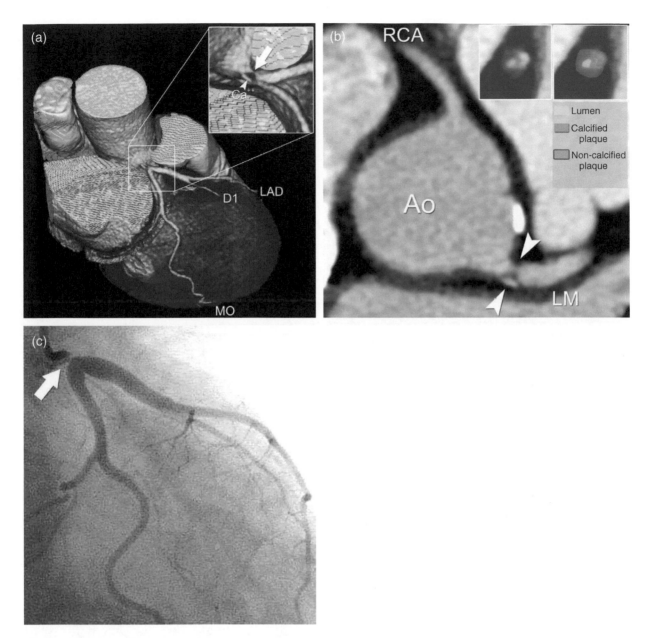

Figure 17.2 Young female patient presenting with chest pain and non-specific T wave abnormalities. (a) Severe stenosis (large arrow) and calcification (arrowhead) of the left main artery (LM). (b) Cross-sectional image of left main artery showing stenosis (between arrowheads). Right upper panels show orthogonal projection at site of left main stenosis. (c) Corresponding invasive coronary angiography demonstrating severe left main stenosis (arrow). LAD, left anterior descending; D1, first diagonal; MO, marginal obtuse; Ao, aorta, RCA, right coronary artery.

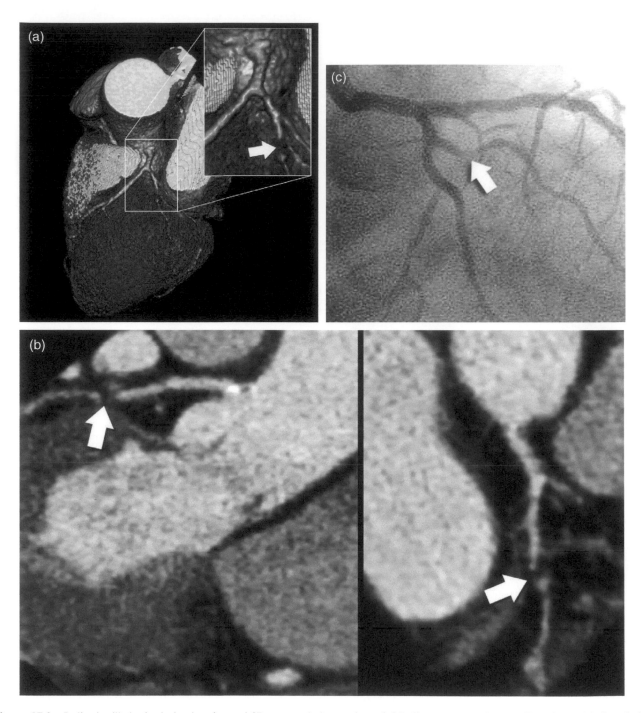

Figure 17.3 Patient with typical chest pain and ST segment depressions. (a) Left coronary artery. Left main and left anterior descending are normal. Left circumflex shows severe lesion at bifurcation (arrow) of obtuse marginal branch. (b) Multiplanar reconstruction showing non-calcific severe lesion at bifurcation (arrows). Calcium is present in the proximal part of the artery (bright spot). (c) Corresponding invasive coronary angiography with lesion in obtuse marginal branch (arrow).

Table 17.1 Value of calcium to predict cardiac death and non-fatal myocardial infarction (MI) in patients presenting at emergency department

| Calcium scan | McLaughlin et al.[2] (n = 134) | | Georgiou et al.[3] (n = 192) | |
	n	Event rate at 30 days (%)	n	Event rate at 50 ± 10 months (%)
Negative	48	0	76	0
Positive	86	4.4 (non-fatal MI n = 4)	116	15.6 (cardiac deaths n = 11, non-fatal MI n = 19)

Annualized rates of cardiovascular events: death, MI, coronary artery bypass graft, percutaneous transluminal coronary angioplasty, hospitalization for angina and ischemic stroke (from Georgiou et al. Am J Coll Cardiol 2001;38:105).

ruled out in 40% of patients. None of these patients were found to have an ACS. Sensitivity to detect ACS on the basis of presence of coronary plaque was 100%, specificity was 49%, positive predictive value was 19%, and negative predictive value was 100%. Patients with an ACS had significantly more coronary segments with plaque as compared with patients without an ACS. Moreover, the extent of coronary atherosclerosis was of additional value as compared with traditional risk stratification based on baseline patient demographics and clinical risk assessment. The presence of a significant (50% or more lumen diameter reduction) stenosis could be ruled out in 71% of patients, and none of these patients were found to have an ACS. Instead, an ACS was diagnosed in 61% of patients with a significant coronary stenosis. Sensitivity to detect ACS on the basis of presence of a significant coronary stenosis was 100%, specificity was 85%, positive predictive value was 46%, and negative predictive value was 100%. It is of note that CT yielded non-diagnostic image quality in 17% of patients, predominantly owing

to the presence of severe coronary calcifications and non-evaluable smaller-sized coronary stents.

CT coronary angiography in low-risk patients with ACS

Two studies have reported on the diagnostic accuracy of CT coronary angiography to detect and exclude the presence of an ACS in low-risk patients in whom myocardial infarction had been ruled out. Non-invasive stress testing is recommended to detect inducible ischemia in such patients before dismissal from the hospital. Goldstein et al randomized 203 patients to a CT coronary angiography group or a standard of care group of patients undergoing nuclear stress testing[7]. No procedure-related complications occurred in both groups. CT found minimal or no coronary artery disease in 67% of patients, allowing immediate dismissal from the emergency department. None of these patients had a major adverse coronary event during the 6-month follow-up. Significant coronary stenoses were found in 8% of patients, as confirmed by conventional coronary angiography. It is of note that 25% of patients in the CT group underwent additional nuclear stress testing owing to presence of intermediate lesions with unclear hemodynamic significance or non-diagnostic CT scans. The proportion of patients with the correct diagnosis was similar in both groups (97% and 98%, respectively). However, the time to diagnosis was significantly shorter with CT as compared with nuclear stress testing (3.5 versus 15 h, p <0.01), and the total cost of care was significantly reduced by CT, primarily as a result of shorter stay at the emergency department. Rubinshtein et al

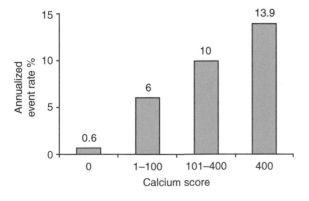

Figure 17.4 Relative risk for cardiac events in relation to calcium score. From reference 5, with permission.

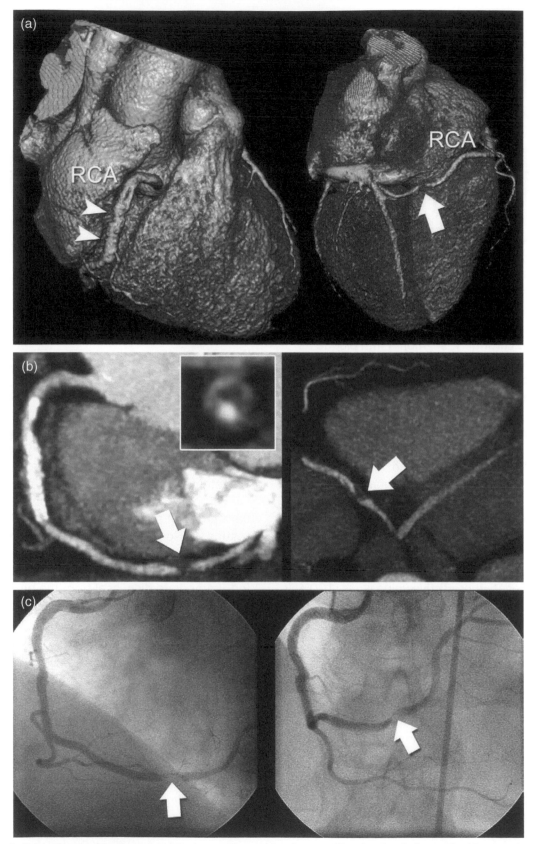

Figure 17.5 Patient with chest pain and no electrocardiographic abnormalities. Previously the patient had undergone a stent implantation in the right coronary artery (RCA). (a) Left panel shows stent in RCA. Right panel shows severe lesion in distal RCA. (b) Multiplanar reconstructions. Left panel shows no calcification. Mid-RCA shows a stent. Distal RCA shows a non-calcific severe lesion (arrow). Insert is an orthogonal view of lesion. Right panel shows severe lesion in distal RCA (arrow). (c) Corresponding invasive diagnostic angiography showing severe lesion (arrow).

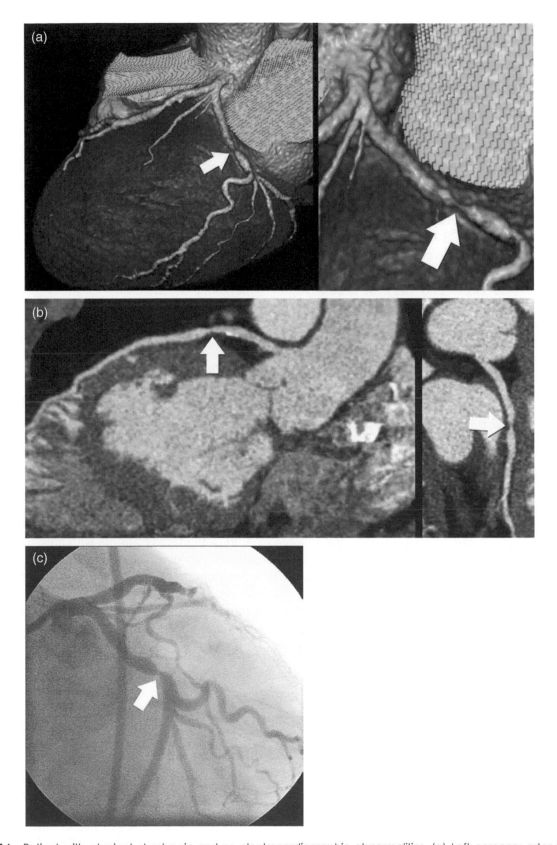

Figure 17.6 Patient with atypical chest pain and no electrocardiographic abnormalities. (a) Left coronary artery showing. normal left anterior descending and a severe lesion (arrows) of the left circumflex. (b) Multiplanar reconstruction showing non-calcific significant lesion in left circumflex (arrows). (c) Corresponding diagnostic invasive angiography showing severe lesion in left circumflex.

evaluated 58 patients at low risk (no biomarkers and no ECG changes) who were followed for 15 months[8]. The CT positive predictive value of death, myocardial infarction, or revascularization was 52% and the negative predictive value was 97%. Gallagher et al performed CT calcium scoring, CT coronary angiography, and nuclear stress testing in low-risk acute chest pain patients without myocardial infarction[9]. Patients with an overall Agatston calcium score of 400 or more, or with one or more significant coronary stenosis were classified as positive by CT. Sensitivity to detect or rule out ACS by CT versus stress nuclear testing was 86% versus 71%, specificity was 92% versus 90%, positive predictive value was 50% versus 38%, and negative predictive value was 99% versus 97%. The authors concluded that CT coronary angiography is at least as good as stress nuclear testing in the detection or exclusion of ACS after myocardial infarction has been ruled out.

Gated chest CT examinations: triple rule out protocol

Currently available CT scanners allow thin-slice, gated examinations of the entire thorax within a reasonable breath-hold time, which allows simultaneous evaluation of the presence of significant coronary artery disease, pulmonary embolism, or aortic dissection. Johnson et al performed such a triple rule out protocol in 55 patients presenting at the emergency department with acute chest pain of unknown origin[10]. Simultaneous evaluation of the coronary arteries, pulmonary arteries, and ascending aorta was possible in 99% of patients. The cause of chest pain was found in 67% of patients by CT. No diagnosis was found by CT or at clinical follow-up in 25% of patients. The correct diagnosis was not diagnosed by CT in 8% of patients, which included severe mitral valve regurgitation, endocarditis, arrhythmia, and a single underestimated coronary stenosis. These results indicate that CT shows promise in the triage of patients with acute chest pain of unknown origin. However, the high radiation exposure related to gated chest CT scans is of concern, especially in younger patients and patients with recurrent symptoms

requiring serial examinations. A recent study reported a radiation exposure as high as 28 ± 7 mSv for gated chest CT examinations[11]. Moreover, multiple diagnoses as the cause of acute chest pain can be found in a single patient in approximately 20% of cases, and it is unclear whether CT can be of use to identify the predominant diagnosis in such patients[12]. Thus, gated CT examinations of the entire chest should be reserved only for highly selected patients with acute chest pain of unknown origin after careful evaluation of risk factors, clinical variables, biomarkers, and ECG test results, and not as a screening method for early triage in all patients with acute chest pain presenting at an emergency department.

CONCLUSION

CT coronary angiography shows promise in the detection or exclusion of ACS and reduces the time to diagnosis, thereby facilitating earlier referral to urgent percutaneous coronary intervention or bypass surgery in patients with a positive CT scan, or direct dismissal from the emergency department in patients with negative CT findings. However, current literature indicates a higher number of non-evaluable CT coronary angiography scans in patients with ACS as compared with stable patients with chronic angina pectoris or atypical chest pain[6,13,14]. Further refinement of CT technology is necessary to reduce both radiation exposure and artifacts related to patient breathing, coronary motion, and severe coronary calcifications in acute chest pain patients.

REFERENCES

1. Pope JH, Aufderheide TP, Ruthazer R et al. Missed diagnoses of acute cardiac ischemia in the emergency department. N Engl J Med 2000; 342: 1163–70.
2. Tosteson A, Goldman L, Udvarhelyi IS, Lee T. Cost-effectiveness of a coronary care unit versus an intermediate care unit for emergency department patients with chest pain. Circulation 1996; 94: 143–50.
3. Laudon DA, Vukov LF, Breen JF et al. Use of electron-beam computed tomography in the evaluation of chest pain patients in the emergency department. Ann Emerg Med 1999; 33: 15–21.
4. McLaughlin VV, Balogh T, Rich S. Utility of electron beam computed tomography to stratify patients presenting to the emergency room with chest pain. Am J Cardiol 1999; 84: 327–8.

5. Georgiou D, Budoff MJ, Kaufer E et al. Screening patients with chest pain in the emergency depar tment using electron beam tomography: a follow-up study. J Am Coll Cardiol 2001; 38: 105–10.

6. Hoffmann U, Nagurney J, Moselewski F et al. Coronary multidetector computed tomograph y in the assessment of patients with acute chest Pain. Circulation 2006; 114: 2251–60.

7. Goldstein JA, Gallagher MJ, O'Neill W et al. A randomized controlled trial of multi-slice coronar y computed tomograph y for evaluation of acute chest pain. J Am Coll Cardiol 2007; 49: 863–71.

8. Rubinshtein R, Halon D, Gaspar T et al. Impact of 64-slice cardiac computed tomography angiography on clinical decision-making in emergency depar tment patients with chest pain of possible myocardial ischemic origin. Am J Cardiol 2007; 100: 1522–6

9. Gallagher M, Ross M, Raff G, Goldstein J, O'Neill W, O'Neil B. The diagnostic accuracy of 64-slice computed tomograph y coronary angiography compared with stress nuclear imaging in emergency department low-risk chest pain patients. Ann Emerg Med 2007; 49: 125–36.

10. Johnson T, Nikolaou K, Wintersperger B et al. ECG-gated 64-MDCT angiography in the differential diagnosis of acute chest pain. AJR Am J Roentgenol 2007; 188: 76–82.

11. Litmanovitch D, Zamboni G, Hauser T, Lin P, Clouse M, Raptopoulos V. ECG-gated chest CT -angiography with 64-MDCT and tri-phasic IV contrast administration regimen in patients with acute non-specific chest pain. Eur Radiol 2008; 18: 308–17.

12. Fruergaard P, Launbjerg J, Hesse B et al. The diagnoses of patients admitted with acute chest pain but without m yocardial infarction. Eur Hear t J 1996; 17: 1028–34.

13. Chersin E, Litmanovitch D, Dragu R et al. 16-MDCT coronar y angiography versus invasive coronary angiography in acute chest pain syndrome: a blinded prospective study . AJR Am J Roentgenol 2006; 166: 177–84.

14. Meijboom WB, Mollet NR, Van Mieghem C et al. 64-Slice CT coronary angiography in patients with non-ST ele vation acute coronary syndrome. Hear t 2007; 93: 1386–92.

CHAPTER 18

Preoperative assessment of the coronary tree before cardiac valve surgery

CORONARY ARTERY DISEASE AND VALVE PATHOLOGY

Patients with aortic stenosis and coronary artery disease have the same pathophysiology, share common risk factors and are of advancing age. The presence of concomitant significant coronary artery disease is found in approximately one-third of these patients with aortic stenosis [1-4]. The presence of obstructive coronary artery disease worsens prognosis [5-7], and combined valve and bypass surgery of significant coronary artery disease, reduces early and late mortality [6,8]. Angina pectoris is present in 25–35% of patients with valvular heart disease. However, angina pectoris is a poor predictor of obstructive coronary artery disease in these patients because angina pectoris can have multiple causes such as left ventricular enlargement, increased wall stress, or wall thickening with subendocardial ischemia [2,9]. The value of non-invasive electrocardiogram (ECG)-stress testing to detect concomitant coronary artery disease is limited owing to the presence of left ventricular hypertrophy and left bundle branch block in patients with valvular disease. Resting or exercise-induced wall motion abnormalities and myocardial perfusion abnormalities, as seen with stress echo and nuclear tests, lack sufficient accuracy for reliable detection of concomitant coronary artery disease [10-13]. As a result of the poor predictive value of angina pectoris and the lack of accuracy of non-invasive tests, the American College of Cardiology (ACC)/American Heart Association (AHA) committee [14] recommends that preoperative invasive coronary angiography (CCA) is indicated in symptomatic patients and/or those with left ventricular dysfunction in:

(1) Men 35 years or older;
(2) Premenopausal women 35 years or older with risk factors for coronary artery disease;
(3) Postmenopausal women.

DIAGNOSTIC PERFORMANCE

Several studies have reported excellent diagnostic accuracy to detect or rule significant coronary artery disease using 16- and 40- or 64-slice scanners [15-19] (Table 18.1). A negative CT scan reliably ruled out the presence of significant coronary artery disease (Figure 18.1). However, a positive CT scan had insufficient reliability and in these cases invasive coronary angiography was necessary to confirm the presence of coronary narrowing (Figures 18.2–18.8). A recent observational study described the clinical use of a 16-slice CT scanner in 132 patients [20]. After exclusion of 16 patients owing to poor image quality, the remaining 116 patients were divided into two groups. Patients without significant coronary artery disease underwent isolated valve surgery without referral to invasive coronary angiography and patients with significant coronary artery disease on CT coronary angiography (CTCA) were referred for invasive coronary angiography. In 30 out of 44 patients in whom significant coronary artery disease was seen on CTCA, percutaneous coronary intervention (PCI) (n = 26) or coronary artery bypass graft (CABG) (n = 4) was performed and in six

210

Table 18.1 Diagnostic performance of 16-, 40-, and 64-slice scanners to detect coronary stenosis with conventional coronary angiography as the standard of reference

	Year	Detectors (n)	Patients (n)	TP	TN	FP	FN	Sensitivity (%)	Specificity (%)	PPV (%)	NPV (%)
Gilard et al[15]	2006	16	55	11	35	9	0	100	80	55	100
Manghat et al[16]	2006	16	35	15	16	4	0	100	80	79	100
Reant et al[17]	2006	16	40	12	21	6	1	92	78	67	95
Pouleur et al[18]	2007	40	82	14	60	7	1	93	90	67	98
Meijboom et al[19]	2006	64	70	18	48	4	0	100	92	82	100

TP, true positive; TN, true negative; FP, false positive; FN, false negative.

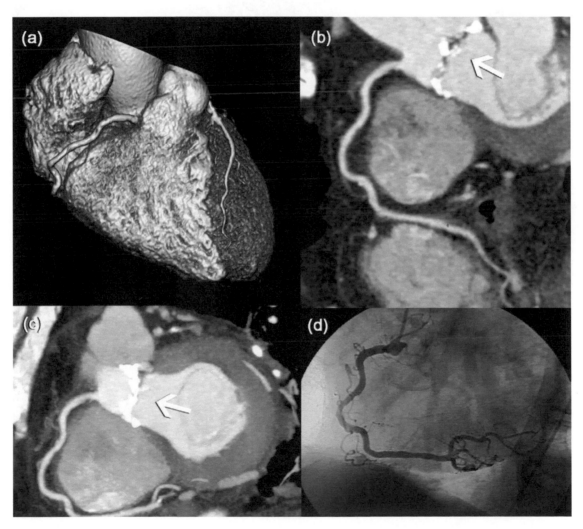

Figure 18.1 Volume-rendered (a), maximum intensity projection (b), and curved multiplanar reconstruction (c) CT images showing a patent right coronary artery which is confirmed by invasive coronary angiogram (d). The bright white spots (arrow) represent calcifications of the stenotic aortic valve. Same patient as in Figures 18.2 and 18.3.

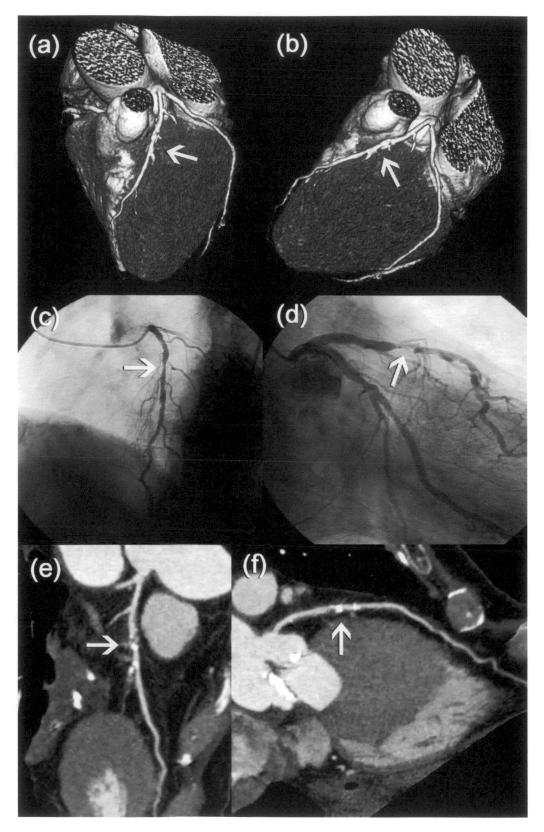

Figure 18.2 Volume-rendered images (a) and (b) and curved multiplanar reconstructions (e) and (f) revealing a significant stenosis (arrow) in the left anterior descending coronary artery, which was also detected by invasive coronary angiogram (c) and (d). Same patient as in Figures 18.1 and 18.3.

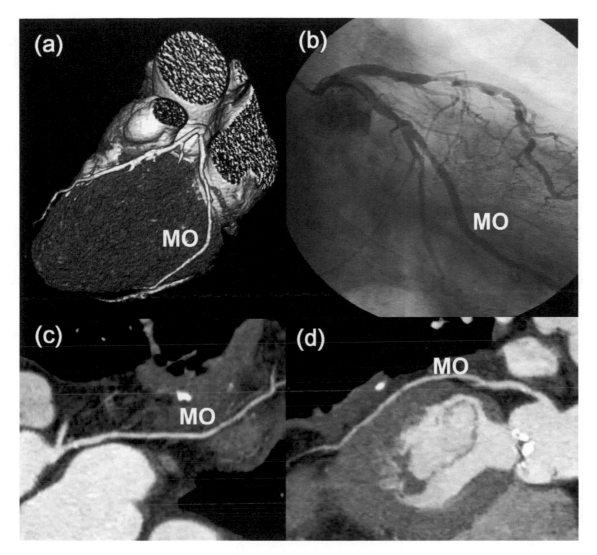

Figure 18.3 Volume-rendered image (a) and curved multiplanar reconstructions (c) and (d) showing non-significant plaque in the marginal obtuse (MO). (b) Invasive coronary angiogram corroborates the CTCA finding of wall irregularities in the MO. Same patient as in Figures 18.1 and 18.2.

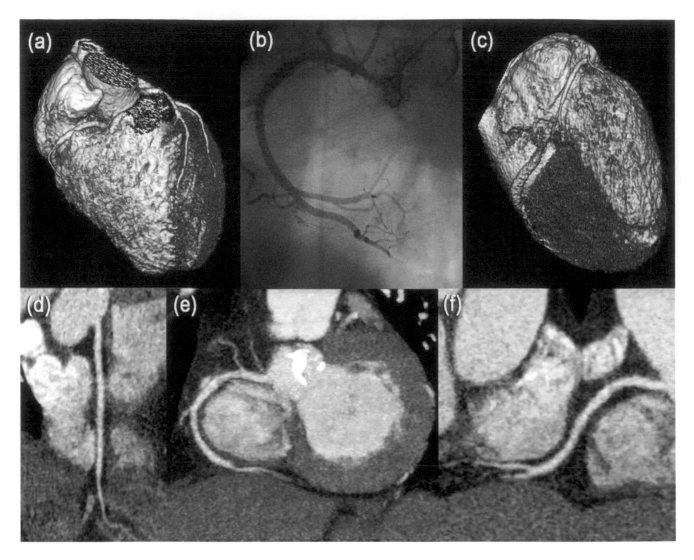

Figure 18.4 (a) and (c) Volume-rendered images of the right conorary artery (RCA). (d)Ð(f) Curved multiplanar reconstructions of the RCA showing no significant coronary lesions as confirmed by invasive coronary angiogram (b). Same patient as in Figures 18.5 and 18.6.

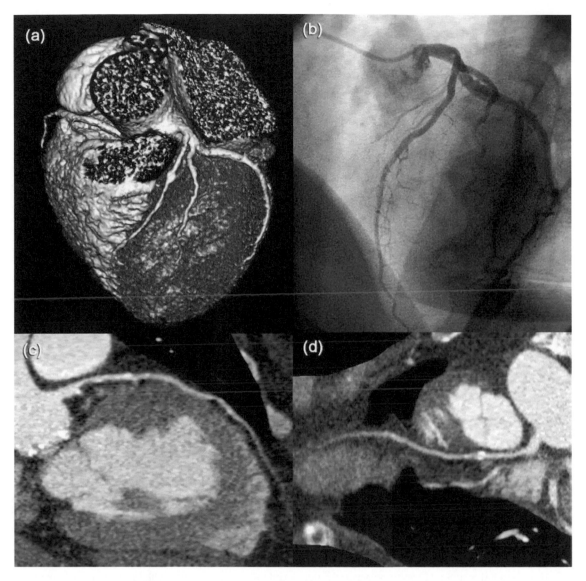

Figure 18.5 Despite the high body mass index of this patient (37.1), resulting in low signal-to-noise giving more noisy images, significant lesions could be excluded. (a) Volume-rendered image of left coronary artery and proximal part of right coronary artery.(c) and (d) curved multiplanar reconstructions of the left anterior descending reveal a mixed plaque in the proximal part which was scored on quantitative coronary angiography as 25% diameter narrowing (b). Same patient as in Figures 18.4 and 18.6.

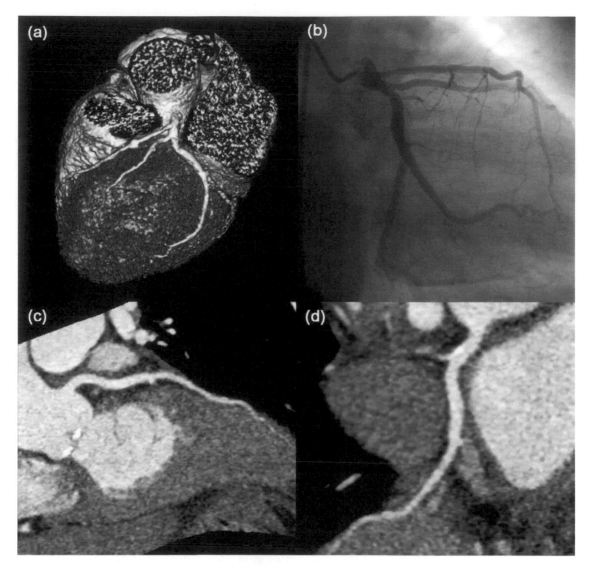

Figure 18.6 The large first marginal branch revealed no significant lesions on curved multiplanar reconstructions and volume-rendered image of left circumflex artery with large first marginal branch (c) and (d) as was confirmed with invasive coronary angiography (b). Same patient as in Figures 18.4 and 18.5.

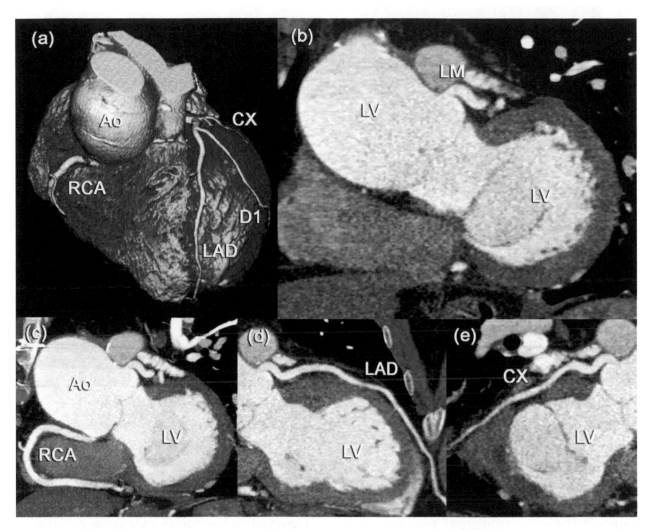

Figure 18.7 Patient with a clinical history of a Ross procedure, presenting with dyspnea owing to an aortic regurgitation. (a) Volume-rendered CT image visualizing the anatomy of the coronary tree and the dilated ascending aorta. (Ao). (b) Maximum intensity projection image showing the dilated ascending aorta (diameter 5.5 cm) and a slightly enlarged left ventricle (LV). Maximum intensity projection image (c) revealing the patent right coronary artery (RCA) and curved multiplanar reconstructions (d) and (e) showing a patent left anterior descending (LAD) and circumflex (CX). D1, first diagonal; LM, left main.

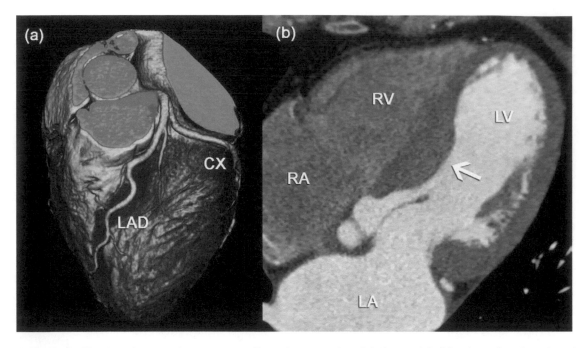

Figure 18.8 Patient with normal coronaries as seen on the volume-rendered CT image(a). (b) A four-chamber view shows the septal thickening (arrow) establishing the diagnosis of hypertrophic cardiomyopathy. LAD, left anterior descending; CX, circumflex; RV, right ventricle; RA, right atrium; LV, left ventricle; LA, left atrium.

patients no revascularization was performed (borderline stenosis in small vessels). In eight patients CTCA o verestimated lesion se verity and only coronar y lesions of less than 50% of luminal diameter w ere detected on in vasive coronary angiography. There were no major cardiac complications in the patients in whom only less than 50% stenosis w as seen on CTCA.

CT CORONARY ANGIOGRAPHY TO PLAN THE SURGICAL APPROACH FOR REDO CARDIAC SURGERY AFTER CORONARY REVASCULARIZATION

Patients with a histor y of CABG, who undergo redo cardiac surger y, have a higher risk for complications than patients undergoing their fir st CABG[21]. Re-opening the thorax has the risk of damaging patent coronar y grafts or injuring other vital mediastinal structures like the aorta

and right ventricle. In a recent study the additive value of preoperative CTCA w as shown[22]. CTCA provided an accurate assessment of the position of various vital mediastinal str uctures and delineated the relationship betw een bypass grafts, right ventricle, aorta, and the posterior sternum.

ASSESSMENT OF VALVES WITH CT CORONARY ANGIOGRAPHY

Besides evaluating the coronaries, other structures of the heart can be seen in great detail using CTCA. Dedicated reconstr uctions can be made to assess both the left ventricle and the valves. Although CTCA does not pro vide flow information it does allow the possibility of visualizing the valvular anatom y and measuring the aortic valve area and the diameter of the annulus. Studies reporting on the cor relation between the aortic valve area as measured b y transthoracic echocardiography (TTE), transesophageal echocardiography (TEE), and cine magnetic resonance (MR) compared with CTCA show good correlations[23,24].

LIMITATIONS

The limited temporal resolution of 16- and 64-slice CT scanner s warrants the use of beta-blockers or benzodiazepines to reduce hear t rates. However, the application of beta-block ers in patients with aor tic stenosis and impaired left ventricular function is frequently contraindicated, making these patients less suitable for CT scanning. However, dual source CT scanners having an increased temporal resolution of 83 ms, may allow high-quality scanning with fast heart rates. Atrial fibrillation remains a contraindication to perfor ming CTCA. The presence of calcium, occurring more often in patients with aortic valve disease, creates blooming ar tifacts, which obscure the visualization of the under lying non-calcified plaque or lumen and comprise precise stenosis e valuation.

CONCLUSION

The diagnostic accuracy of 64-slice CT scanner s is clinically reliable for r uling out the presence of significant coronar y lesions in patients undergoing elective valve surgery, and CTCA implementation as a gatekeeper in these patients might be indicated.

REFERENCES

1. Vandeplas A, Willems JL, Piessens J, De Geest H. F requency of angina pectoris and coronary artery disease in severe isolated valvular aor tic stenosis. Am J Cardiol 1988; 62: 117-20.
2. Alexopoulos D, Kolovou G, Kyriakidis M et al. Angina and coronary artery disease in patients with aor tic valve disease. Angiology 1993; 44: 707-11.
3. Olofsson BO, Bjerle P, Aberg T, Oster man G, Jacobsson KA. Prevalence of coronar y artery disease in patients with valvular heart disease. Acta Med Scand 1985; 218: 365-71.
4. Ramsdale DR, Bennett DH, Bray CL et al. Angina, coronary risk factors and coronar y artery disease in patients with valvular disease. A prospective study . Eur Hear t J 1984; 5: 716-26.
5. Lytle BW. Impact of coronar y artery disease on valvular hear t surgery. Cardiol Clin 1991; 9: 301-14.
6. Mullany CJ, Elveback LR, Frye RL et al. Coronary artery disease and its management: influence on sur vival in patients undergoing aortic valve replacement. J Am Coll Cardiol 1987; 10: 66-72.
7. Iung B, Drissi MF, Michel PL et al. Prognosis of valve replacement for aor tic stenosis with or without coexisting coronar y heart disease: a comparative study. J Heart Valve Dis 1993; 2: 430-9.
8. Lund O, Nielsen TT, Pilegaard HK, Magnussen K, Knudsen MA. The influence of coronar y artery disease and b ypass grafting on early and late sur vival after valve replacement for aor tic stenosis. J Thorac Cardio vasc Surg 1990; 100: 327-37.
9. Green SJ, Pizzarello RA, Padmanabhan VT, Ong LY, Hall MH, Tortolani AJ. Relation of angina pectoris to coronar y artery disease in aor tic valve stenosis. Am J Cardiol 1985; 55: 1063-5.
10. Rask P, Karp K, Edlund B, Eriksson P, Mooe T, Wiklund U. Computer-assisted evaluation of dip yridamole thallium-201 SPECT in patients with aor tic stenosis. J Nucl Med 1994; 35: 983-8.
11. Samuels B, Kiat H, Friedman JD, Berman DS. Adenosine pharmacologic stress myocardial perfusion tomographic imaging in patients with significant aortic stenosis. Diagnostic efficacy and comparison of clinical, hemodynamic and electrocardiographic variables with 100 age-matched control subjects. J Am Coll Cardiol 1995; 25: 99-106.
12. Kettunen R, Huikuri HV, Heikkila J, Takkunen JT. Preoperative diagnosis of coronar y artery disease in patients with valvular heart disease using technetium-99m isonitrile tomographic imaging together with high-dose dip yridamole and handgrip exercise. Am J Cardiol 1992; 69: 1442-5.
13. Kupari M, Virtanen KS, Turto H et al. Exclusion of coronar y artery disease b y exercise thallium-201 tomograph y in patients with aortic valve stenosis. Am J Cardiol 1992; 70: 635-40.
14. Bonow RO, Carabello B, de Leon A C Jr et al. Guidelines for the management of patients with valvular hear t disease: executive summary. A report of the American College of Cardiology/American Heart Association Task Force on Practice Guidelines (Committee on Management of P atients with Valvular Heart Disease). Circulation 1998; 98: 1949-84.
15. Gilard M, Cornily JC, Pennec P et al. Accuracy of multislice computed tomography in the preoperative assessment of coronary disease in patients with aor tic valve stenosis. J Am Coll Cardiol 2006; 47: 2020-4.
16. Manghat NE, Kakani N, Morgan-Hughes GJ. 64-slice cardiac computed tomography: appearance of a complex coronar y to pulmonary arterial fistula with conus ar tery aneurysm. Heart 2006; 92: 1308.
17. Reant P, Brunot S, Lafitte S et al. Predictive value of noninvasive coronary angiography with multidetector computed tomography to detect significant coronar y stenosis before valve surgery. Am J Cardiol 2006; 97: 1506-10.
18. Pouleur AC, le Polain de Waroux JB, Kefer J et al. Usefulness of 40-slice multidetector row computed tomograph y to detect coronary disease in patients prior to cardiac valve surger y. Eur Radiol 2007; 17: 3199-207.
19. Meijboom WB, Mollet NR, Van Mieghem CA et al. Pre-operative computed tomography coronary angiography to detect significant coronary artery disease in patients referred for cardiac valve surgery. J Am Coll Cardiol 2006; 48: 1658-65.
20. Russo V, Gostoli V, Lovato L et al. Clinical value of multidetector CT coronar y angiography as a pre-operative screening test before noncoronar y cardiac surger y. Heart 2006; 93: 1591-8.
21. Salomon NW, Page US, Bigelow JC, Krause AH, Okies JE, Metzdorff MT. Reoperative coronar y surgery. Comparative analysis of 6591 patients undergoing primar y bypass and 508 patients undergoing reoperative coronary artery bypass. J Thorac Cardio vasc Surg 1990; 100: 250-9.

22. Gasparovic H, Rybicki FJ, Millstine J et al. Three dimensional computed tomographic imaging in planning the surgical approach for redo cardiac surgery after coronary revascularization. Eur J Cardiothorac Surg 2005; 28: 244–9.

23. Feuchtner GM, Dichtl W, Friedrich GJ et al. Multislice computed tomography for detection of patients with aortic valve stenosis and quantification of severity. J Am Coll Cardiol 2006; 47: 1410–17.

24. Pouleur AC, le Polain de Waroux JB, Pasquet A, Vanoverschelde JL, Gerber BL. Aortic valve area assessment: multidetector CT compared with cine MR imaging and transthoracic and transesophageal echocardiography. Radiology 2007; 244: 745–54.

CHAPTER 19

Assessment of left ventricular function and viability

LEFT VENTRICULAR FUNCTION

CT scanning of the heart permits evaluation of both the coronary arteries and left ventricular function, if data sets are reconstructed throughout the cardiac cycle (e.g. every 5% or 10% of the R-to-R interval). These data sets can be used to reconstruct images at different levels (e.g. apical, mid, and basal) of the left ventricle at different phases of the cardiac cycle (Figure 19.1).

Left ventricular volumes can be computed by dedicated software after automated contouring of the left ventricular cavity. These software algorithms either apply Simpson's rule (summation of the short-axis images) or calculate left ventricular volumes based on the actual number of voxels within the left ventricular cavity. Volume–time curves are automatically obtained, which allow reliable identification of the end-systolic and end-diastolic phase, and calculation of stroke volume, ejection fraction, and (time-to) peak filling rate. Quantitative information regarding left ventricular wall motion, thickening, and thickness can be derived after additional contours of the epicardium are obtained (Figure 19.2 and Table 19.1). Earlier studies comparing the results of CT with magnetic resonance imaging (MRI), bi-plane angiography, echocardiography, or gated single photon emission CT (SPECT)[1-4] demonstrated good correlation between both left ventricular volumes and ejection fractions. However, these studies reported an overestimation of end-systolic volumes resulting in a slight underestimation of ejection fractions owing to insufficient temporal resolution of CT to capture the relatively short end-systolic phase.

Moreover, these studies reported moderate accuracy of CT in the assessment of left ventricular regional wall motion abnormalities, especially in the evaluation of hypokinetic myocardial segments (Figure 19.3). However, more recent studies using CT scanners with improved temporal resolution (up to 43 ms) reported that CT not only provides accurate assessment of global left ventricular functional parameters, but also allows time-dependent variables and reliable evaluation of regional wall motion[5,6]. In addition, these scanners may not require administration of beta-blockers prior to CT coronary angiography scans, which is of importance since beta-blockers may have a negative effect on left ventricular function. It is of note that sequential ('step-and-shoot') CT scanning or spiral CT scanning using prospective electrocardiogram (ECG) X-ray tube modulation with a minimum tube current of less than 20% of the reference tube current excludes reliable assessment of left ventricular function. However, these scan protocols significantly reduce the radiation exposure associated with CT coronary angiography. Thus, a combined evaluation of the coronary arteries and left ventricular function is only feasible at the cost of a higher radiation exposure and the necessity of having functional CT information should be carefully weighted on an individual patient basis.

VIABILITY IMAGING AFTER MYOCARDIAL INFARCTION

Myocardial perfusion imaging is of interest in the evaluation of patients suspected of having

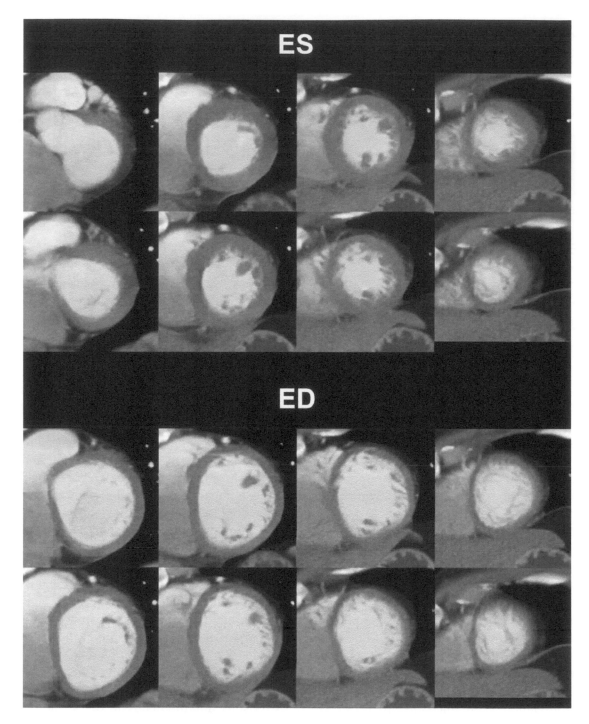

Figure 19.1   Reconstruction of short-axis images of the left ventricle obtained at the end-systolic (ES) and end-diastolic (ED) phase allows quantification (after semiautomatic contouring of the endocardial and epicardial border of the left ventricle) of stroke volume, ejection fraction, and peak filling rate. This patient, with a history of acute myocardial infarction, had an impaired thickening of the apical part of the septum.

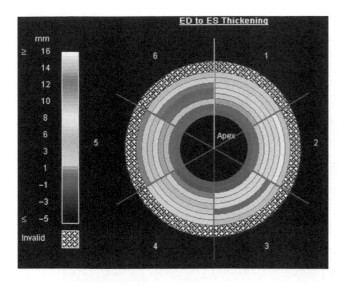

Figure 19.2 Bull© eye view of left ventricular wall thickening. (1)£{6) Anterior, anterolateral, inferolateral, inferoseptal, septal, and anteroseptal sectors, respectively. ED, end-diastole; ES, end-systole.

Table 19.1 Left ventricular function (see Figure 19.1)

Cardiac f nction		Normal range (M) (CT)
Ejection fraction (EF) (%)	55.0	56.00Đ78.00
End-diastolic volume (EDV) (ml)	228.6	77.00Đ195.00
End-systolic volume (ESV) (ml)	102.9	19.00Đ72.00
Stroke volume (CO) (l/min)	125.6	51.00Đ133.00
Cardiac output (CO) (l/min)	5.90	2.82Đ882
Myocardial mass (at ED) (g)	124.1	118.00Đ238.00
Myocardial mass (g)	122.1 ± 11.8	118.00Đ238.00

ED, end-diastole.

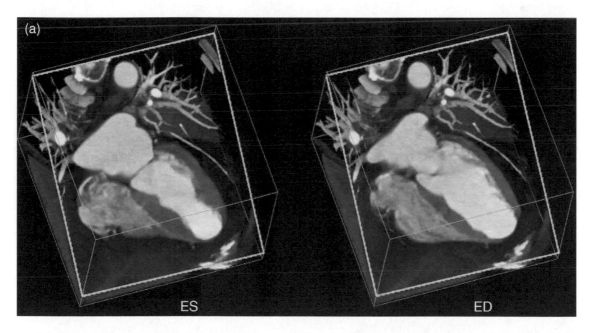

Figure 19.3 (a) Cross-sections of the heart showing a four-chamber view in the end-systolic (ES) and end-diastolic (ED) phase, while the remaining volume remains visible. This patient had a previous myocardial infarction resulting in an aneurysm of the left ventricle.

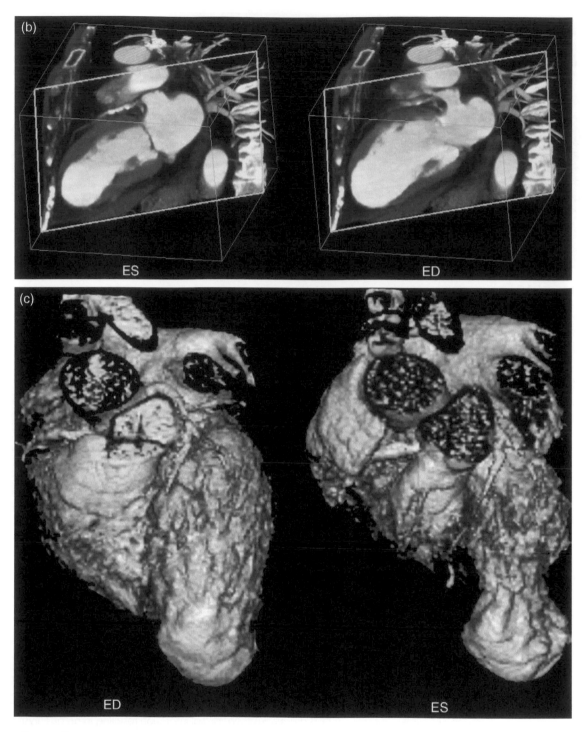

Figure 19.3Ñ(Contɑ̃l) (b) Cross-sections of the heart showing a two-chamber view in the end-systolic and end-diastolic phase of the same patient. (c) Volume-rendered images of the end-systolic and end-diastolic phase of the same patient. The presence of a left ventricular aneurysm is visualized, and the apex is not contracting.

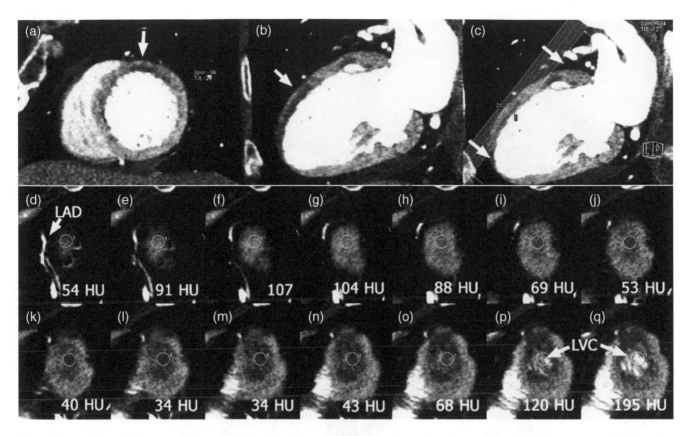

Figure 19.4 (a) and (b) Quantitative analysis of transmural CT attenuation values in a case of anterior myocardial infarction (arrows). (c) Thin slices (0.8 mm at 0.5-mm intervals) are reconstructed in parallel alignment to the infarcted myocardial wall, starting from the epicardial border inward (arrows). In 14 consecutive slices (d)–(q), a region of interest is placed at the same in-plane position to measure average attenuation. (d) Low attenuation values were found in the pericardium, and (o)–(q) high values in the ventricular cavity (LVC). (e)–(n) Cross-sections of myocardium from the epicardial to endocardial border. (l) and (m) Lowest attenuation (dark areas) is found near the endocardium (34 HU) compared with (f) highest attenuation (bright areas) toward the epicardial border (107 HU). LAD, left anterior descending coronary artery.

coronary artery disease since it may reflect the hemodynamic impact of a coronary stenosis. CT perfusion imaging is limited by several technical issues. The main problem is that the scan protocol should be adapted to a stationary, volume covering, and dynamic acquisition to assess the myocardial uptake of contrast material over time. However, such a protocol would result in an unacceptably high radiation exposure and contrast material load for the patient. A few studies have reported on the potential of CT myocardial perfusion imaging using a scan protocol optimized for CT coronary angiography in patients after myocardial infarction[7,8]. These studies indicate that patients with (semi)acute or chronic myocardial infarction can be distinguished on the basis of myocardial enhancement patterns[8,9] (Figures 19.4 and 19.5). However, it does not appear to be possible to distinguish between recent myocardial infarctions with normal wall thickness and myocardial perfusion deficits only on the basis of regional hypoperfusion using a standard CT coronary angiography scan protocol.

Several studies have reported on the potential of delayed-enhanced CT scanning to detect and quantify infarct size after myocardial infarction. Such information has important prognostic value because infarct size predicts long-term clinical outcome in patients with an acute myocardial infarction. Acute and chronic myocardial infarctions are

225

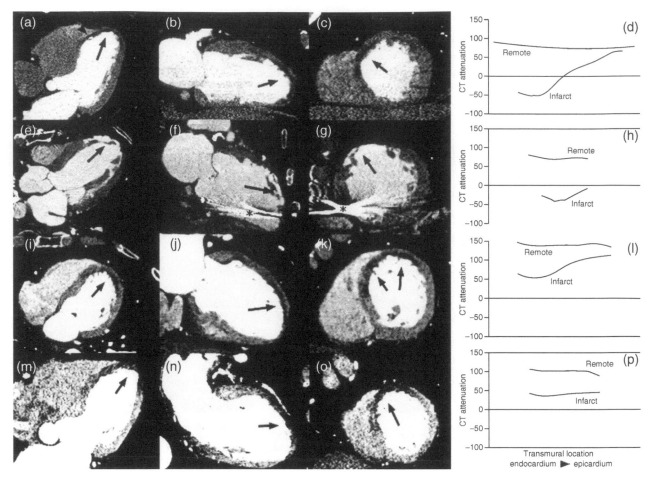

Figure 19.5 Four cases of anterior infarction (arrows) shown in four-chamber (a), (e), (i), and (m), two-chamber (b), (f), (j), and (n) and short-axis (c), (g), (k) and (o) cross-sections. (d), (h), (l), and (p) For each case, a graph shows the attenuation (Hounsfield units) at consecutive transmural locations from the endocardium toward the epicardial border for infarcted and normal remote myocardium (a)Đ(d). The first case is a long-standing infarct with a perfusion defect toward the subendocardial side (arrow a,b) and a small calcitication (arrowhead In. (c) in the septum (e)Đ(h). The second case of long-standing myocardial infarction shows transmural low attenuation, aneurysm formation (arraws) and a pacemaker wire (asterisk) in the right ventricle (f)Đ(g). The third case is a recent myocardial infarction (primary percutaneous coronary intervention approximately 4 hours after onset of symptoms, maximum creatinine kinase level 2.384 U/l) with a perfusion defect that extends half way through the myocardium (m)Đ(p). The fourth case of acute myocardial infarction (primary percutaneous coronary intervention approximately 4 hours after onset of symptoms, maximum creatinine kinase level 3.163 U/l) shows decreased attenuation transmurally. Examples of long-standing myocardial intarction (cases 1 and 2) show lower minimal CT attenuation values compared with acute cases (3 and 4).

characterized by myocardial hyperenhancement, whereas areas of microvascular obstruction ('no reflow areas') are characterized by regional hypoenhancement [10,11]. Peak hyperenhancement occurs approximately 5 minutes after contrast administration [10,11] (Figure 19.6).

The majority of the studies were performed in animal models, and a close correlation between

infarct size quantified by CT and MRI was found [10,12]. However, CT has a limited contrast-to-noise ratio as compared with MRI, and a relatively high amount of contrast material was used to overcome this issue. Moreover, a second CT scan adds further radiation exposure to the already high dose associated with CT coronary angiography. Application of a low-dose delayed-enhanced

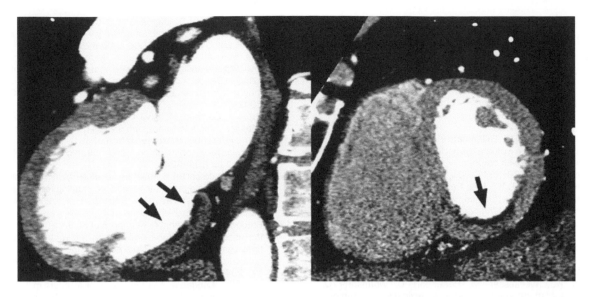

Figure 19.6 Acute inferior myocardial infarction without a known history of acute coronary syndrome. Nevertheless, very low subendocardial attenuation (−79 HU) was observed in the inferior wall (arrows), suggesting a previous subclinical event.

CT scan protocol using a tube voltage of 80 kV seems promising[13]. Another study used contrast material administered during primary percutaneous interventions in patients with acute myocardial infarction to detect viable myocardial tissue with CT delayed enhancement[14].

EVALUATION OF CARDIAC VALVES

Crude anatomical information regarding cardiac valve function can be derived from the same data used for left ventricular function evaluation (Figure 19.7). Recent literature has reported a

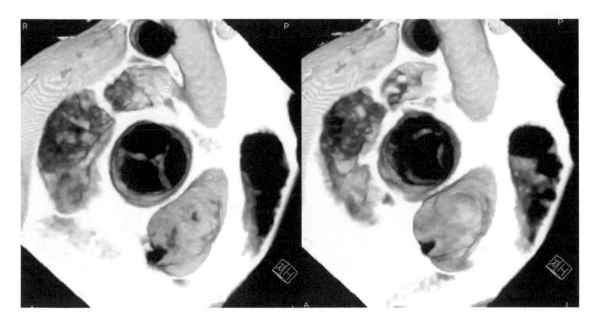

Figure 19.7 Reconstruction of the end-diastolic and end-systolic phase at the level of the aortic root shows the opening and closing of the aortic valve and allows assessment of valve function.

good correlation between CT planimetr y, Doppler echocardiography, and cine MR for the e valuation of aortic valve stenosis [15-17].

REFERENCES

1. Juergens KU, Grude M, Fallenberg EM et al. Using ECG-gated multidetector CT to e valuate global left ventricular m yocardial function in patients with coronar y artery disease. AJR Am J Roentgenol 2002; 179: 1545–50.
2. Grude M, Juergens KU, Wichter T et al. Evaluation of global left ventricular myocardial function with electrocardiogram-gated multidetector computed tomograph y: comparison with magnetic resonance imaging . Invest Radiol 2003; 38: 653–61.
3. Dirksen MS, Bax JJ, de Roos A et al. Usefulness of dynamic multislice computed tomograph y of left ventricular function in unstable angina pectoris and comparison with echocardiography. Am J Cardiol 2002; 90: 1157–60.
4. Juergens KU, Weckesser M, Bettendorf O, Wormanns D. Duodenal somatostatinoma and gastrointestinal stromal tumor associated with neurofibromatosis type 1: diagnosis with PET/CT. AJR Am J Roentgenol 2006; 187: W233–4.
5. Brodoefel H, Kramer U, Reimann A et al. Dual-source CT with improved temporal resolution in assessment of left ventricular function: a pilot study . AJR Am J Roentgenol 2007; 189: 1064–70.
6. Busch S, Johnson TR, Wintersperger BJ et al. Quantitative assessment of left ventricular function with dual-source CT in comparison to cardiac magnetic resonance imaging: initial findings. Eur Radiol 2008; 18: 570–5.
7. Nikolaou K, Sanz J, Wintersperger B et al. Assessment of myocardial perfusion and viability from routine contrast-enhanced 16-detector-row computed tomograph y of the hear t: preliminary results. Eur Radiol 2005; 15: 864–71.
8. Nieman K, Cury RC, Ferencik M et al. Differentiation of recent and chronic m yocardial infarction b y cardiac computed tomography. Am J Cardiol 2006; 98: 303–8.
9. Gerber B, Belge B, Legros G et al. Characterization of acute and chronic m yocardial infarcts b y multidetector computed tomography. Circulation 2006; 113: 823–33.
10. Mahnken AH, Koos R, Katoh M et al. Assessment of myocardial viability in reperfused acute myocardial infarction using 16-slice computed tomography in comparison to magnetic resonance imaging. J Am Coll Cardiol 2005; 45: 2042–7.
11. Lardo A, Cordeiro M, Silva C et al. Contrast-enhanced multidetector computed tomograph y viability imaging after m yocardial infarction: characterization of m yocyte death, microvascular obstruction, and chronic scar. Circulation 2006; 113: 394–404.
12. Baks T, Cademartiri F, Moelker AD et al. Multislice computed tomography and magnetic resonance imaging for the assessment of reperfused acute m yocardial infarction. J Am Coll Cardiol 2006; 48: 144–52.
13. Brodoefel H, Reimann A, Klumpp B et al. Sixty-four-slice CT in the assessment of global and regional left ventricular function: comparison with MRI in a porcine model of acute and subacute myocardial infarction. Eur Radiol 2007; 17: 2948–56.
14. Habis M, Capderou A, Ghostine S et al. Acute m yocardial infarction early viability assessment b y 64-slice computed tomography immediately after coronar y angiography: comparison with low-dose dobutamine echocardiograph y. J Am Coll Cardiol 2007; 49: 1178–85.
15. Habis M, Daoud B, Roger VL et al. Comparison of 64-slice computed tomography planimetry and Doppler echocardiography in the assessment of aor tic valve stenosis. J Hear t Valve Dis 2007; 16: 216–24.
16. Feuchtner GM, Müller S, Bonatti J et al. Sixty-four slice CT evaluation of aor tic stenosis using planimetr y of the aor tic valve area. AJR Am J Roentgenol 2007; 189: 197–203.
17. Alkadhi H, Wildermuth S, Plass A et al. Aor tic stenosis: comparative evaluation of 16-detector row CT and echocardiograph y. Radiology 2006; 240: 47–55.

CHAPTER 20

Computed tomography and electrophysiology

INTRODUCTION

CT imaging has become a useful imaging tool in the electrophysiological management of patients with atrial fibrillation and hear t failure. CT imaging provides important information to plan and guide radiofrequency catheter ablation of the pulmonary veins and e valuate potential complications. Imaging of the cardiac veins aids the percutaneous placement of left ventricular pacing leads as par t of resynchronization therap y in patients with heart failure. In this chapter the use of CT in the context of pulmonar y vein ablation and biventricular pacing is discussed.

PULMONARY VEIN ABLATION

Electrical isolation of the pulmonar y veins b y circumferential radiofrequency catheter ablation is one of the in vasive therapeutic options in atrial fibrillation. CT can pro vide detailed infor mation about the anatomy of the atrium, antrum, and pulmonary veins, including the venous ostium diameters (Figures 20.1 and 20.2). Clinically rele vant variations include common veins, in which the superior and inferior pulmonar y vein on one side are not separated; accessor y veins, which enter the left atrium separately from the four main branches; and ostial branches, which drain into the pulmonary vein close to the atriopulmonar y venous junction (F igure 20.3). Fur thermore, the position (of the ostium) of the atrial appendage is important (Figure 20.1). Occasionally pulmonar y veins drain into the right atrium. The relationship between the esophagus and the left atrium is important (Figure 20.4), as ablation in the proximity of the esophagus can on rare occasions result in the se vere complication of an atrioesophageal fistula. The esophagus can be readily identified on CT images, or may even be augmented by swallowing of barium contrast or placement of a nasogastric tube. Although transesophageal echocardiography is routinely performed for this pur pose, CT may allow detection of thrombotic material in the left atrial appendage, particularly when the patient is in sinus rhythm (Figure 20.5).

CT images can be integrated to enhance electromagnetic mapping during ablation procedures. The ability to na vigate catheters and register ablation lesions using the individual anatom y may improve the result of the procedure. Co-registration of the catheter position and the CT images is limited b y the contractile motion, respiration, hemodynamic status, and gross displacement of the hear t between the imaging and ablation procedure.

After pulmonary vein ablation CT can be used for follow-up to identify complications, such as venous stenosis or thrombosis, which occur in 1–10% of patients, sometimes many months after the procedure[1].

To synchronize the acquisition with opacification of the left atrium and pulmonar y veins contrast enhancement can be monitored in the left atrium during bolus tracking or test bolus injection. If the aor ta is used for contrast timing , as in coronary CT angiograph y, sufficient contrast medium needs to be used to allow for the dela y.

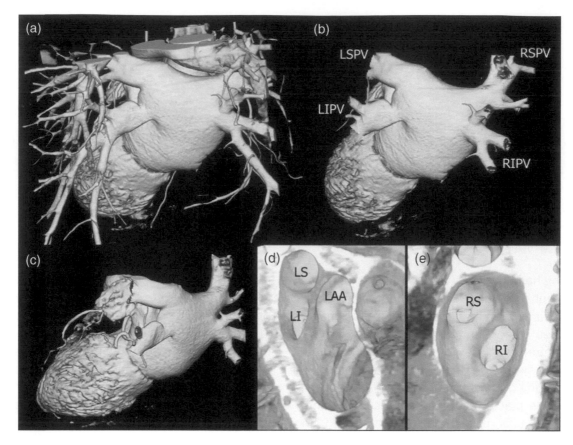

Figure 20 .1 Cardiac CT of pulmonary veins. Three-dimensional volume-rendered images show the anatomy of the left atrium and pulmonary veins. In (a) the aorta and spine have been removed from the image, in (b) and (c) the pulmonary veins have been clipped and the proximal segments of the pulmonary artery have been removed. (d) and (e) Endovascular views show the anatomy of the individual pulmonary vein ostia and the left atrial appendage (LAA). LS, Left superior; LI, left inferior; RS, right superior; RI, right inferior; PV, pulmonary vein.

Electrocardiogram (ECG) gating will improve image quality in patients in sinus rh ythm. In case of atrial fibrillation at the time of CT examination, ECG gating ma y not be necessar y as it often does not substantially impro ve image quality . Acquisition of the CT data at the end of quiet respiration has been recommended for co-registration of the images in the electroph ysiology laboratory[2]. Images are generally reconstr ucted during end-diastole and processed using multiplanar reformation to create or thogonal views at the le vel of the ostium of the individual pulmonar y veins for vessel size measurements (F igure 20.2). Additionally, three-dimensional (endovascular)

reconstr uctions can be made to create an overview of the pulmonar y vein anatom y (Figure 20.1).

CARDIAC VEINS AND BIVENTRICULAR PACING

In selected patients with se vere symptomatic heart failure cardiac resynchronization therap y improves symptoms and exercise tolerability . Biventricular pacing can be achie ved by percutaneous placement of an electrode in a cardiac vein over the epicardial surface of the left ventricle,

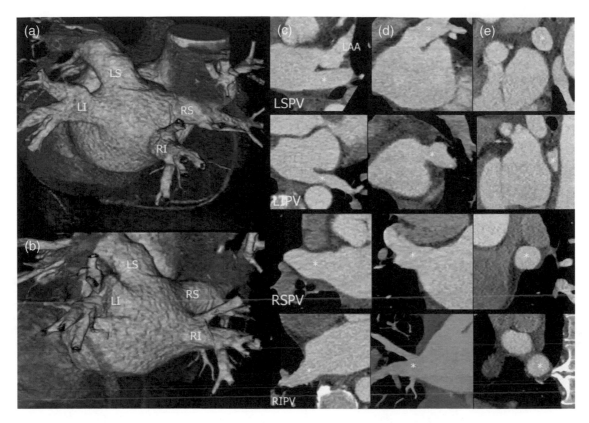

Figure 20 .2 (a) and (b) Volume-rendered images of pulmonary veins. Orthogonal cross-sections, longitudinally (c) and (d) and short-axis (e), can be created using multiplanar reformation and maximum intensity projection to measure the pulmonary vein dimensions. LS, left superior; LI, left inferior; RS, right superior; RI, right inferior; PV, pulmonary vein; LAA, left atrial appendage.

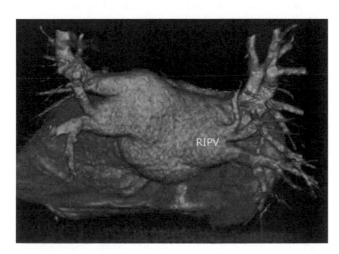

Figure 20 .3 The right inferior pulmonary vein (RIPV) appears to be absent, several branches drain directly into the antrum of the left atrium.

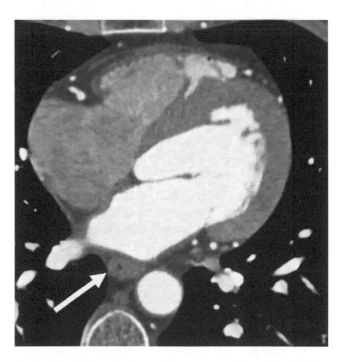

Figure 20 .4 The esophagus is often readily identified in the posterior mediastinum (arrow).

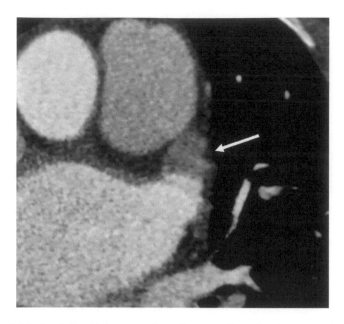

Figure 20.5 Low-density material in the left atrial appendage is suggestive of a thrombus (arrow). Particularly during atrial fibrillation incomplete mixture of contrast medium can cause the appearance of thrombus material in the atrial appendage.

preferably at the location of latest activation. To image the venous system of the heart, CT serves as an alternative to invasive retrograde venography, which is moderately effective and can be complicated by excessive use of contrast medium or damage to the coronary sinus related to balloon occlusion [3].

The coronary sinus in the diaphragmatic part of the left atrioventricular groove continues as the great cardiac vein alongside the left circumflex coronary branch (Figures 20.6 and 20.7). At the anterior surface of the heart this vein continues into the anterior interventricular groove along the left anterior descending coronary artery. Marginal veins of variable size drain into the great cardiac vein in the left atrioventricular groove. The middle cardiac vein or posterior interventricular vein runs parallel to the posterior descending artery in the posterior interventricular groove and usually drains directly into the coronary sinus.

CT can provide information regarding the availability, location, and size of the individual cardiac veins and the options for lead placement [4,5]. The take-off angle of the venous branch from the great cardiac vein, which may complicate positioning of the lead, can be assessed prior to the procedure. The distance from the venous side branches to the coronary sinus. CT images may also be used for electromagnetic navigation of wires into technically challenging venous anatomy[6]. Variant sinus anatomy and the presence of rudimentary valvular structures (Thebesian valves) at the sinus orifice can be detected by CT. While venous enhancement used to be an unavoidable phenomenon with earlier CT technology, current (dual-source) 64-slice scanners require prolongation of the time between aortic enhancement and data acquisition to allow sufficient opacification of the cardiac veins. In patients with implanted pacing devices CT imaging (of the coronary arteries) can be complicated by artifacts caused by the pacemaker wires and, particularly, the distal electrodes (Figure 20.8).

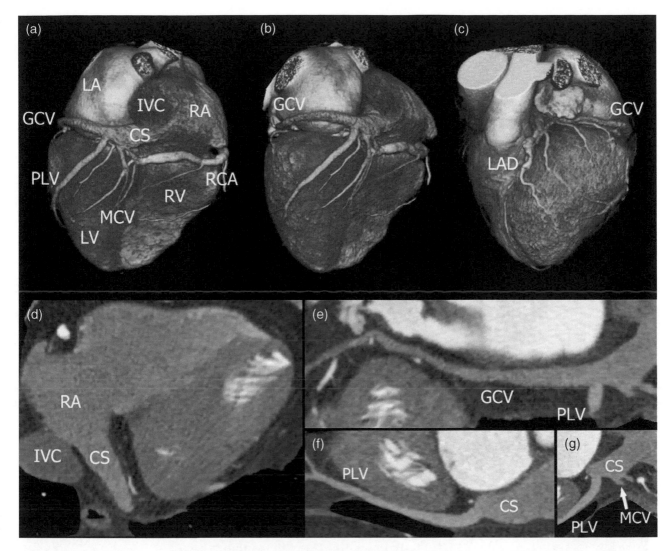

Figure 20 .6 Cardiac vein anatomy on three-dimensional volume-rendered images (a)Đ(c) (rotated from the diaphragmatic to the anterolateral surface of the heart) and curved multiplanar reformations (d)Đ(g). There is a (double) medial cardiac vein (MCV) as well as a substantial posterolateral cardiac vein (PLV) that could easily accommodate a left ventricle (LV) electrode. In addition to the vein diameters, CT also displays the coronary sinus anatomy, the angle between the vein branches and the coronary sinus (CS) or great cardiac vein (GCV). RV, right ventricle; LA, left atrium; RA, right atrium; IVC, inferior vena cava; RCA, right coronary artery; LAD, left anterior descending coronary artery.

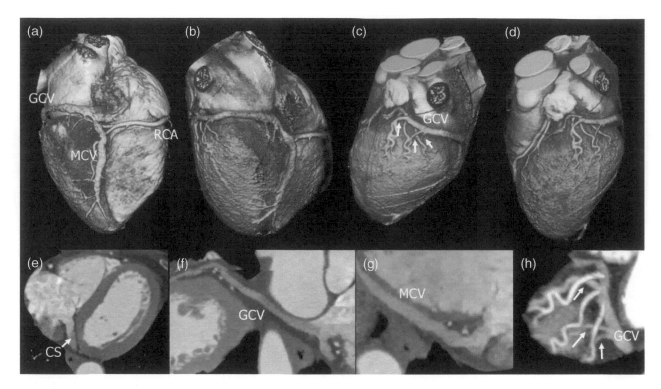

Figure 20.7 Cardiac vein anatomy. In this case there is a large middle cardiac vein (MCV) but only small marginal and posterolateral veins (arrows), which limits the options for left ventricular electrode placement. GCV, great cardiac vein; RCA, right coronary artery; CS, coronary sinus.

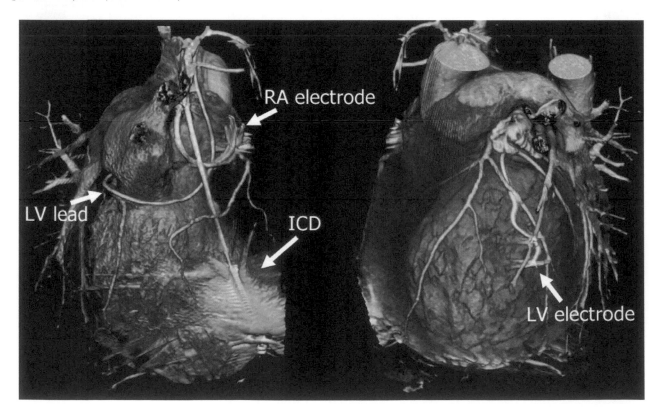

Figure 20 .8 CT imaging after placement of a dual-chamber biventricular pacemaker with intracorporal defibrillator. Electrodes can be observed in the roof of the right atrium (RA), the right ventricle, and on the epicardial surface (within a cardiac vein branch). The implantable cardioverter defibrillator (ICD) electrode causes the most severe image artifacts.

REFERENCES

1. Lacomis JM, Goitein O, Deible C, Schwartzman D. CT of the pulmonary veins. J Thorac Imaging 2007; 22: 63–76.
2. Malchano ZJ, Neuzil P, Cury RC et al. Integration of cardiac CT/MR imaging with three-dimensional electroanatomical mapping to guide catheter manipulation in the left atrium: implications for catheter ablation of atrial fibrillation. J Cardiovasc Electrophysiol 2006; 17: 1221–9.
3. Meisel E, Pfeiffer D, Engelmann L et al. Investigation of coronary venous anatomy by retrograde venography in patients with malignant ventricular tachycardia. Circulation 2001; 104: 442–7.
4. Jongbloed MR, Lamb H, Bax JJ et al. Noninvasive visualization of the cardiac venous system using multislice computed tomography. J Am Coll Cardiol 2005; 45: 749–53.
5. Abbara S, Cury RC, Nieman K et al. Noninvasive evaluation of cardiac veins with 16-MDCT angiography. AJR Am J Roentgenol 2005; 185: 1001–6.
6. Rivero-Ayerza M, Thornton AS, Theuns DA et al. Left ventricular lead placement within a coronary sinus side branch using remote magnetic navigation of a guide wire: a feasibility study. J Cardiovasc Electrophysiol 2006; 17: 128–33.

CHAPTER 21

Non-cardiac findings on cardiac computed tomography

Cardiac CT not only provides information about the heart, great vessels, and coronary arteries, but also about a portion of the lungs, mediastinum, chest wall, spine, and upper abdomen. Inevitably examinations of these additional structures will produce incidental findings that may be clinically insignificant but which may also be of clinical importance such as early cancer (Figures 21.1–21.6). Expertise is required to interpret accurately both cardiac and non-cardiac incidental findings.

Several studies have reported the prevalence of significant non-cardiac findings on CT calcium screening examinations [1-7]. Hunold et al were the first to report on accidental cardiac and non-cardiac findings (Table 21.1)[2]. The mean age of the patients was 59 ± 16 years (range 20–86 years) and 78% were males. The most frequent findings

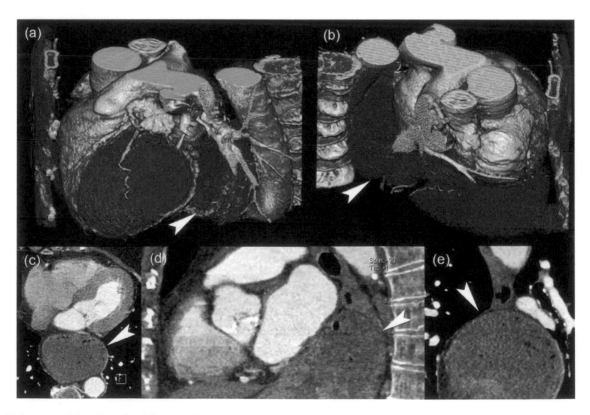

Figure 21.1 Large hiatal hernia. (a) and (b) Volume-rendered images of thorax showing the heart and a large mass in close proximity to the heart (arrowheads). (c) and (d) Multiplanar reconstructed images revealed a mass posterior (c) to the heart contours (d) (arrowheads) compressing the left atrium. (e) Coronal reformatted plane of hernia (arrowhead).

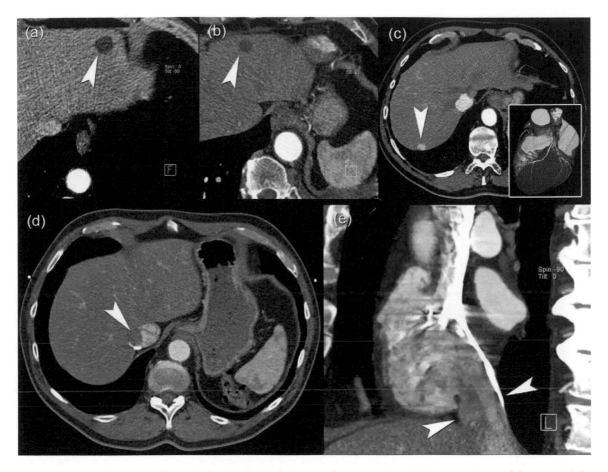

Figure 21.2 Liver abnormalities: (a) and (b) hypodense liver cysts (arrowheads); (c) hemangioma of liver; and (d) and (e) pseudothrombus of vena cava inferior due to non-homogeneous distribution of contrast material (arrowhead) and pseudo-obstruction of vena cava inferior (arrowheads (e)).

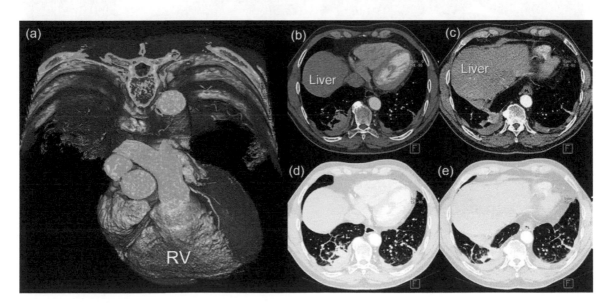

Figure 21.3 Pleural atelectasis. (a) Volume-rendered image of heart, posterior thoracic cavity with spine, and ribs. (b)–(e) Axial images showing heart and liver. The posterior pleura is thickened and posterior lower lobes of lung show areas of atelectasis on both sides. RV, right ventricle.

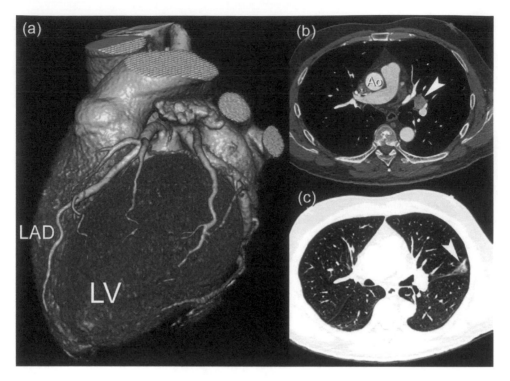

Figure 21.4 Lung carcinoma. (a) Volume-rendered image of the heart with normal left coronary arteries. (b) Axial image with tumor at left lung hilum (arrowhead). (c) Axial image with segmental lung atelectasis (arrowhead). L AD, left anterior descending; LV, left ventricle.

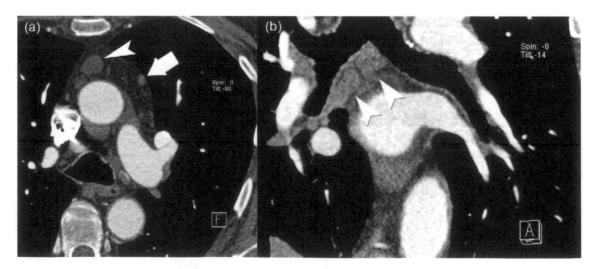

Figure 21.5 Lymph nodes in mediastinum. (a) and (b) Axial images demonstrating small lymph nodes (thick arrow) and large lymph node below the trachea carina (large arrowheads) in the anterior mediastinum.

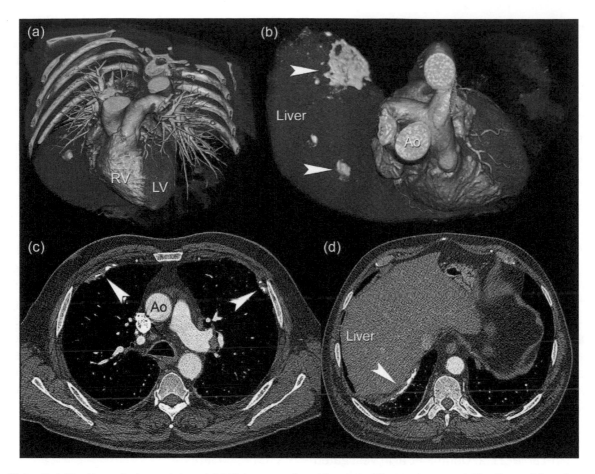

Figure 21.6 Calcifications of pleura. (a) and (b) Volume-rendered images of thorax. Large calcifications of the pleura at the right diaphragmatic site (arrowheads). (c) and (d) Calcifications of pleura at various localizations (arrowheads). RV, right ventricle; LV, left ventricle; Ao, aorta.

Table 21.1 Incidence of non-coronary findings on electron beam CT coronary calcium screening in 1812 consecutive patients. A total of 2055 accidental findings were present in 953 (53%) of patients[2]

	Incidental f idings (%)	Number of incidental f idings	Diagnostic consequences (n)*	Therapeutic consequences (n)*
Heart (pericardium, valves, cavities)	33	676	136	11
Aorta	28	564	9	6
Lung	28	564	13	3
Mediastinum	4	72	12	1
Abdominal organs	2	71	16	1
Spinal column	5	101	0	0

*Number of patients.

Table 21.2 Significant non-cardiac findings on CT coronary calcium examinations in 1326 patients[1]

	n
Non-calcified long nodules <1 cm	53
Lung nodules ≥1 cm	12
Infiltrates	24
Indeterminate liver disease	7
Sclerotic bone lesions	2
Breast abnormalities	2
Polycystic liver disease	1
Esophogeal thickening	1
Ascites	1
Total number with non-cardiac findings	103 (7.8%)

were calcifications of various organs, in particular, aortic and heart valve calcifications. The majority of these incidental findings w ere not clinically significant. Horton et al examined 1326 consecutive patients with an a verage age of 55.4 year s (range 23–87 year s), 60% of whom w ere males and 75% non-smok ers[1]. The abnor mal findings are listed in Table 21.2. Onuma et al in vestigated the frequency of non-cardiac findings in 503 patients who underw ent multislice CT (MSCT) coronary angiography[5]. Cardiologists assessed the heart, while radiologists re viewed the other organs. The mean age of the patient group was 66 ± 9.9 years and 76% w ere males. The incidental non-cardiac findings are listed in Table 21.3.

Several other studies ha ve reported similar findings. In a pooled analysis of all studies concer ning 8083 patients major non-cardiac and cardiac findings requiring specific treatment occurred in 2% of patients (T able 21.4)[1-7]. The occurrence of malignant disease was 0.4%. These studies raise a n extremely important question concerning the responsibility for inter-pretation of the cardiac CT scan. Who should read the scans: the cardiologist or the radiologist? The radiologist is specifically trained in the detection and interpretation of thoracic and abdominal scans, whereas the cardiologist is more specifically trained in the inter pretation of the cardiovascular scan and much less so in other areas. W e therefore belie ve that it is in the best interest of the patient that the examinations are interpreted in close cooperation betw een cardiologist and the radiologist.

CONCLUSION

The incidence of significant non-cardiac incidental findings on cardiac CT scan w as on average 7.1%, and the incidence of cardiac findings w as 7.5%.

Table 21.3 Non-cardiac findings on MSCT coronary angiography in 503 patients

	n	Further investigations (n)*	Therapeutic consequences (n)*
Pulmonary nodules <1 cm	49	25	2
Pulmonary nodules >1 cm	12	8	1
Pulmonary infilbration	16	10	4
Pleural effusion	17	16	6
Extrapleural mass	1	1	0
Breast abnormalities	3	3	1
Lymph node swelling	3	1	0
Aortic disease	8	7	2
Other	5	4	2
Total	114 (23%)	75 (15%)	18 (3.6%)

*Number of patients.

Table 21.4 Frequency and consequences of incidental findings on cardiac CT: a pooled analysis

	Patients (n)	Incidence (%)
Major non-cardiac findings	6271	7.1 (2–15)
Major cardiac findings	1812	7.5
Findings requiring specific treatment		2 (40/2315)
Occurrence of malignant disease		0.4 (9/2481)

Subsequent treatment was deemed necessary in approximately 2%. Correct identification and interpretation of incidental findings requires specific expertise which is best guaranteed by combined reading of the CT scans by a radiologist and cardiologist.

REFERENCES

1. Horton KM, Post WS, Blumenthal RS, Fishman EK. Prevalence of significant noncardiac findings on electron-beam computed tomography coronary artery calcium screening examinations. Circulation 2002; 106: 532–4.
2. Hunold P, Schmermund A, Seibel RM, Gronemeyer DH, Erbel R. Prevalence and clinical significance of accidental findings in electron-beam tomographic scans for coronary artery calcification. Eur Heart J 2001; 22: 1748–58.
3. Elgin EE, O'Malley PG, Feuerstein I, Taylor AJ. Frequency and severity of "incidentalomas" encountered during electron beam computed tomography for coronary calcium in middle-ages army personnel. Am J Cardiol 2002; 90: 543–5.
4. Schragin J, Weissfeld J, Edmundowicz D, Strollo D, Fuhrman C. Non cardiac findings on coronary electron beam computed tomography scanning. J Thor Imaging 2004; 19: 82–6.
5. Onuma Y, Tanabe K, Nakazawa G et al. Noncardiac findings in cardiac imaging with multidetector computed tomography. J Am Coll Cardiol 2006; 48: 402–6.
6. Haller S, Kaiser C, Buser P, Bongartz G, Bremerich J. Coronary artery imaging with contrast-enhanced MDCT: extracardiac findings. AJR Am J Roentgenol 2006; 187: 105–10.
7. Dewey M, Schapauff D, Teige F, Hamm B. Non-cardiac findings on coronary computed tomography and magnetic resonance imaging. Eur Radiol 2007; 17: 2038–43.

CHAPTER 22

Artifacts

An artifact is defined as a distortion or error in an image that is not related to the structure being imaged[1]. Artifacts can be divided into two main categories:

(1) Artifacts that are inherent to the technical design of the scanner or inherent to the physics of the technique. For instance, using a black and white film creates black and white images. This generates an artifact because the color is missing owing to the technical limitation of film that can only create black and white images.

(2) Artifacts that are generated in the application of the technique. For instance, the shutter speed of a camera falls short if the object to be photographed moves faster than the shutter speed which results in a blurred image.

Artifacts may also be defined as an inaccurate representation of the structure being imaged. The degree of inaccuracy may be small and have no impact on the diagnostic information of the image or may be large and severely distort the diagnostic information.

Coronary imaging is considered to be the ultimate challenge to CT because the coronary arteries are small, tortuous, and subject to significant motion owing to cardiac contraction and inspiration[2,3]. This places optimal demands on the techniques in terms of temporal, spatial, and contrast resolution, that cannot always be met. For instance, the speed of motion during systole is too fast for the specifications of the CT scanner. Thus, to achieve optimal 'artifact-free' coronary images the acquisition should be fast (short temporal resolution), the voxels should be small (high x-y-z axis resolution), and the attenuation value should be high (optimal contrast resolution)[4].

Adequate knowledge about artifacts is necessary to prevent their generation, or if they do occur should help to identify and interpret the artifact. In the following paragraphs temporal, spatial, and contrast resolution, and other parameters are discussed.

TEMPORAL RESOLUTION

Temporal resolution is of paramount importance in imaging of moving organs (Figure 22.1). An object can move at a certain speed and a sharp image of the object can be obtained only if the time required to obtain the image is faster than the speed of motion of the object. In cardiac CT, temporal resolution is the time required for the acquisition of data that are used to generate one image.

Temporal resolution in CT imaging depends mainly on the gantry rotation time and on the algorithm for image reconstruction. The algorithms for image reconstruction are defined based on the number of segments that they can use to reconstruct one image. The 180° of gantry rotation that are required to generate one image can be obtained from the same cardiac cycle (e.g. single segment) or from more than one consecutive cardiac cycle (e.g. multisegment). In principle, single-segment algorithm should be preferred at low heart rates (<70 bpm) and whenever possible. For high heart rates (>70 bpm), multisegment algorithms may improve image quality.

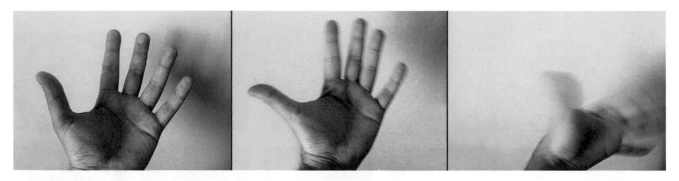

Figure 22.1 Temporal resolution. The relationship between speed of image acquisition and the speed of motion of the object to be imaged determines the amount of blurring that will be displayed. Ideally, the speed of image acquisition is much faster than the speed of the object. In cardiac CT these two factors are equally dependent on the heart rate and the reconstruction algorithm.

It is obvious that the slower the motion of the object the better the images. Therefore, using a fixed temporal window, the balance between the speed of acquisition and the speed of the object can be improved by slowing down the motion of the object. This is the reason why several centers suggest using negative chronotropic drugs prior to the scan to reduce the heart rate. Respiratory or other voluntary or non-voluntary motion artifacts can only be reduced by other measures, including breath hold and lying still on the couch.

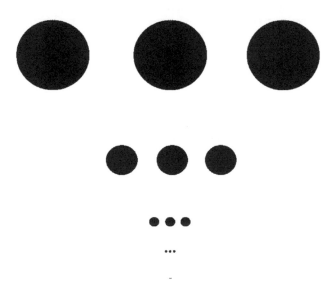

Figure 22.2 Spatial resolution. The capability of a technique to separate two neighboring objects defines its spatial resolution

SPATIAL RESOLUTION

Spatial resolution is the capability to discern two small objects (Figure 22.2). It depends on several different parameters related to the CT scanner. Most of the parameters that affect spatial resolution cannot be modified by the operator (focal spot size, detector size, distance between focal spot and detector ring, number of projections, etc.). The operator instead can modify other parameters in the scan and reconstruction phases (e.g. collimation, reconstruction increment, field of view, filtering, etc.) to exploit the maximal spatial resolution allowed by the CT scanner.

CONTRAST RESOLUTION

The degree of contrast to differentiate between tissues with varying attenuation characteristics is defined as contrast resolution (Figure 22.3). Because CT has a much better contrast resolution than conventional radiography, tissues with only very small differences in density can be distinguished. The contrast resolution is affected by a number of fixed factors such as the detector sensitivity and patient size. Factors that can be influenced include the radiation intensity (the X-ray tube's current and voltage), slice thickness, reconstruction filtering, and image noise. Additionally, the display of the tissue contrast is affected by the window settings. The display size and the distance between the

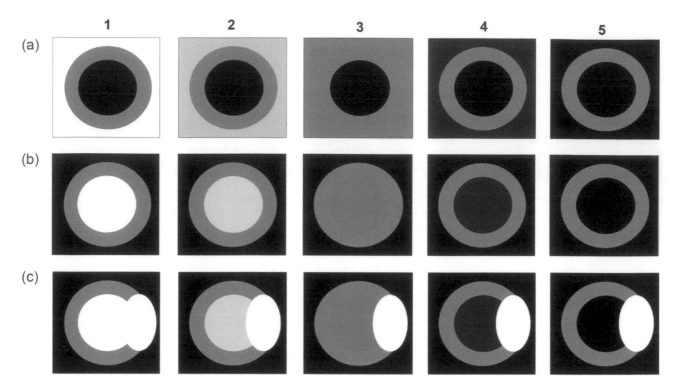

Figure 22.3 Contrast resolution. Contrast resolution defines the capability of a technique to discriminate between objects when their imaging properties are similar. In the first example (row a, 1Ð5) a round object with a black core surrounded by a gray ring is set into a background that varies from white (1) to black (5). In the middle panel (3), the background is similar to the ring of the object so that it disappears, while the black core remains visible. In the second example (row b, 1Ð5) a rounded object with a white core and a gray ring is set into a black background. The color of the core varies from white (1) to black (5). This causes the core of the object to merge with the surrounding ring when their colors become similar. In the third example (row c, 1Ð5) the same object as in row B is displayed, that in this case can be regarded as a cross-sectional view of a coronary vessel. The background is black because it is fat tissue, the ring around the object is gray like the vessel wall (i.e. endothelium, tunica media, adventitia, and eventually plaque tissue) and the core of the object (i.e. vessel lumen) is of variable color depending on the vascular enhancement. In addition, a white object (i.e. calcification in the vessel wall) is added to the gray ring. The variation of the colour of the lumen from white (1) to black (5) shows how the respective components of the coronary artery are visualized. In particular, too high an enhancement in the lumen prevents an adequate depiction of the borders of the calcification in the vessel wall (1), while the absence of enhancement prevents the visualization of the lumen (3). The ideal situation occurs when the vessel enhancement has a value that is in between that of the calcification and the vessel wall. The cases represented in (4) and (5) are not of clinical use because they presuppose the presence of a negative contrast within the vessel lumen.

observer and the screen influence the perception of contrast resolution. Image noise, which is the fluctuation of the measurement compared with the nominal density, affects contrast resolution. The amount of noise is related to a number of the factors mentioned above, including the radiation intensity, the slice thickness, and detector size.

NOISE

Noise can be exemplified as the 'fog' when looking out of the window. Depending on the amount and density of the water particles in the air the image that is seen becomes progressively fuzzy and contours are more difficult to detect.

The noise in the CT image is the variability of the attenuation value between two neighboring voxels compared with the average attenuation measured in that area (Figure 22.4). Ideally, a perfect scanner would produce images with extremely low noise so that when the operator measures the attenuation in the vessel lumen the resulting value would be almost the same in neighboring voxels. Commercially available scanners can produce images with very low noise but

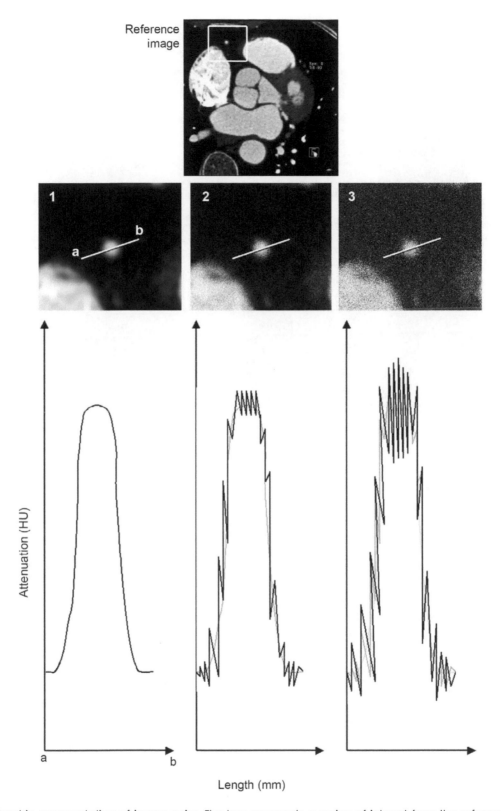

Figure 22.4 Graphic representation of image noise. The box represents a region of interest from the reference axial image obtained at the mid-segment of the right coronary artery. In (1)–(3) noise is progressively added. The attenuation values along the line a–b are then plotted in the length–attenuation graphs. The first example (1) shows the case of very low noise and the corresponding graph displays a smooth curve in the transition between a and b. In the examples (2) and (3), the increase in noise causes a progressively larger oscillation of the attenuation values. This example explains why images with noise are more difficult to evaluate.

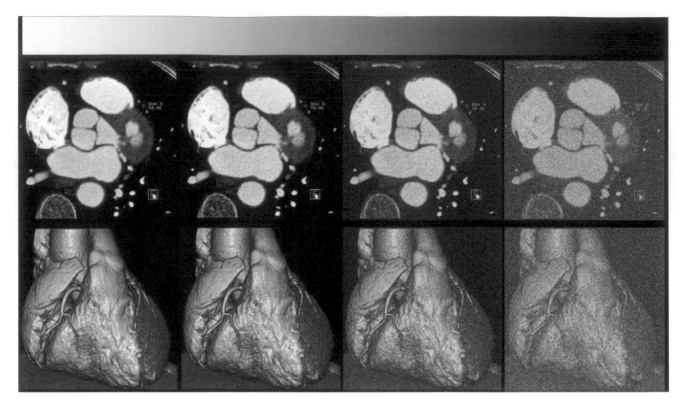

Figure 22.5 Increasing image noise exemplified in the visualization of the right coronary artery

at the 'price' of a high dose of radiation. One of the main factors that deter mine the noise in the image is the number of milliamperes per second produced by the X-ra y tube. Increasing the milliamperes per second will increase the number of photons that can hit the detector , thereby increasing the ratio betw een signal and noise.

When noise increases in the images (Figure 22.5) the ability to discer n objects is impaired regardless of the spatial resolution.

PARTIAL VOLUME, INTERPOLATION, AND FILTERING

Partial volume (also known as 'volume a veraging') is an ar tifact that occur s in all voxels of all images. It depends on the fact that voxels are much larger than the str uctures that the y

represent. For instance, in a voxel of 0.3 x 0.3 x 0.3 mm, a submillimetric str ucture such as endothelium cannot be represented (F igure 22.6). Therefore, it will be a veraged with other sur rounding structures such as the vessel lumen and the inner layers of the vessel wall (i.e. adventitia). The final appearance of the voxel where the endothelium lies will be the result of the averaged attenuation of all the str uctures that are present.

Interpolation averages the attenuation across neighboring and distant pixels/voxels. It is used to create data and fill the gap betw een two known points. This becomes par ticularly evident in areas of the image where there is a very large attenuation gradient. Examples of these areas are the edge betw een air and soft tissues in the lung parenchyma, or the edge betw een calcium and soft tissue in the coronar y artery walls.

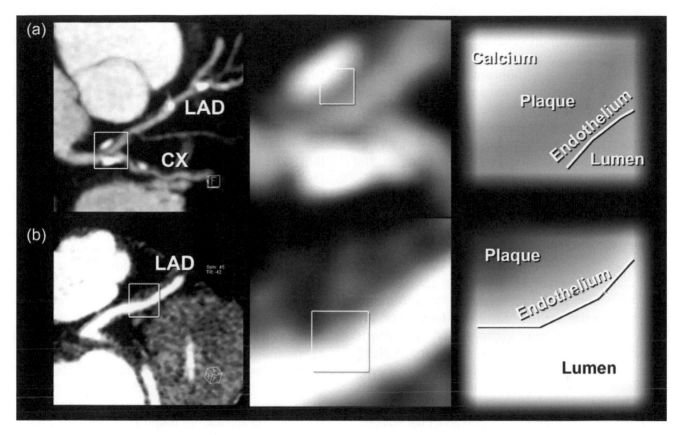

Figure 22.6 Volume averaging. Volume averaging is an artifact that affects all images in the data set. (a), Mixed plaque (calcific and non-calcific plaque) in the left anterior descending artery (LAD). The progressive magnification of the plaque in the transition area between calcium, plaque, and lumen displays how the microscopic structures such as endothelium cannot be distinguished. This is also the case in a non-calcific plaque (b). CX, circumflex artery

Partial volume and interpolation causes the so-called 'blooming' effect as can be seen in calcium, contrast material, and surgical clips in the coronary arteries. These highly attenuating structures appear much larger than their actual size because of the averaging within the voxel and interpolation between all the neighboring voxels.

Filtering reduces this effect. Filters are designed to enhance the edges between structures with different attenuation. This procedure tries to restore the balance between the need for an adequate interpolation (that smooths the image) and the need for adequate detection of edges (that sharpens the image). Unfortunately, filtering increases the noise of the image.

Therefore, the operator should identify the correct balance between filtering and noise to obtain sharper images.

BEAM-HARDENING ARTIFACTS

Beam-hardening artifacts occur when the radiation is completely absorbed by an object with extremely high attenuation. The effect can be compared to a shield for the X-ray beam. The human body modifies the photon spectrum of the heterochromic X-ray beam. High-energy photons are absorbed to a lesser extent, while low-energy photons are highly absorbed. Therefore, the average energy level of absorbed photons is shifted to the higher energies, that strike the detector array. This phenomenon causes beam-hardening artifacts.

In cardiac imaging different objects have a high X-ray absorption: pacemaker wires, prosthetic valves, surgical clips, indicators at the anastomosis site of bypass grafts, sternal wires, and stents. The pooling of high concentrations of contrast material in the superior vena cava and right atrium and ventricle can also cause beam-hardening artifacts.

CLASSIFICATIONS

The classification of artifacts in coronary CT can be based on the physics that create the artifact, on the source of the artifact, or on the appearance of the artifacts. A pragmatic approach would be to follow a 'chronological' classification. This implies that the sequence of the scan procedure is followed and the artifacts that are generated in each phase are explained. When available, solutions and practical advice are given to compensate or prevent the occurrence of the respective artifacts.

MOTION ARTIFACTS

Motion artifacts are caused by motion of the patient or one of his/her parts in an unexpected or exaggerated manner (Table 22.1). In the first case, a typical example is respiratory motion when the patient is not supposed to breathe (Figure 22.7). In the second case, a typical example is the motion of the coronary artery because of an inadequate ratio between the acquisition speed (e.g. temporal resolution) and the speed of the vessel (Figure 22.8).

The correct approach to motion artifacts starts before the scan. Most sources of motion artifacts can be managed properly with thorough patient selection and preparation.

High heart rates (>70 bpm) should be avoided (Figure 22.9), although, it may be possible to achieve sufficient image quality with a high heart rate, the success is lower and parts of the coronary tree cannot be visualized.

Irregular heart rates are not an absolute contraindication to coronary CT angiography. While irregular heart rates characterized by a high ventricular response (>70 bpm) amplify the problems described for high heart rates, mild heart rhythm irregularities with an average heart rate <70 bpm can be managed in most cases (if the software allows electrocardiogram (ECG) editing) during the reconstruction of the images (see below).

Extrasystoles can be considered as mild heart rhythm irregularities, and are not a contraindication for coronary CT angiography unless they are very frequent (more than one in two heart beats). It can be wise to look for the occurrence or disappearance of extrasystoles during breath hold prior to scan. This can be tested with a test 15 s breath hold.

Patient breathing during the scan can cause scan failure (Figure 22.10). Therefore, the patient should be thoroughly instructed and tested in his/her breath holding prior to the scan. The operator should check that the patient performs an inspiratory breath hold without performing a Valsalva maneuver. The higher pressure generated during this maneuver can reduce the inflow of contrast material through the subclavian vein and the pressure can also impair the ability of the patient to stay still. Patients can also have difficulties in maintaining a still position when the breath hold is too deep (Figure 22.11). Moreover, with a required apnea of about 15–18 s, a deeper breath hold will provide a significant advantage. When the required apnea is longer the patient should be trained accordingly. It is then recommended to teach the patient to perform an inspiratory breath hold without Valsalva maneuver.

In some cases the patient can move voluntarily during the scan because of the sudden heat sensation that rushes through the whole body (owing to the intravenous administration of contrast material), and which may cause coughing or sneezing. The operator should explain to the patient the type of feeling he/she will experience to prevent coughing or sneezing.

Another source of involuntary motion, different from the one determined by heart contraction, is

Table 22.1 Type, cause, and management of artifacts

Type	Problem	Cause	Solution	Practical advice
Motion (Think well, talk well, and act well BEFORE the patient starts the procedure)	High heart rate	Insufficient temporal resolution	Scan heart rate <70bpm for the visualization of the entire coronary tree	At heart rate >70bpm the scan can be performed but the complete visualization of the coronary tree will not be possible. If the indication of the scan is proximal coronary obstructive disease scan with heart rate <90bpm can be performed even though with a lower rate of success when compared to lower heart rate
	Irregular heart rate	Atrial fibrillation Other irregularities Insufficient temporal resolution Too short diastolic phase	Scan regular heart rate Medication ECG editing Abort ECG editing	For irregularities characterized by a defined QRS complex and at least intermittent diastolic periods >500ms it is still possible to perform ECG editing Before the scan evaluate the presence of extrasystole. When extrasystole are present on a sinus rhythm <65 bpm the ECG editing it is always feasible
		Extrasystole triggered during breath hold	Test the apnea prior to the scan and look for extrasystole	Test the apnea prior to the scan
	Patient breathing	Poor patient instructions Stressed patient	Instruct thoroughly the patient Perform more than one test apnea	
		Language barrier	Adapt language	The referring physician should properly address this type of patient Ensure the technician talks to the patient prior to the scan
		Partial or total deafness	Trigger breath hold with a visual signal (if available on the scanner)	
	Breath-hold control	Valsalva maneuver	Instruct and test the patient to prevent Valsalva maneuver	Valsalva maneuver impairs the ability to remain still and also prevents the inflow of contrast material from the subclavian vein because of the increased intrathoracic pressure
		Too deep inspiratory breath hold	Instruct and test the patient to perform a normal inspiratory breath hold	Too deep an inspiratory breath hold impairs the ability to remain still
	Patient voluntary motion	Hot sensation from contrast material	Warn the patient about the heat he/she will experience during the scan	
		Coughing/sneezing	Warn the patient about the importance of staying still during breath hold and eventually use medication to reduce the symptoms	
	Patient non-voluntary motion	Diaphragmatic drift	Reduce scan time	With a scan time of 15⊠20s a certain amount of diaphragmatic drift cannot be avoided. With a scan time of <10s the impact of diaphragmatic drift will be significantly reduced

(Continued)

Table 22.1 Type, cause, and management of artifacts—cont'd

Type	Problem	Cause	Solution	Practical advice
Image contrast/noise (Owing to 'tube current/patient absorption')	'Large' patient	High tissue absorption throughout the data set	Increase mA/s	The overwhelming noise in the image can prevent adequate diagnostic evaluation of coronary arteries. For patients >100kg use the maximum dose allowed by the scanner compatible with patient's age
	'Very large' breast	High tissue absorption in the distal part of the data set	Increase mA/s	The overwhelming noise in the image can prevent adequate diagnostic evaluation of the distal part of the coronary arteries. Use the maximum dose allowed by the scanner compatible with patient's age
Beam hardening (Owing to scan and reconstruction geometry)	Streak artifacts	Contrast materia (SVC and right heart) Calcium, stents, clips	Use bolus chaser Increase mA/s Use higher convolution filters	Use the most 'diagnostic' radiation dose. A low dose of radiation is still too high if the diagnosis cannot be made
Volume averaging (Owing to interpolation)	'Blooming'	Contrast material Calcium, stents, clips	Use bolus chaser Increase mA/s Use higher convolution filters	Use the most 'diagnostic' radiation dose. A low dose of radiation is still too high if the diagnosis cannot be made
Temporal window	Misregistration of data in one isolated stack of images	Patient motion	Improve patient instructions	
	Motion in segment 2 (mid-RCA)	Suboptimal selection of temporal window	Try a different reconstruction (±50ms/10%)	Think ahead: optimization should be 'per vessel' rather than per data set
	Diffuse but not heavy motion especially on the RCA	Suboptimal selection of temporal window	Try a different reconstruction window (±50ms/10%)	
	Heavy motion artifact in one isolated stack of images	Extrasystole/premature heart beat	Exclude extrasystole with ECG editing	
	Heavy motion artifact in multiple stacks of images	Irregular ECG wave or irregular heart rhythm	Check ECG automatic triggering and edit if necessary	
Missing data (The software cannot find the information regarding a certain moment in time and you have to understand why)	Lack of information at a defined level of the scan range	Irregular ECG baseline	ECG editing	
		Mistriggering Very low heart rate (<40bpm)	ECG editing ECG editing	

Category	Problem	Cause	Solution
	Extrasystole with borderline ECG editing heart rate		Perform dummy apnea
	Missed LM	Scan start too low; Patient apnea during topogram was different from that during the angiography scan	Re-scan the small proximal range after administering a 60 ml bolus of contrast material
	Missed PDA	Scan ends too high; Patient apnea during topogram was different from that during the angiography scan	Re-scan the small distal range after administering a 60-ml bolus of contrast material; Use a scan range longer than required and end the scan manually when the real-time images show the PDA
Vessel enhancement (For stenosis assessment high is better)	Poor enhancement	Extremely fast circulation time (young patients, congenital anomalies of the great vessels of the thorax and heart)	Start the scan visually and increase injection parameters (volume/rate/iodine)
		Early-triggering bolus tracking	Streak artifacts from the SVC and projecting into the ROI, trigger the scan; Position carefully the ROI in the middle of the ascending aorta and select the monitoring level not too close to the heart
		Late-triggering bolus tracking	Start the scan visually when the contrast material appears in the ascending aorta
		Low rate	Use >3 ml/s
		Low iodine	Use >350 mg/ml
		Low volume	Use no less than 100 ml
		Wrist IV	Use antecubital access
		Partial extravasation	Use large veins; Test veins with saline
	No enhancement	Injector not connected	Connect injector
		Injector-tube disconnection	Tight injector-tube connection
		Extravasation	Use large veins
Image quality	Noisy images	Too low mA/s	Reduce filtering (will decrease confidence in stenosis evaluation)
		⌀large ⌀patient/breast	Reduce filtering (will decrease confidence in stenosis evaluation)

ECG, electrocardiogram; SVC, superior vena cava; RCA, right coronary artery; LM, left main coronary artery; PCA, posterior descending artery; ROI, region of interest; IV, intravenous; LAD, left anterior descending coronary artery.

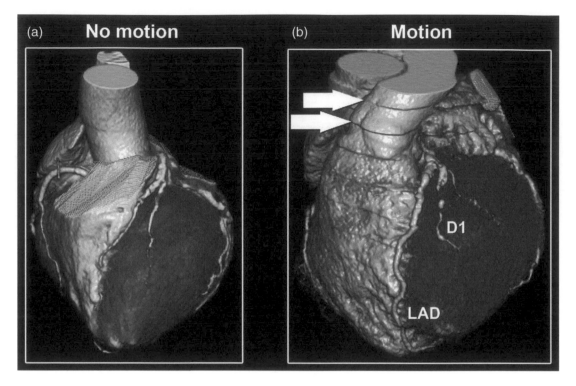

Figure 22.7 Voluntary motion. Two examples are displayed with three-dimensional volume rendering. (a) No voluntary motion is present. (b) Voluntary motion is present (arrows). LAD, left anterior descending; D1, first diagonal branch.

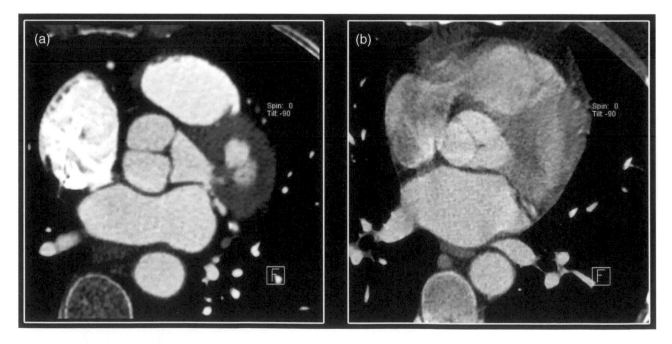

Figure 22.8 Involuntary motion. Two example axial images are displayed. (a) No motion is present and the structures of the heart are sharp. (b) Motion from heart beat is present and all the relevant structures of the heart are blurred.

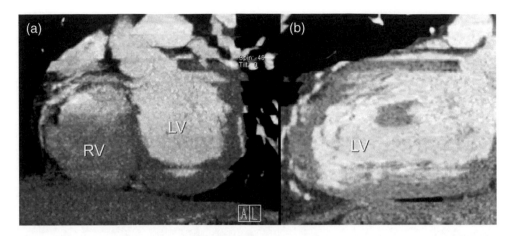

Figure 22.9 Motion artifacts resulting from high heart rate. High heart rates may cause deterioration of image quality. (a) Short-axis view of the right coronary artery. (b) Long-axis view from the left anterior descending artery. The images were obtained from a patient with a heart rate of 120 bpm. LV, left ventricle; RV, right ventricle.

the 'diaphragmatic drift'. This phenomenon occurs 8–10 s after the initiation of a standard breath hold. It consists of a slow and progressive motion of the diaphragm in the caudocranial direction. Usually, because it is slow and progressive, and it runs in one direction, it does not significantly affect the diagnostic quality of the images. It only enhances the misregistration between consecutive stacks of images, creating steps. There is no means to avoid it; however, a shorter scan time (<10 s) will probably reduce significantly the occurrence of diaphragmatic drift.

IMAGE SIGNAL TO NOISE RATIO

Image noise impairs image quality, which can result in non-diagnostic image quality and, therefore, scan failure (Table 22.1). The radiation dose (i.e. mA/s) should be modified according to the ratio between) the X-ray dose and the absorption of the patient. In patients with normal weight and length, the X-ray dose should be adjusted depending on the specific scanner. Preset protocols and experience usually allow identification of the appropriate dose. A low X-ray dose is desirable;

however, this reduces image quality. When the ratio between the X-ray dose and the patient's absorption is too low the scan can be too noisy and therefore not assessable (Figure 22.12).

There are two situations in which the radiation dose must be increased. The first is in a large patient with a significant amount of soft tissue surrounding the thorax (Figure 22.13). More soft tissue means that the radiation is absorbed and fewer photons strike the detector array, which results in increased noise. The second is in a woman with large breasts (Figure 22.14). Here the presence of a large amount of fat tissue absorbs photons again causing increased noise. In both cases, a physical examination and/or scans that precede the coronary CT angiography would identify the situation and a higher X-ray dose should be given.

Definite values of milliamperes cannot be provided because they depend on the specific characteristics of a specific scanner (e.g. rotation time, X-ray tube power, etc.). As a guideline, once the operator has defined a protocol that provides an optimal image quality in 'standard patients', the milliamperes should be increased by 15–20% in large-sized patients or women with large breasts. In cases of extremely large patients or

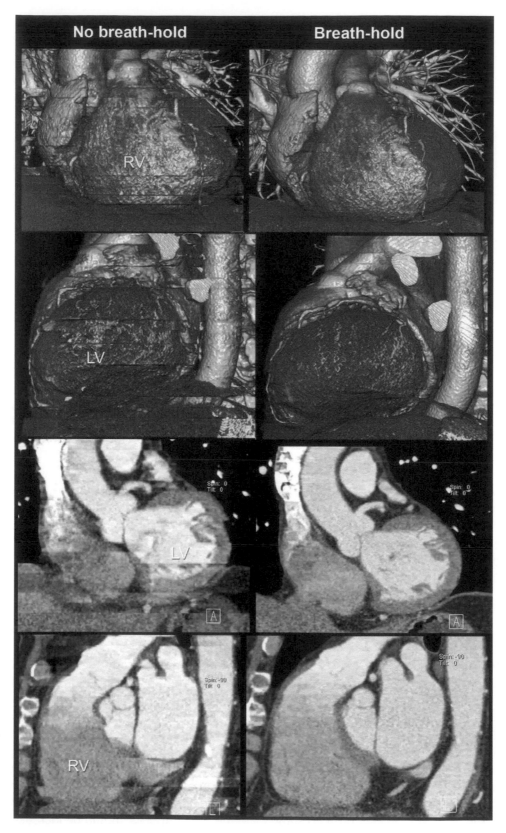

Figure 22.10 Cardiac CT scan without and with breath hold. The images obtained during a non-breath hold acquisition cannot be evaluated. The only solution is to repeat the scan as displayed in the right panels. LV, left ventricle; RV, right ventricle.

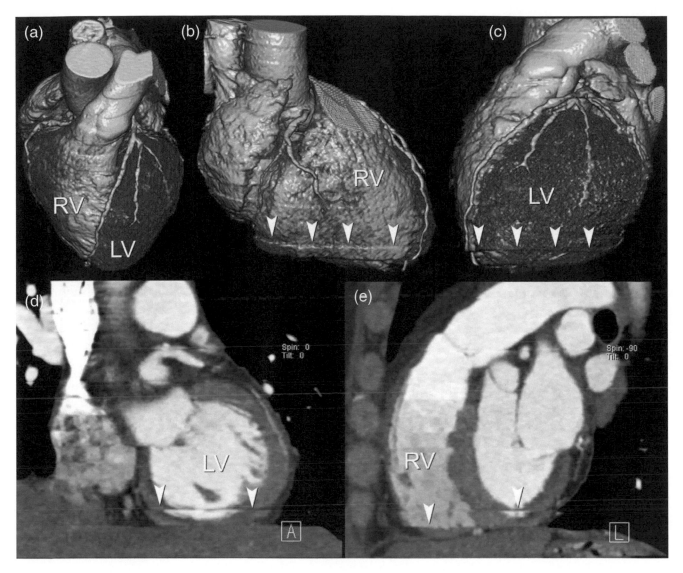

Figure 22.11 Respiratory-motion artifacts. In some cases the patient cannot perform a steady breath hold during the scan. At the end of the scan some motion artifacts may be observed. Volume rendering of the proximal part of the data set shows a very good image quality (a). In the distal part of the data set, there is misregistration between the stacks of images (arrowheads in (b) and (c)). Also, in the coronal (d) and sagittal (e) multiplanar views the presence of misregistration (arrowheads) can be appreciated. LV, left ventricle; RV, right ventricle.

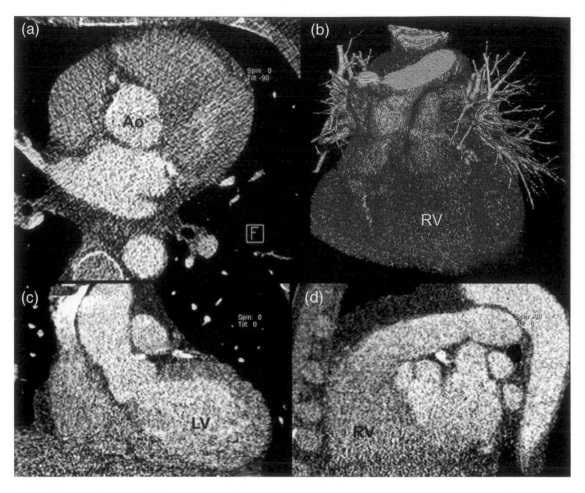

Figure 22.12 Noise causing scan failure. The cardiac CT scan result may be too noisy when the ratio between the X-ray attenuation by the patient and the X-ray dose is too high. The images reconstructed from a data set with excessive noise cannot be improved. The noise in the axial image (a) does not allow adequate images to be achieved with volume rendering (b), or with coronal (c), or sagittal (d) multiplanar views. LV, left ventricle; RV, right ventricle.

breasts, the number milliamperes should be set to the maximum allowed by the scanner.

BEAM-HARDENING ARTIFACTS

Beam-hardening artifacts are always present when a high-density object is imaged in the data set (Table 22.1). The importance of the artifact progressively increases with the degree of attenuation of the object until it creates a true 'shadow' of low attenuation on the opposite side of the object.

Beam-hardening artifacts are annoying because they prevent adequate visualization of the surrounding structures (Figures 22.15 and 22.16). Unfortunately, to date, there is no good solution to avoid or handle this type of artifact.

VOLUME AVERAGING ARTIFACTS

Volume averaging occurs in all cases when large differences in attenuation are present between two neighboring structures (Table 22.1). In cardiac CT this occurs most often around structures with high attenuation such as calcium, stents, surgical clips, and pooling of contrast material. The appearance of an object with high attenuation is enlarged (Figure 22.17).

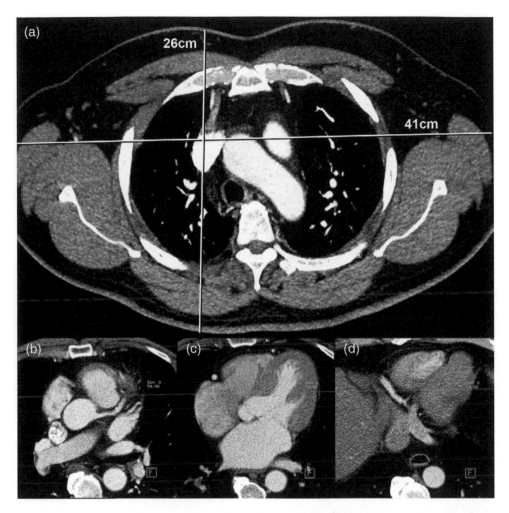

Figure 22.13 Coronary CT of a large patient. In patients with a high body weight or body mass, the scan power has to be set to a maximum to produce images of diagnostic quality. In this example a patient weighing >100 kg was scanned with a tube load of 725 mA/s and a rotation time of 375 ms (a). The generated axial images at different levels (b)–(d) are of diagnostic image quality.

TEMPORAL WINDOW

The correct positioning of the temporal window within the cardiac cycle to obtain motion-free images is mandatory for a data set of good quality. Unfortunately, there are only a few rules to identify the position within the diastolic phase where the motion of all coronary segments is minimized (Table 22.1). Often, especially when the heart rate is not stable or with high heart rates, it is not possible to identify one single data set in which all segments are motion-free.

The basic approach can be summarized as follows. After the end of the scan procedure the operator should perform a reconstruction in the mid-to-end-diastolic phase starting at −400 ms before the R wave or at 60% of the R-to-R interval. When the images are not optimal in this data set there are two possibilities: the data set is of good quality but one or more segments still have residual motion, or the data set is not of diagnostic quality and there is residual motion along the entire coronary tree. In the first case, the operator should perform additional reconstruction with similar settings (e.g. −350/−450 ms or 55/65%). In the second case, the operator should perform a multiphasic reconstruction (i.e. 10–20 reconstructions at each 5–10% of

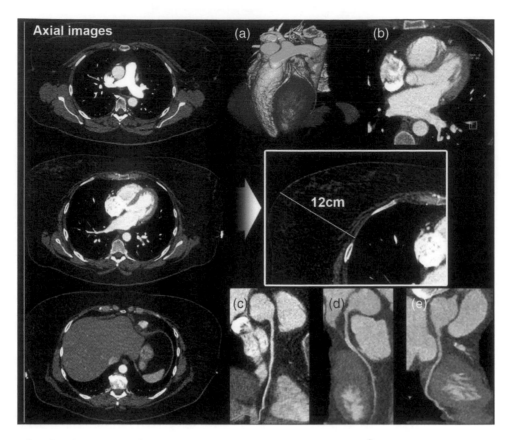

Figure 22.14 Cardiac CT of a woman with large breasts. The ratio between patient's X-ray absorption and X-ray dose should be optimized in the presence of a large breast. In this example the patient was scanned with a tube load of 720 mA/s and a rotation time of 375 ms. The panoramic axial images in the left panel show the amount of tissue that surrounds the thorax (see thickness in the white box). The three-dimensional volume rendering (a) and the axial images (b) are of sufficient image quality. The curved multiplanar reconstruction of the right coronary artery (c), left anterior descending (d), and left circumflex, (e) although noisy, are also of diagnostic image quality.

the R-to-R interval) throughout the cardiac cycle to sample the best position for the temporal window.

In some cases the image quality of the data set is good even though one single stack of images is misregistered (Figure 22.18). A small amount of misregistration can often be observed (Figure 22.19). In these cases no further data sets are required.

When residual motion is confined to the mid-right coronary artery a further data set should be reconstructed with slightly earlier and slightly delayed temporal window settings.

When residual motion affects the entire right coronary artery a reconstruction should be performed at around 30% of the R-to-R interval.

When a stack of images looks completely out of registration while in others no major motion artifact has been observed, the operator should inspect the ECG for the presence of premature beats (Figure 22.20).

MISSING DATA

When the ECG signal is low and noisy, the automatic triggering software can have problems in properly detecting the R wave (Table 22.1). Therefore, the quality of the ECG signal and proper ECG triggering should always be checked by the operator before starting the reconstructions.

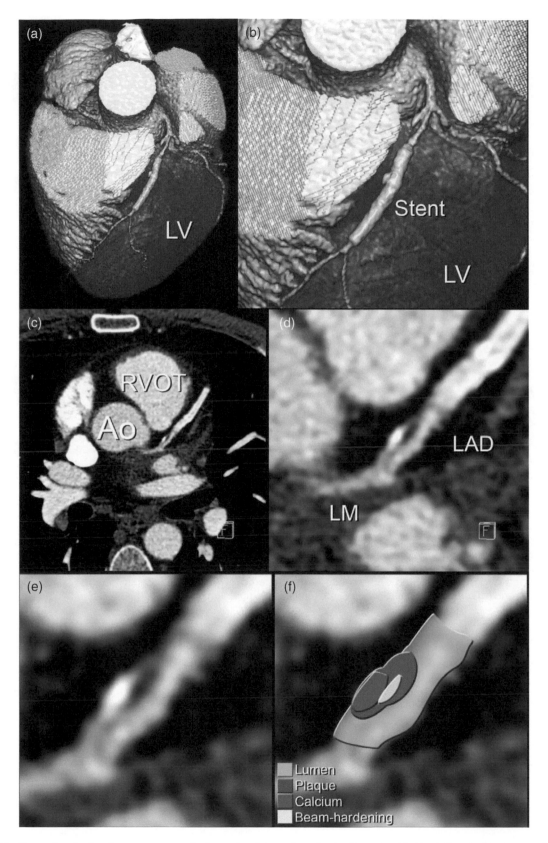

Figure 22.15 Beam hardening from coronary stents and calcium. A patient with a stent in the left anterior descending (LAD) is displayed with three-dimensional volume rendering (a) and (b). On the original axial images at the level of the proximal left anterior descending (c) and especially after magnification (d) a plaque can be visualized with both calcific and non-calcific parts. After further magnification (e), and labeling (f) several different components of the plaque can be identified. In particular, it is possible to see the dark region (yellow colour in (f)) close to the calcific region (blue in (F)) of the plaque and projecting towards the lumen of the vessel (green in (F)). This region is not an actual low-attenuation region owing to the presence of lipid material but it is a shadow owing to beam-hardening artifact. Ao, ascending aorta; LM, left main coronary artery; LV, left ventricle; RV, right ventricle.

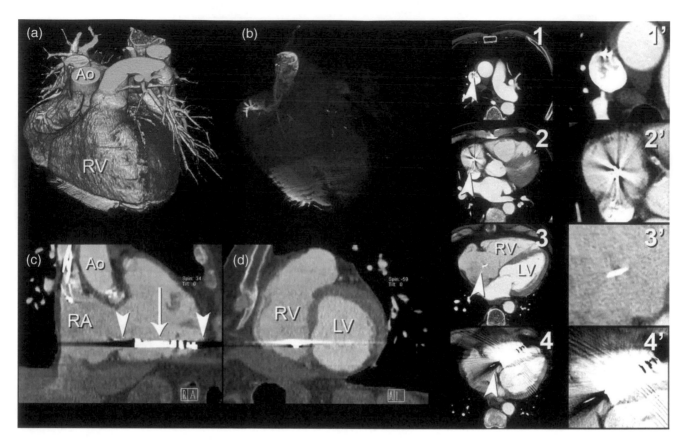

Figure 22.16 Beam hardening from pacemaker wires. A patient with a pacemaker is displayed with three-dimensional volume rendering with solid settings (a) and transparent settings (b). In the coronal (c) and sagittal (d) multiplanar planes the pacemaker wire (arrow) and the beam-hardening artifacts (arrowheads) in the right heart are clearly displayed. In the right panel of the figure, axial images in a craniocaudal direction (1–4) are displayed and the position of the pacemaker wire is indicated (arrowheads). The magnification of the same images in the region of the pacemaker (1'–4') shows how large the artifacts can become depending on the orientation of the wire compared with that of the X-ray beams. In addition, volume averaging effects also play a role. The appearance of the pacemaker wire is much larger than the actual size owing to this artifact. Ao, ascending aorta; RA, right atrium; LV, left ventricle; RV, right ventricle.

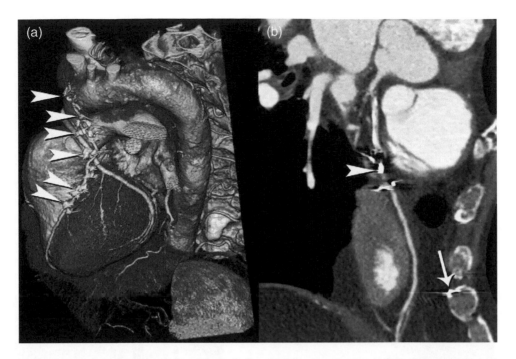

Figure 22.17 Volume averaging from surgical clips. Surgical clips used to close the branches of the left internal mammary artery are clearly displayed in the three-dimensional volume-rendering image (a). They appear to be much larger than their actual size because of the volume-averaging effect (arrowheads). In a curved multiplanar reconstruction (b) showing the left anterior descending artery the presence of the surgical clips causes artifacts at the anastomoses between the vessel and the left internal mammary artery (arrowhead). The wires used to fix the sternum after sternotomy generate the same type of artifact (arrow)

At high heart rates (>70 bpm) some residual motion can often be observed. In these cases a multisegment reconstruction algorithm should be applied to reduce the effective temporal resolution. These algorithms differ slightly between manufacturers but they are all based on the reconstruction of one image from two or more heart cycles. The use of these algorithms can improve image quality; however, the improvement is not always sufficient to guarantee sufficient image quality (Figures 22.21 and 22.22).

Data can be missed when the scan range is not adequately set (Table 22.1). The main reasons for missing data are related to a too short a scan range or to a discrepancy in the depth of patient's breath hold between the topogram and the angiographic scan.

The worst case occurs when the cranial part of the scan is missing, making it impossible to evaluate the left main coronary artery and the proximal branches. Missing data can also occur when the scan range ends too early and part of the entire posterior descending artery is missing.

The scan range should be set a little larger than actually needed to prevent these problems. When real-time display of the actual position of the table is available, the operator should use a longer scan range and stop the scan when the entire heart has been scanned.

VESSEL ENHANCEMENT

A high vascular enhancement is required to improve the visualization of small vessels (Table 22.1). In some cases the enhancement will not be satisfactory regardless of an optimal intravenous administration protocol.

Poor vascular enhancement can occur when the patient has an extremely fast veno-arterial circulation time or the position of the region of interest in the ascending aorta that is used to

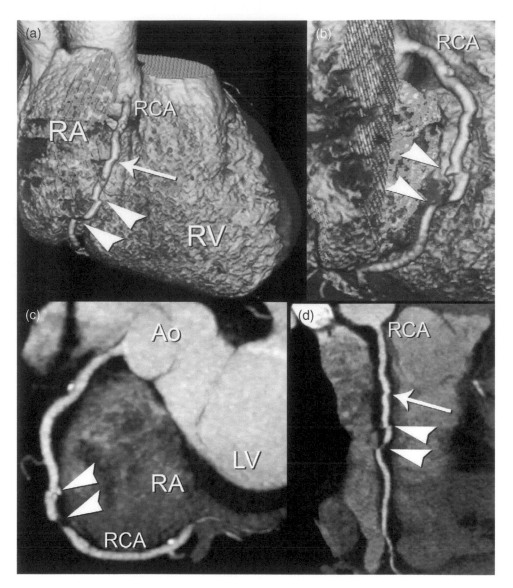

Figure 22.18 *Severe misregistration artifact. In some cases, even though the heart rate is optimal and there are no evident irregularities, one or more stacks of images can be misregistered. (a) Three-dimensional volume rendering displaying the right coronary artery (RCA). A high (arrowheads) and a lower (arrow) degree of misregistration are displayed. In the magnification of the image (b), the misregistration clearly causes an interruption in the continuity of the RCA (arrowheads). Using maximum intensity projection (c) in a plane parallel to the atrioventricular groove the configuration of the vessel also appears to be altered (arrowheads). In the curved multiplanar reconstruction (d) the appearance of the two sites of misregistration (arrowheads and arrow) is displayed. Ao, ascending aorta; RA, right atrium; LV, left ventricle; RV, right ventricle.*

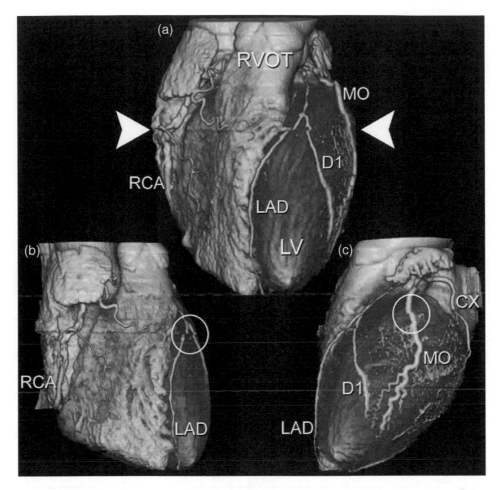

Figure 22.19 Subtle misregistration artifact. In some case misregistration artifacts may be subtle. (a) Left anterior view using three-dimensional volume rendering. The location of the misregistration artifact is highlighted by the arrowheads and the horizontal white line. The impact of this artifact on the integrity of the left anterior descending (LAD) (b) (white circle) and on the large marginal branch (MO) of the left circumflex (CX) (c) (white circle) is displayed. This artifact should not be mistaken for a stenosis. D1, first diagonal branch; RCA, right coronary artery; LV, left ventricle; RVOT, right ventricle outflow tract.

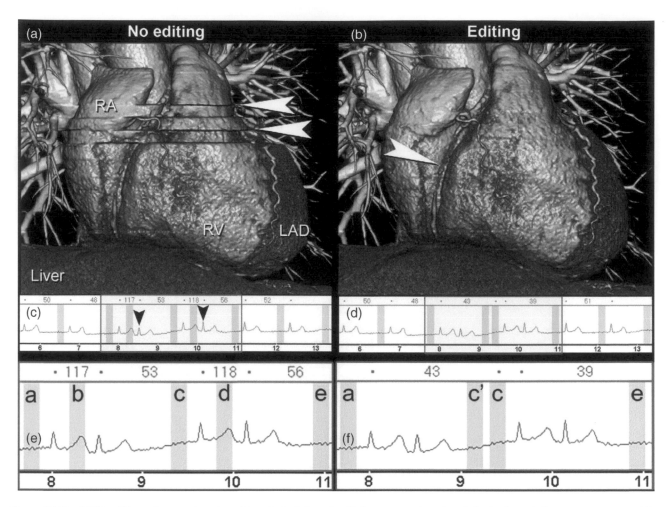

Figure 22.20 ECG editing of premature heart beat. A data set with two premature beats is displayed. The appearance of the data set before and after ECG editing is displayed with an anterior view using three-dimensional volume rendering (a) and (b). The premature beats cause a complete misregistration of the stacks of images (arrowheads in (a)), while after editing the spatial relationship is restored and the chronic total occlusion of the right coronary artery becomes more clearly visible (arrowhead in (b)). The corresponding ECG signals are displayed in (c) and (d). The premature beats (black arrowheads in (c)) in the blue box are the targets for ECG editing. The software generally uses all R waves to determine the temporal windows (A–E in (e)). This causes the temporal windows to fall in the very short diastolic phase just before the premature beat (B and D in (e)). This phase does not match with the others (A, C, and E in (e)). After ECG editing (d and (f)) the temporal windows located in the diastolic phase that preceded the premature beats (B and D in (e)) are deleted (f), and an additional temporal window (C' in (f)) is added to provide the software with enough information to reconstruct one image between adjacent temporal windows. RA, right atrium; LAD, left anterior descending; LV, left ventricle; RV, right ventricle.

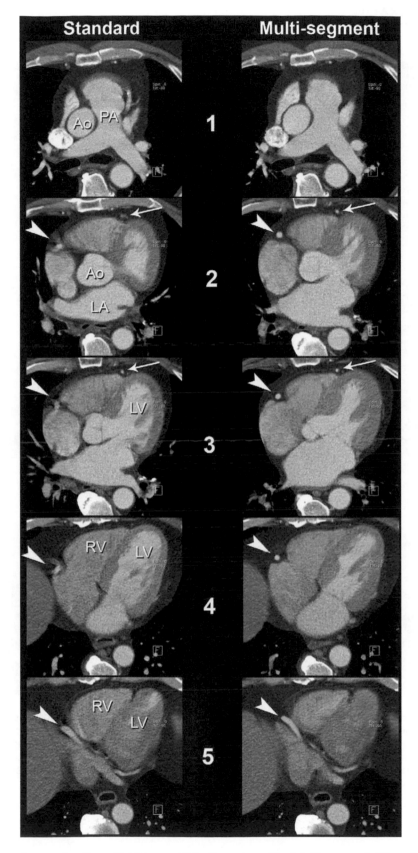

Figure 22.21 Multisegment reconstruction with improvement of image quality. Axial images at different levels (1Đ5) of the heart are shown using standard reconstruction (left panels) and multisegment reconstruction (right panels) in a patient with a heart rate of 85 bpm. In this case, higher image quality was obtained using multisegment reconstruction which is illustrated for the right (arrowheads) and left anterior descending (arrows) coronary artery. Ao, aorta; PA, pulmonary artery; RA, right atrium; LA, left atrium; LV, left ventricle; RV, right ventricle.

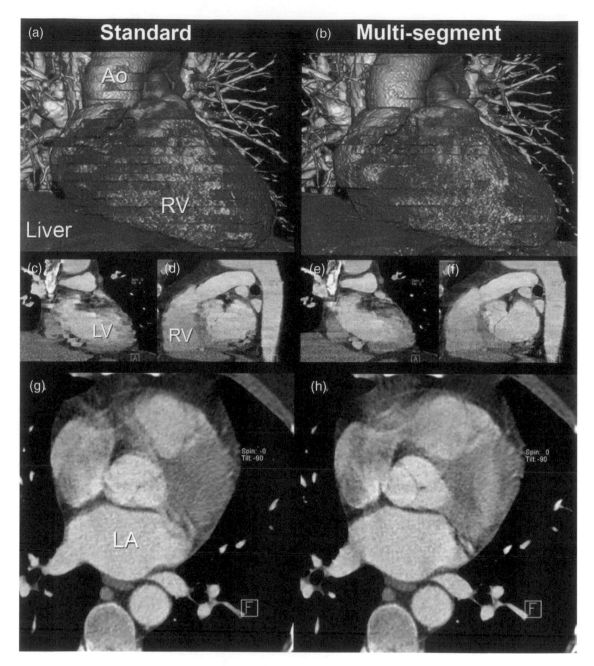

Figure 22.22 Multisegment reconstruction without significant improvement of image quality. Image quality did not significantly improve using multisegment reconstruction (right panels) when compared with that of standard reconstruction (left panels) in a patient with a mean heart rate of 92 bpm. Panels (a) and (b) are volume-rendered images showing better delineation of the left ventricle (LV) using multisegment reconstruction, which is also the case on the multiplanar reconstructed images (c)–(f). However, the coronary angiographic image quality did not significantly improve using multisegment reconstruction which is illustrated on the axial images (g) and (h). Ao, aorta; LA, left atrium; RV, right ventricle.

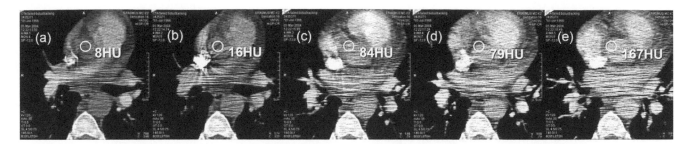

Figure 22.23 Failed bolus tracking. The circle highlights the region of interest which is positioned within the ascending aorta. Using a bolus tracking technique, scans are made at the same level to monitor the arrival of contrast material within the ascending aorta (a)⊟(e). These scans are not made during apnea and the position of the ascending aorta can differ within the monitoring scans. In this case, the region of interest was moved out the region of the ascending aorta in several scans (c) and (d). Therefore, the arrival of the contrast material was not accurately detected and the angiography scan was started too late.

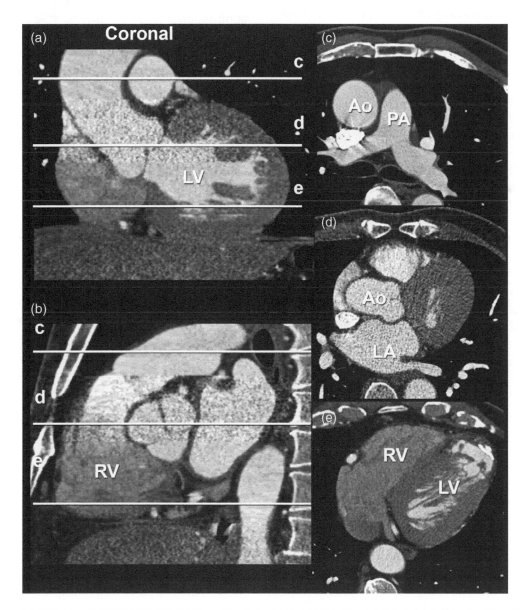

Figure 22.24 Incorrect use of X-ray tube modulation. The use of prospective X-ray tube modulation significantly reduces the radiation exposure during CT coronary angiography. However, this technique should not be used in patients with arrhythmia, because this can result in inaccurate synchronization timing and, consequently, a lower radiation output during the important diastolic phase. The effect of inaccurate tube modulation on image quality is clearly visible on the coronal (a) and sagittal (b) images (illustrated by the arrow) which was caused by a premature beat during the CT scan. High-quality axial images are shown at the levels with correct timing of the tube modulation (a) and (c), whereas image quality suffers from noise at the level of incorrect timing (b). Ao, aorta; PA, pulmonary artery; LA, left atrium; LV, left ventricle; RV, right ventricle.

trigger the bolus tracking is not optimal (Figure 22.23). Other causes of poor enhancement are usually related to suboptimal contrast material administration. When the great vessels of the thorax do not show contrast visualization a technical failure of the contrast material administration procedure is usually the cause.

IMAGE QUALITY

An image is of high quality when the contours of the objects are sharp and it is easy to recognize the vessel contours and coronary plaques (Table 22.1).

To obtain sharp images the residual motion should be minimized, enhancement inside the lumen should be high (~300 HU), and image noise should be minimized.

Image noise may not be evenly distributed in the data set when a premature heartbeat occurs and the prospective tube current modulation is active, which causes the modulation to be activated during the diastolic phase (Figure 22.24). To prevent this artifact it is recommended that the ECG of the patient prior to the scan and during a test apnea should be carefully observed to check for the presence of premature heartbeats. When premature heartbeats are present the operator should switch off the prospective tube current modulation.

In Table 22.1 the various artifacts are summarized with reasons why the problems occur, and what these problems cause, and how they can be resolved, all of which is followed by practical advice.

CONCLUSION

Finally, one should be aware that artifacts are always present in CT imaging, related to the basics of the CT technique, while in cardiac CT imaging, there are the additional cardiac contraction motion artifacts. It is expected that newer scanners with improved spatial and temporal resolution, more refined reconstruction algorithms, and, eventually, different hardware resolutions will minimize the impact of artifacts in coronary CT imaging.

REFERENCES

1. Morgan CL. Basic Principles of Computed Tomography. Baltimore: University Park Press, 1983.
2. Nieman K, Cademartiri F, Lemos PA et al. Reliable noninvasive coronary angiography with fast submillimeter multislice spiral computed tomography. Circulation 2002; 106: 2051–4.
3. Ropers D, Baum U, Pohle K et al. Detection of coronary artery stenoses with thin-slice multi-detector row spiral computed tomography and multiplanar reconstruction. Circulation 2003; 107: 664–6.
4. Hu H, He HD, Foley WD, Fox SH. Four multidetector-row helical CT: image quality and volume coverage speed. Radiology 2000; 215: 55–62.

CHAPTER 23

Contrast enhancement in coronary angiography

To perform CT coronary angiography it is mandatory to obtain prominent vascular enhancement. Because contrast material is administered intravenously, the scan has to be performed during the first pass of contrast material within the vessels of interest, which is usually defined as the arterial phase of contrast passage [1].

The presence of contrast-material inside the artery generates a high contrast between the artery lumen and the adjacent structures (including vessel wall, perivascular soft tissues, or neighboring veins). Appropriate arterial enhancement significantly improves the quality of image postprocessing and increases confidence in the evaluation of coronary abnormalities. To obtain the optimal arterial enhancement for the purpose of CT coronary angiography several issues need to be addressed.

BOLUS GEOMETRY

Bolus geometry is the pattern of enhancement represented as a time–density curve (Figure 23.1) in a given vessel after the administration of a bolus of contrast material. Optimal bolus geometry is characterized by a rectangular shape with a steep rise of the curve to a maximum plateau which lasts a little longer than the CT time followed by a steep descent. However, such bolus geometry cannot be achieved in clinical practice. Instead, the bolus geometry observed in vivo is characterized by a slow increase of the curve, a delay to reach the peak rather than a plateau, and is followed by a slow decrease of enhancement.

It is important to recognize this and that timing and duration of CT scanning should be synchronized to the timing and duration of the actual bolus geometry.

Optimization of the bolus geometry

Actual bolus geometry is influenced by several parameters, that are patient related such as age, body weight, cardiac output[2-8], or are related to the modality of contrast-material administration, which is operator controlled. Contrast-injection parameters and synchronization of bolus geometry and CT scan timing play a significant role in bolus geometry.

Contrast-material injection parameters

Contrast-material injection parameters are contrast-material volume, injection rate, and iodine concentration (Figure 23.2).

Contrast-material volume An increase in contrast-injection volume produces an increase in arterial enhancement. However, there is also a delay in the time to peak of maximum enhancement[9-11] (Figure 23.2a).

It is of note that a higher patient weight is associated with a poorer performance of the contrast administration protocol. This is partly as a result of the larger blood pool of heavier patients, which decreases the contrast enhancement and partly owing to the higher attenuation of X-rays, which decreases the signal to noise ratio. It is recommended that the volume of contrast material be

(a)

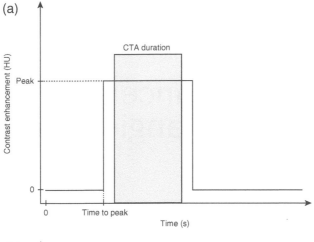

(b)

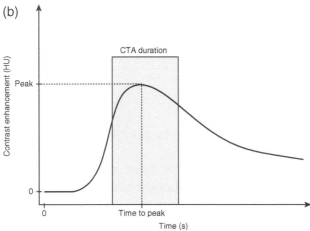

Figure 23.1 Bolus geometry. (a) Optimal bolus geometry. Enhancement in the vessel of interest rises with a very steep slope up to the peak, and then remains steady for the whole plateau, which ideally is a little longer than the scan time. (b) Actual bolus geometry. In actual bolus geometry there is a slow increase in vascular enhancement up to a peak. Then, the enhancement starts to drop. There is no real plateau of enhancement. CTA, computed tomography angiography.

increased by 20–25% when the patient's weight is more than 90 kg.

Contrast-injection rate An increase in injection rate produces an increase in arterial enhancement. In addition, there is an earlier peak of maximum enhancement[7,9,10,12-14] (Figure 23.2b). However, the effects of the increase of the injection rate are limited because higher rate of injection into a cubital vein may be associated with a higher chance of contrast-material extravasation. Therefore, in practice the injection rate used ranges between 4 and 5 ml/s.

(a)

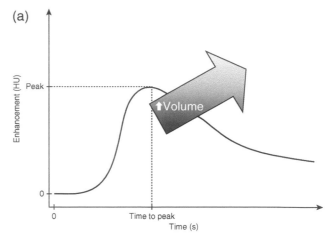

(b)

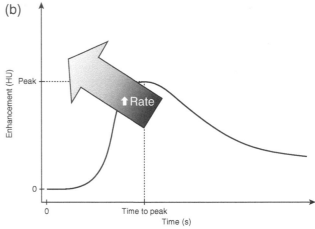

(c)

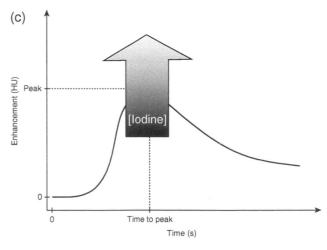

Figure 23.2 Injection parameters. (a) Effect of contrast-material volume. An increase in the volume of contrast material produces a concomitant increase in the peak of maximum enhancement and a delay in the time to peak. (b) Effect of contrast-material rate. An increase in the rate of contrast-material injection produces a concomitant increase in the peak of maximum enhancement and an anticipation of the time to peak. (c) Effect of contrast-material iodine concentration. An increase in contrast-material iodine concentration produces an increase in the peak of maximum enhancement without any influence on the time to peak.

Contrast-material iodine concentration An increase in iodine concentration of the contrast material produces an increase in arterial enhancement[10,15], while the peak of maximum enhancement remains unaffected (Figure 23.2c). It is of note that owing to the higher viscosity of compounds with a high iodine concentration they should be heated to 38 °C before injection. Also, a higher iodine concentration is associated with a higher chance of renal dysfunction.

It has been suggested that multiphasic protocols using varying injection rates during the injection of contrast material should improve the homogeneity of the plateau of arterial enhancement[8,16-19]. However, modern 16-row multislice scanners have reduced the scan time to less than 20 s, thereby obviating the need for such protocols.

Contrast-material synchronization techniques

Contrast-material synchronization techniques are fixed delay, test bolus technique, and bolus tracking technique. With these techniques the operator tries to synchronize optimally the peak of maximum arterial enhancement with the CT angiography scan (Figure 23.3).

Fixed delay technique A fixed delay between the start of intravenous administration of contrast material and the start of the scan is not optimal. The variability in the delay of peak maximum enhancement is substantial, mainly owing to patient-related parameters (Figure 23.3a). For instance, in patients with an impaired left ventricular dysfunction a delay of typically 18–20 s as in normal situation is too short and will result in scanning of coronary arteries that are not yet enhanced.

Test bolus technique The test bolus technique is based on the calculation of the transit time between the site of injection and the ascending aorta using a small volume of contrast material as a test bolus (10–15 ml)[1,6,7] (Figure 23.3b).

This technique has been demonstrated to be reliable; however, it is not perfect. It has been reported that there is a correlation between the delay calculated by means of the test bolus and a point in the up slope of the curve of bolus geometry, but no correlation with the peak of maximum enhancement[4,7].

Bolus tracking technique The bolus tracking technique is based on the real-time monitoring of the arrival of contrast material in the ascending aorta. During the intravenous injection, the arrival of contrast material is monitored by a dynamic acquisition of a single slice at the level of the ascending aorta. When a predetermined density threshold of enhancement is achieved within the lumen of ascending aorta, the CT scan is automatically triggered[1] (Figure 23.3c).

The threshold used for an optimal triggering of the scan is 100 HU above the baseline value of attenuation of the ascending aorta sampled in a non-enhanced premonitoring scan. Therefore, the actual value of attenuation that triggers the scan will vary between 50 and 100 HU.

The arrival of contrast material triggers the scan, and the table automatically moves to the previously set starting position; in the meantime the instructions for breath hold are given to the patient. This step usually requires 4–5 s. The scan can then be started. Bolus tracking has been demonstrated to produce better results in terms of vascular enhancement when compared with other techniques[22,23].

Other parameters

In addition to the main parameters already discussed, there are additional measures that can improve the modality of administration and the use of contrast material in cardiac CT, such as bolus chaser. Bolus chaser is a volume of saline that is injected immediately after the bolus of contrast-material (Figure 23.4). Usually it is administered at the same rate as the contrast-material bolus. To administer a bolus chaser it is necessary to use either two parallel injectors or a single double-head injector[23,24]. The rationale behind the use of a bolus chaser is based on flushing of the contrast material after the end of the injection. With the bolus chaser the contrast material is pushed at a predetermined speed, while without it the contrast material slows down to the speed provided by the venous flow.

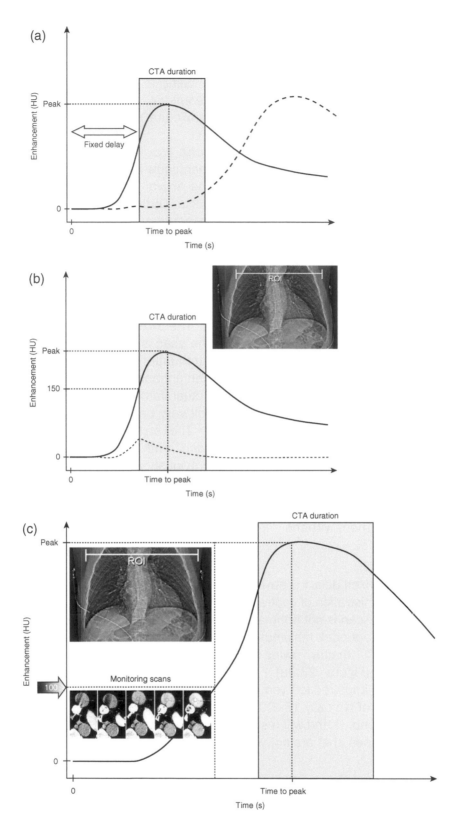

Figure 23.3 Synchronization techniques. (a) Fixed delay technique. The use of a fixed delay is very practical because it does not require any technical optimization; however, it is not sutiable for every patient. The major risk is that in a patient with slow venoarterial circulation, the scan is performed when the contrast material has not yet arrived in the coronary arteries (dashed line). (b) Test bolus technique. The use of a test bolus allows calculation of the transit time between the injection site (e.g. antecubital vein) and the ascending aorta. The calculated delay of 4–6 s should be added in order to fit with the bolus geometry of the angiographic bolus. (c) Bolus tracking technique. The use of a real-time bolus tracking technique allows the delay to be tailored to each patient without the use of additional contrast material and it is based on the actual bolus geometry of the main angiographic bolus rather than on a smaller test bolus. During the injection of contrast material, a series of monitoring scans sample the enhancement in the ascending aorta, and when the trigger threshold is reached (+100 HU), the scan is automatically started after the 4 s that are necessary to give the patient the breath-hold instructions. CTA, CT angiography; ROI, region of interest.

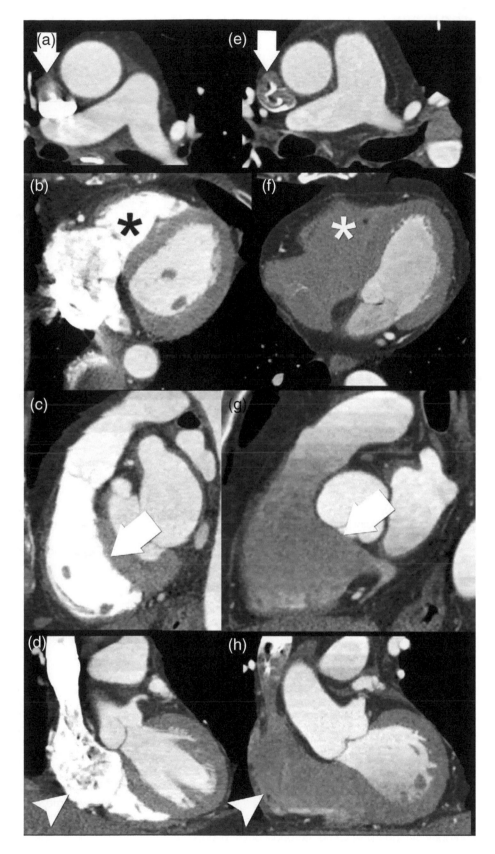

Figure 23.4 Effect of bolus chaser on bolus geometry. In the images a protocol with the same volume of contrast material is compared without (a)E(d) and with bolus chaser (e)E(h). Several different images are displayed to highlight the presence or reduction of vascular enhancement owing to the administration of bolus chaser. In (a) and (e) the two different protocols are compared in an axial image at the level of the ascending aorta and pulmonary artery. The superior vena cava at this level (arrows) is very bright in (a), where there is no bolus chaser, and is almost un-enhanced in (b), where a bolus chaser follows the main bolus. In (b) and (f) the two different protocols are compared in an axial image at a midventricular level. The right chambers of the heart are hyper-dense (asterisk)(b) or hypodense (asterisk)(f) depending on the absence or presence of a bolus chaser. The same patterns are clearly displayed in a sagittal plane passing through the right ventricle and the pulmonary artery (arrows) (c) and (g), and in a coronal plane passing through the right ventricle and the superior vena cava (arrowheads) (d) and (h).

Table 23.1 Recommendations for contrast enhancement in CT coronary angiography

Parameters	Coronary CTA	Comment	Non-coronary CT	Comment
Injection				
Volume (ml)	100	Increase when the scan range, and therefore the scan time, increases (e.g. CABG)	100	Increase when the scan range, and therefore the scan time, increases (e.g. study of the entire thorax)
Rate (ml/s)	4	Increase to 5 ml/s when scan time is below 15 s and the antecubital vein is large	3	A lower rate is preferable and allows a longer enhancement
Iodine concentration (mg/ml)	350Ð400	Preferably 400 mg/ml	300Ð400	Ñ
Synchronization				
Fixed delay (s)	18Ð20	Increase of 5Ð10 s in patients with reduced cardiac output	18Ð20	Increase of 5Ð10 s in patients with reduced cardiac output
Test bolus				
volume (ml)	15Ð20	Or 15Ð20% of the main contrast-material bolus	15Ð20	Or 15Ð20% of the main contrast-material bolus
rate (ml/s)	4		4	
delay (s)	TT + 4Ð6		TT + 4Ð6	
Bolus tracking				
ROI	Ascending aorta	Positioned in the center of the vessel as seen on axial premonitoring images	Ascending aorta	Positioned in the center of the vessel as seen on axial premonitoring images
threshold (HU)	+100	No less than 75 HU to avoid anticipated triggering from beam-hardening artifacts in the superior vena cava	+100	No less than 75 HU to avoid anticipated triggering from beam-hardening artifacts in the superior vena cava
Others				
Bolus chaser				Not required
volume (ml)	40	Or 35Ð40% of the contrast-material bolus	Ñ	Ñ
rate (ml/s)	4	Or same rate as contrast-material	Ñ	Ñ
Contrast-material administration				
site	Antecubital	Recommended because it reduces the chances of contrast-material extravasation and the diffusion of contrast material in collateral venous pathways	Antecubital	Recommended because it reduces the chances of contrast-material extravasation and the diffusion of contrast material in collateral venous pathways
side	Right	It is recommended because the right subclavian and innominate veins are not crossing the aortic arch	Right	It is recommended because the right subclavian and innominate veins are not crossing the aortic arch

CTA, computed tomography angiography; CABG, coronary artery bypass graft; TT, transit time; ROI, region of interest.

The use of bolus chaser has been repor ted to provide benefits in ter ms of reduction of contrast-material volume and beam-hardening ar tifacts at the level of the thoracic outlet, superior vena cava, and right atrium and ventricle [23,27], which is desirable for a better e valuation of the right coronary artery.

Injection site and device

Usually a large and proximal antecubital vein is used for CT coronar y angiography. An 18–20-gauge intravenous cannula allows the desired injection rate to be acheived without complications (e.g. vein r upture and contrast extravasation). We found that in near ly all men the 18-gauge cannula can be inser ted without much difficulty, while in women or o verweight patients the 20-gauge cannula is easier .

NON-CORONARY STUDIES

In the e valuation of cardiac thrombi, cardiac/pericardial and mediastinal masses, and the visualization of cardiac veins, a high vascular enhancement is not necessar y and a low er injection rate with the same contrast-material volume will produce longer vascular enhancement. A dela yed scan phase can be helpful to depict the patter n of vascularization of a cardiac mass. Cardiac veins can be visualized b y simply increasing the scan dela y by 10 s or by using a higher trigger threshold (e.g . 150–175 HU) in bolus tracking.

RECOMMENDATIONS

Adequate vascular enhancement is of paramount importance to the success of coronar y CT angiography. The injection parameter s and the resulting synchronization protocols should be optimal (Table 23.1).

In clinical practice, 16-row (or higher) multi-slice CT scanner s require an injection volume of approximately 100 ml for sufficient enhancement during the entire duration of the CT angiograph y scan. Because the recommended injection rate is 4 ml/s, the contrast-material administration time will be 25 s, which is a little longer than the average scan time.

The ideal iodine concentration for coronar y CT angiography should be 350 mg/ml or more. With this concentration, a high vascular enhancement can be produced without a cor responding increase in injection rate. When using high iodine concentration contrast material (monomeric 350 mg/ml or dimeric 320 mg/ml), it should be noted that, because of their high viscosity , they must be administered only after appropriate heating at 38 °C.

The optimal technique for contrast-material synchronization is bolus tracking , which is a vailable on current multislice CT scanner s with cardiac imaging capabilities. The trigger threshold of attenuation for the region of interest in the ascending aorta should be chosen around +100 HU. A low er threshold will be too sensitive to the beam-hardening artifacts in the superior vena ca va resulting in early triggering and scan failure.

The test bolus technique can also be used, but a better vascular enhancement is achie ved by addition of 4–6 s to dela y the transit time of the test bolus betw een the injection site and the ascending aorta.

REFERENCES

1. Cademartiri F, van der Lugt A, Luccichenti G, Pavone P, Krestin GP. Parameters affecting bolus geometr y in CT A: a re view. J Comput Assist T omogr 2002; 26: 598–607.
2. Handlin LR, Kindred LH, Beauchamp GD, Vacek JL, Rowe SK. Reversible left ventricular dysfunction after subarachnoid hemorrhage. Am Hear t J 1993; 126: 235–40.
3. Kono T, Morita H, Kuroiwa T et al. Left ventricular w all motion abnormalities in patients with subarachnoid hemorrhage: neurogenic stunned myocardium. J Am Coll Cardiol 1994; 24: 636–40.
4. van Hoe L, Marchal G, Baert AL, Gryspeerdt S, Mertens L. Determination of scan dela y time in spiral CT -angiography: utility of a test bolus injection. J Comput Assist T omogr 1995; 19: 216–20.
5. Bae KT, Heiken JP, Brink JA. Aor tic and hepatic contrast medium enhancement at CT. Part II. Effect of reduced cardiac output in a porcine model. Radiolog y 1998; 207: 657–62.
6. Nakajima Y, Yoshimine T, Yoshida H et al. Computerized tomography angiography of r uptured cerebral aneur ysms: factors affecting time to maximum contrast concentration. J Neurosurg 1998; 88: 663–9.
7. Platt JF, Reige KA, Ellis JH. Aor tic enhancement during abdominal CT angiography: correlation with test injections, flow rates, and patient demographics. AJR Am J Roentgenol 1999; 172: 53–6.
8. Fleischmann D, Rubin GD, Bankier AA, Hittmair K. Impro ved uniformity of aor tic enhancement with customized contrast medium injection protocols at CT angiograph y. Radiology 2000; 214: 363–71.

9. Garcia P, Genin G, Bret PM et al. Hepatic CT enhancement: effect of the rate and volume of contrast medium injection in an animal model. Abdom Imaging 1999; 24: 597–603.

10. Han JK, Kim AY, Lee KY et al. Factors influencing vascular and hepatic enhancement at CT: experimental study on injection protocol using a canine model. J Comput Assist Tomogr 2000; 24: 400–6.

11. Yamashita Y, Komohara Y, Takahashi M et al. Abdominal helical CT: evaluation of optimal doses of intravenous contrast material—a prospective randomized study. Radiology 2000; 216: 718–23.

12. Bae KT, Heiken JP, Brink JA. Aortic and hepatic peak enhancement at CT: effect of contrast medium injection rate—pharmacokinetic analysis and experimental porcine model. Radiology 1998; 206: 455–64.

13. Kim T, Murakami T, Takahashi S et al. Effects of injection rates of contrast material on arterial phase hepatic CT. AJR Am J Roentgenol 1998; 171: 429–32.

14. Luboldt W, Straub J, Seemann M, Helmberger T, Reiser M. Effective contrast use in CT angiography and dual-phase hepatic CT performed with a subsecond scanner. Invest Radiol 1999; 34: 751–60.

15. Bluemke DA, Fishman EK, Anderson JH. Effect of contrast concentration on abdominal enhancement in the rabbit: spiral computed tomography evaluation. Acad Radiol 1995; 2: 226–31.

16. Hittmair K, Fleischmann D. Accuracy of predicting and controlling time-dependent aortic enhancement from a test bolus injection. J Comput Assist Tomogr 2001; 25: 287–94.

17. Fleischmann D, Hittmair K. Mathematical analysis of arterial enhancement and optimization of bolus geometry for CT angiography using the discrete fourier transform. J Comput Assist Tomogr 1999; 23: 474–84.

18. Bae KT, Heiken JP, Brink JA. Aortic and hepatic contrast medium enhancement at CT. Part I. Prediction with a computer model. Radiology 1998; 207: 647–55.

19. Bae KT, Tran HQ, Heiken JP. Multiphasic injection method for uniform prolonged vascular enhancement at CT angiography: pharmacokinetic analysis and experimental porcine model. Radiology 2000; 216: 872–80.

20. Kopka L, Rodenwaldt J, Fischer U, Mueller DW, Oestmann JW, Grabbe E. Dual-phase helical CT of the liver: effects of bolus tracking and different volumes of contrast material. Radiology 1996; 201: 321–6.

21. Kirchner J, Kickuth R, Laufer U, Noack M, Liermann D. Optimized enhancement in helical CT: experiences with a real-time bolus tracking system in 628 patients. Clin Radiol 2000; 55: 368–73.

22. Cademartiri F, Nieman K, van der Lugt A et al. IV contrast administration for CT coronary angiography on a 16-multidetector-row helical CT scanner: test bolus vs. bolus tracking. Radiology 2004; 233: 817–23.

23. Haage P, Schmitz-Rode T, Hubner D, Piroth W, Gunther RW. Reduction of contrast material dose and artifacts by a saline flush using a double power injector in helical CT of the thorax. AJR Am J Roentgenol 2000; 174: 1049–53.

24. Cademartiri F, Mollet N, van der Lugt A et al. Non-invasive 16-row multislice CT coronary angiography: usefulness of saline chaser. Eur Radiol 2004; 14: 178–83.

25. Hopper KD, Mosher TJ, Kasales CJ, TenHave TR, Tully DA, Weaver JS. Thoracic spiral CT: delivery of contrast material pushed with injectable saline solution in a power injector. Radiology 1997; 205: 269–71.

26. Sadick M, Lehmann KJ, Diehl SJ, Wild J, Georgi M. Bolus tracking and NaCl bolus in biphasic spiral CT of the abdomen. Rofo 1997; 167: 371–6. [in German]

27. Bader TR, Prokesch RW, Grabenwoger F. Timing of the hepatic arterial phase during contrast-enhanced computed tomography of the liver: assessment of normal values in 25 volunteers. Invest Radiol 2000; 35: 486–92.

CHAPTER 24

The future

Coronary imaging remains the ultimate challenge for any non-invasive imaging technique. Great strides have been made in CT technology, including the introduction of dual-source 64-slice CT technology; however, various problems remain to be resolved before CT coronary angiography becomes a mainstream diagnostic tool within the clinical arena (Figures 24.1 and 24.2). The main problems concern spatial and temporal resolution, radiation exposure, and coronary calcification (Table 24.1).

Invasive coronary angiography is still considered to be the standard reference technique and will probably remain so for the foreseeable future. The advantages and disadvantages of CT coronary angiography compared with invasive coronary angiography are listed in Table 24.2.

Current CT technology has been demonstrated to be useful in various applications, most notably the prognostic value of CT coronary calcium. Furthermore, CT coronary angiography has also gained clinical acceptance in various clinical situations (Figures 24.3–24.5). Recently, the combination of functional and anatomical imaging has become regarded as an option to provide the most optimal information for patient management and for patients referred for medical treatment, percutaneous coronary intervention, or bypass surgery (Table 24.3).

However, it must be understood that the real value of new diagnostic technology should represent an advance compared with existing diagnostic tests and that evidence must be provided that non-invasive CT coronary angiography will change patient management and lead to improved prognosis. Currently, showing that CT coronary angiography is safe, feasible, and cost-effective, and indeed, leads to a decrease in cardiac mortality and morbidity is still some distance away. Multislice CT (MSCT) coronary imaging has enormous potential, and in the future volumetric acquisition of the entire heart in one breath hold and one heart beat may permit comprehensive cardiac imaging with assessment of coronary

Table 24.1 Future challenges of multislice CT coronary angiography

Problem	Current limitation	Possible solution
Small vessels (tight lesion)	Spatial resolution 0.4 × 0.4 × 0.4	Improved detector technology
Cardiac motion artifacts	Insufficient temporal resolution (83–165 ms)	Non-mechanical configuration
Calcification	Blooming, beam-hardening overestimation, obscuring stenosis	Dual energy
Irregular rhythm	Acquisition 5–10 heartbeats	256-detector row i-heart beat acquisition
Radiation exposure	64-slice CT: 15–20 mSv	ECG-triggered X-ray modulation prospective
		ECG-triggered scanning adaptive mA/s settings
Stenosis severity	Visual assessment	Contour detection algorithms

Table 24.2 Comparison of multislice CT (MSCT) with diagnostic coronary angiography

	Diagnostic coronary angiography	64-CT
Patient friendly	Invasive	Non-invasive
Facility	Daycare	Outpatient clinic
Serious complication	<0.1%	Very rare
Reading examination	Cardiologist	Cardiologist/ radiologist
Cost of procedure	High	Low
Procedural time	30 min	10 min
Post-processing time	0	20 min
Throughput	Low	High
Performance investigation	Cardiologist/ nurse/ technician	Technician
Resolution	High	Acceptable
Installation costs	No difference	No difference
Obstruction estimation	QCA	Visual
Non-obstructive plaque	–	+
Calcified plaque	+	+++
Collaterals	High	Minimal
Motion artifacts	None	Unacceptable at high R-to-R interval
Radiation exposure	6Đ8 mSv	10Đ16 mµ
Availability	Worldwide	Limited

QCA, quantitative coronary angioraphy.

Table 24.3 Usefulness of coronary imaging

CT coronary plaque imaging

Risk evaluation
    calcium score
    obstructive and non-obstructive plaques

CT coronary angiography

Exclusion significant coronary artery disease
    evaluation before (major) surgery
    evaluation of low-risk acute coronary syndrome in
        emergency department
    evaluation post-CABG/stents

Diagnostic work-up in chronic stable chest pain syndromes
    evaluation coronary anomalies
    evaluation coronary artery disease in dilated
        cardiomyopathy

Integrated imaging SPECT, PET/CT

Evaluation for referral to revascularization
    CT anatomy
    Blood-flow limiting lesion

SPECT, single photon emission CT; PET, positron emission tomography; CABG, coronary artery bypass graft.

lumen, wall, and left ventricular function and perfusion (Table 24.4).

CONCLUSION

Non-invasive high-quality CT coronary angiography has enormous potential for the evaluation of the absence or presence of coronary atherosclerosis and its consequences which may significantly impact on patient management (Figures 24.6–24.9).

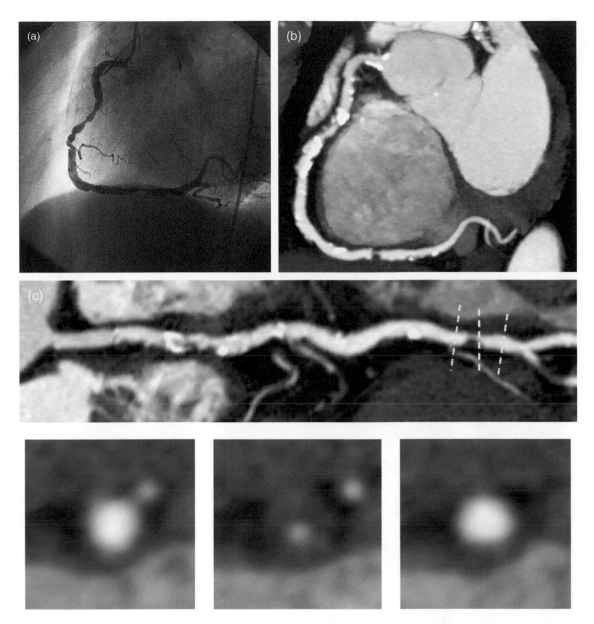

Figure 24.1 (a) Invasive coronary angiography showing serial stenoses in mid-segment of the right coronary artery (RCA) and severe stenosis in distal segment. (b) Dual-source CT coronary angiography of the RCA showing calcific and non-calcific severe obstruction of distal segment of RCA. (c) Multiplanar reconstruction of RCA. The dashed lines indicate the site of the three cross-sectional images proximal, at and distal to the severe non-calcific obstruction (lower row of images). The non-calcific obstruction at the site of narrowing shows expansile remodelling.

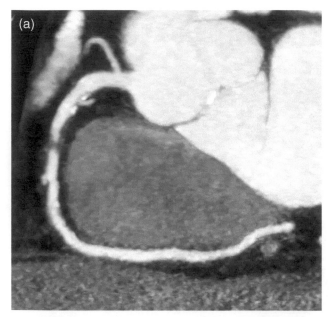

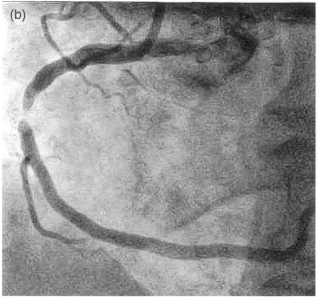

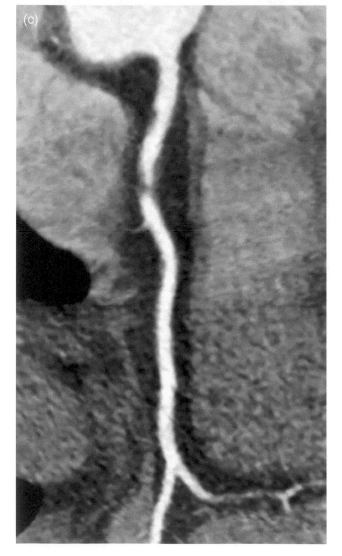

Figure 24.2 (a) Multiplanar reconstruction (MPR) of right coronary artery (RCA). Few calcific small plaques are visible. Mid-segment shows a severe non-calcific stenosis. (b) Invasive coronary angiogram confirms presence of severe stenosis in RCA. (c) Curve MPR of RCA.

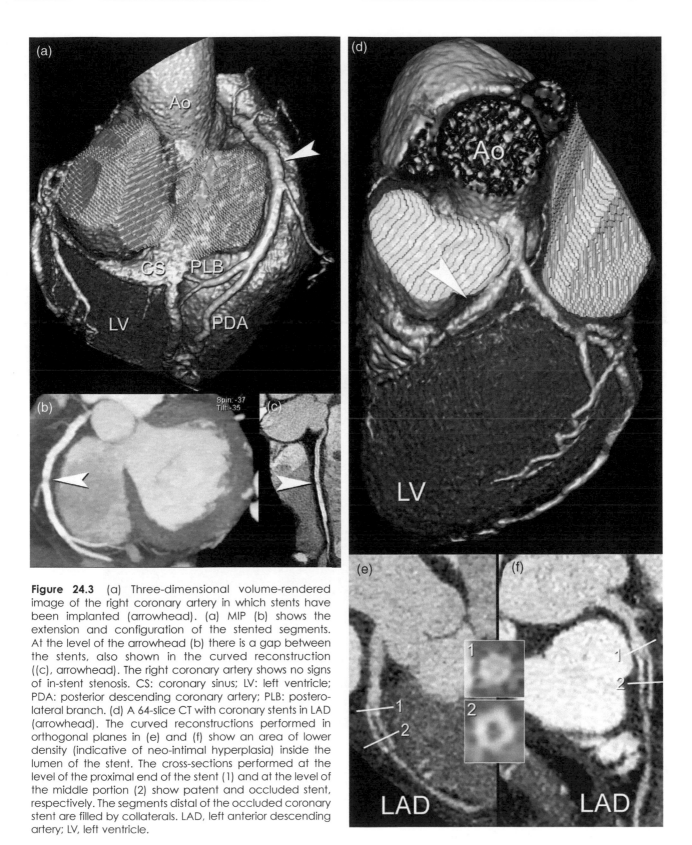

Figure 24.3 (a) Three-dimensional volume-rendered image of the right coronary artery in which stents have been implanted (arrowhead). (a) MIP (b) shows the extension and configuration of the stented segments. At the level of the arrowhead (b) there is a gap between the stents, also shown in the curved reconstruction ((c), arrowhead). The right coronary artery shows no signs of in-stent stenosis. CS: coronary sinus; LV: left ventricle; PDA: posterior descending coronary artery; PLB: postero-lateral branch. (d) A 64-slice CT with coronary stents in LAD (arrowhead). The curved reconstructions performed in orthogonal planes in (e) and (f) show an area of lower density (indicative of neo-intimal hyperplasia) inside the lumen of the stent. The cross-sections performed at the level of the proximal end of the stent (1) and at the level of the middle portion (2) show patent and occluded stent, respectively. The segments distal of the occluded coronary stent are filled by collaterals. LAD, left anterior descending artery; LV, left ventricle.

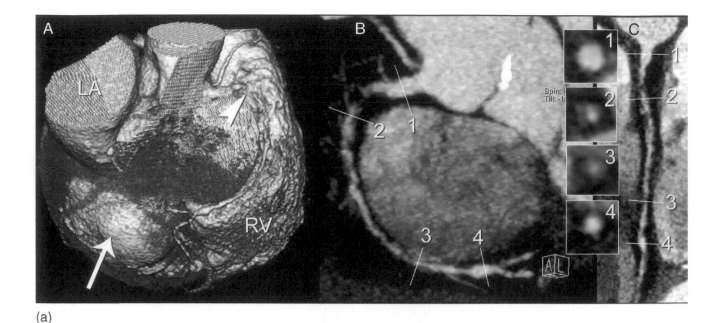

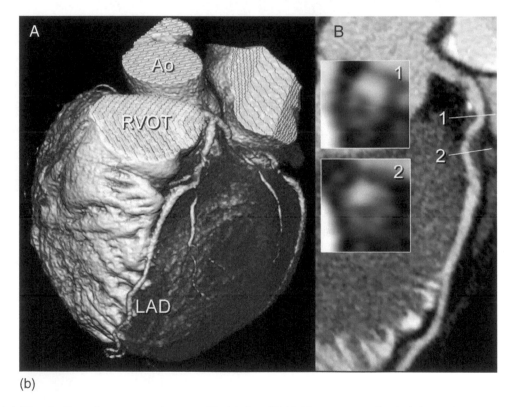

Figure 24.4 (a) Visualization of coronary plaques with 64-slice CT (right coronary artery). (a) The right coronary artery with atherosclerotic involvement of the entire vessel. The left ventricle shows a large area of thinning in the inferior wall due to a previous infarction (thin arrow). The MIP (b) and the curved reconstruction (c) show the diffusely diseased right coronary artery. Cross-sections along the vessel (1-4) demonstrate the different degrees of lumen stenosis and coronary wall thickening. LA, left atrium; RV, right ventricle. (b) Visualization of coronary plaques with 64-slice CT (left anterior descending coronary artery). A diffusely diseased left anterior descending coronary artery is displayed (A). The curved reconstruction (B) shows the presence of large predominantly non-calcified plaques in the proximal left anterior descending coronary artery. The cross-sections (1-2) show positive remodelling. Ao, ascending aorta; LAD, left anterior descending; RVOT, right ventricle outflow tract.

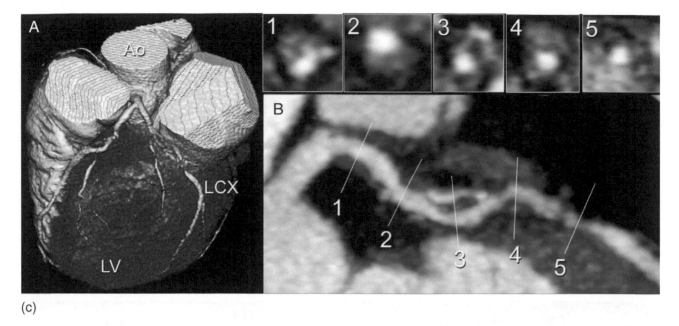

(c)

Figure 24.4, cont'd (c) Visualization of coronary plaques with 64-slice CT (left circumflex coronary artery). A diffusely diseased left circumflex coronary artery is displayed (A). The curved reconstruction (B) shows the presence of large predominantly non-calcified plaques in the proximal left circumflex coronary artery. The cross-sections (1-5) show positive remodelling. Ao, ascending aorta; LCX, left circumflex coronary artery; LV, left ventricle.

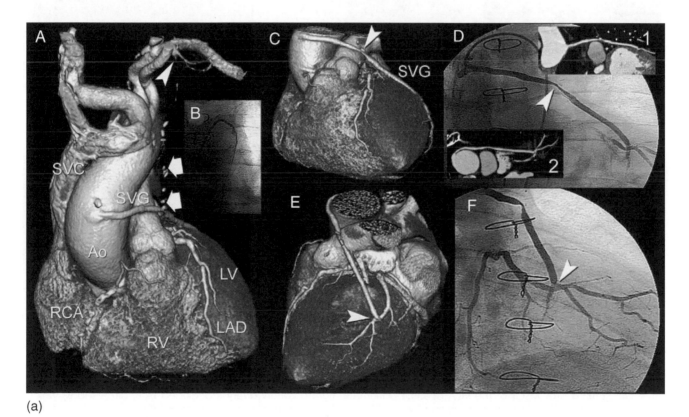

(a)

Figure 24.5 (a) Visualisation of the thoracic cardiovascular system in patient with previous CABG with 64-slice CT. Specifications: 100ml of intravenous contrast material and a scan of 18-20 seconds with a voxel size of 0.4mm3. The left internal mammary artery is visible only at its origin (A Đ arrowhead) while the remaining segments are occluded (A Đ thick arrows). A conventional coronary angiography confirmed these findings (B). The single saphenous vein graft was patent but showed a stenosis in the middle segment (arrowhead in C-D) both evident at three-dimensional volume rendering (C) and at curved reconstructions (1-2 in D). The conventional coronary angiography confirmed these findings (D). The distal anastomosis of the saphenous vein graft (arrowhead in E-F) was patent. Ao, ascending aorta; LAD, left anterior descending coronary artery; LV, left ventricle; RV, right ventricle; SVC, superior vena cava; SVG, saphenous vein graft; CABG, coronary artery bypass grafting.

Continued

283

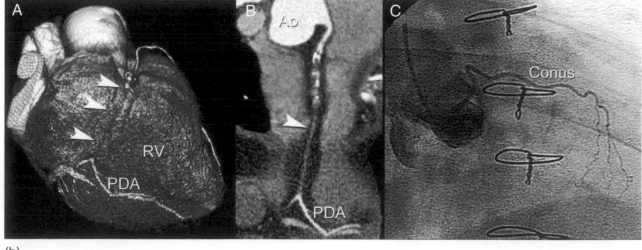

(b)

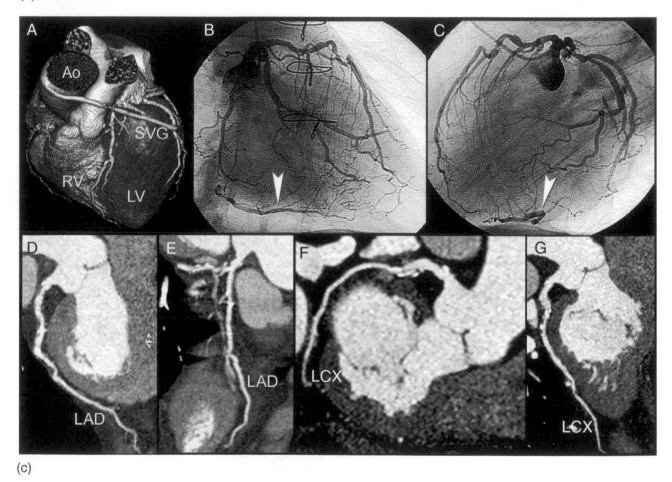

(c)

Figure 24.5, cont'd (b) MSCT of the RCA of same patient. The right coronary artery is occluded (A-B, arrowheads) which is confirmed by conventional coronary angiography (C). PDA, posterior descending coronary artery; RV, right ventricle. (c) MSCT of the left coronary artery of same patient. The left coronary artery, (LAD, LCX) although severely diseased does not have a significant lumen stenosis (A, D-G), as was confirmed by conventional coronary angiography (B,C). The posterior descending artery is filled by collaterals from the left coronary artery (arrowhead in B-C). Ao, ascending aorta; LAD, left anterior descending coronary artery; LCx, left circumflex coronary artery; LV, left ventricle; RV, right ventricle; SVG, saphenous vein graft.

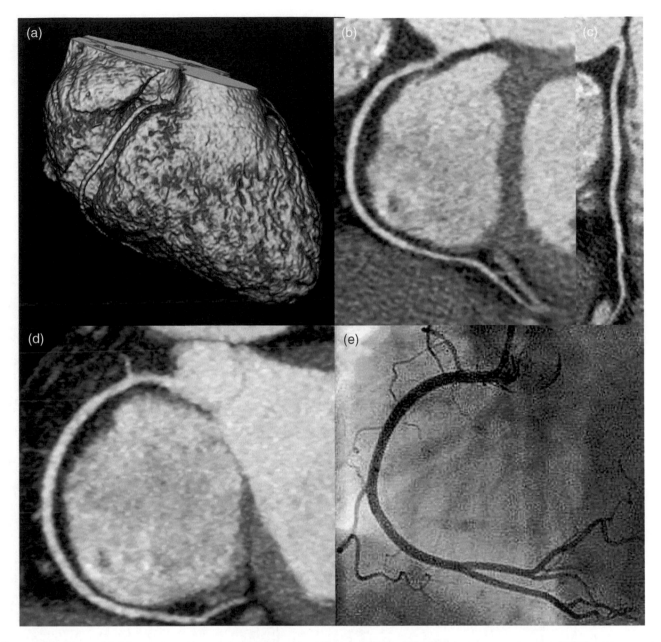

Figure 24.6 Normal right coronary artery. (a) volume rendered image of RCA. (b) Multiplanar reconstruction (MPR) and curved MPR (right panel) of RCA. (c) Maximum intensity projection of RCA. (d) corresponding invasive coronary angiography.

Table 24.4 MSCT comprehensive cardiac imaging

CT coronary artery lumen	Wall motion
Obstructions/occlusion	Wall thickening
Coronary artery wall	LV volume/ejection fraction

Plaque imaging
  non-calcified
  lipid
  fibrous
  calcified
	LV perfusion
	
	Functional ischemia
	
	LV infarct size
	Late enhancement

LV function	

LV, left ventricular.

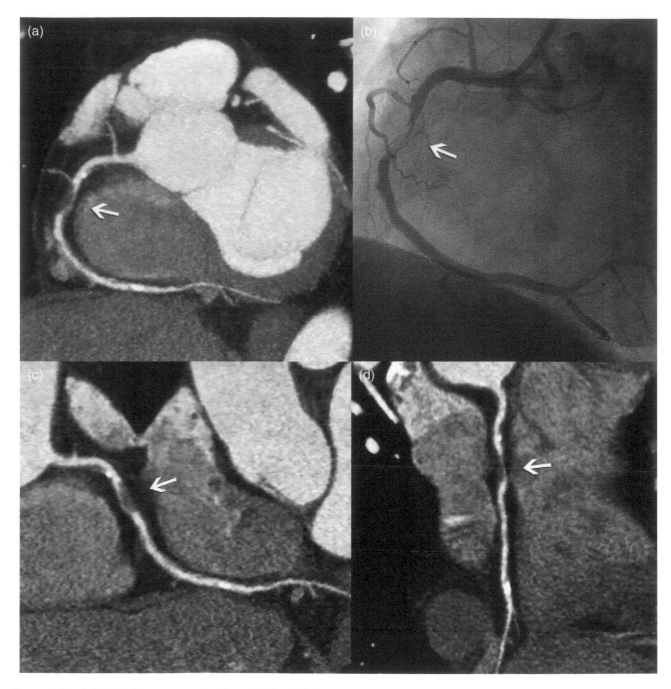

Figure 24.7 (a) Multiplanar reconstruction (MPR) of right coronary artery with severe non-calcified obstruction (arrow). (b) Invasive coronary angiography confirming presence of severe obstruction in RCA (arrow). (c,d) curved MPR's of RCA with severe obstructive disease (arrows).

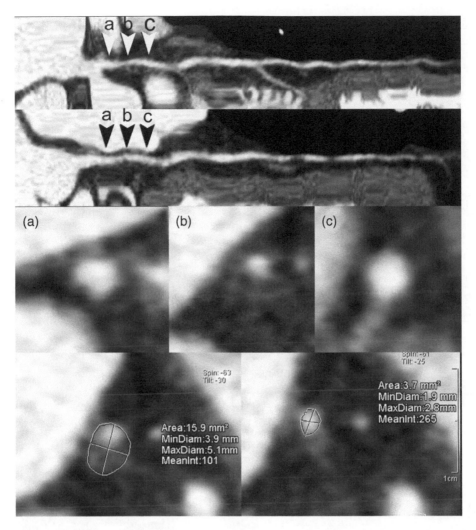

Figure 24.8 Quantification of stenosis. Upper 2 panels: multiplanar reconstruction of left descending coronary artery with proximal obstruction. (a,b,c) cross-sectional image proximal (a) at lesion (b) and distal (c) of obstruction. Lower panel: quantification of stenosis.

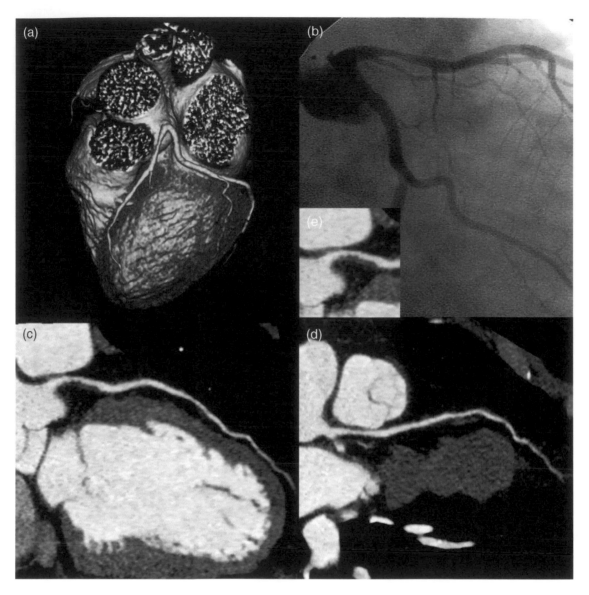

Figure 24.9 (a) Volume rendered image of left coronary artery, with narrowing proximal segment of left anterior descending artery (LAD). (b) Invasive coronary angiography confirming obstruction in proximal LAD. (c,d) Curve MPR's (2 orthogonal views) showing obstruction in LAD.

Index

T - #0569 - 071024 - C304 - 279/216/14 - PB - 9780367452568 - Gloss Lamination